Atlas of HEART DISEASES

ARRHYTHMIAS: ELECTROPHYSIOLOGIC PRINCIPLES

Volume IX

Atlas of HEART DISEASES

ARRHYTHMIAS: ELECTROPHYSIOLOGIC PRINCIPLES

Volume IX

VOLUME EDITOR

Melvin Scheinman, MD

Professor of Medicine
Division of Cardiology
Chief, Cardiac Electrophysiology
The Medical Center at
The University of California, San Francisco
San Francisco, California

SERIES EDITOR

Eugene Braunwald, MD, MD (Hon), ScD (Hon)

Hersey Professor of the Theory and Practice of Medicine
Harvard Medical School
Chairman, Department of Medicine
Brigham and Women's Hospital
Boston, Massachusetts

Mosby

St. Louis Baltimore Boston Carlsbad Chicago Naples New York Philadelphia Portland
London Madrid Mexico City Singapore Sydney Tokyo Toronto Wiesbaden

Developed by Current Medicine Inc., Philadelphia

CURRENT MEDICINE

400 MARKET STREET, SUITE 700 • PHILADELPHIA, PA 19106

Development Editors .... *Marian Bellus, Miriam McCauley*

Design and Layout .... *Jerilyn Bockorick, Lisa Caro*

Illustrators .... *Beth Ann Starkey, Sue Ann Fung-Ho, Wendy Jackelow, Lisa Antonucci Messina, Gary Welch*

Managing Editor .... *Lori Bainbridge*

Art Director .... *Paul Fennessy*

Illustration Director .... *Ann Saydlowski*

Production .... *David Myers, Lori Holland*

Indexing .... *Alexandra Nickerson*

Distribution rights for North America and territories not listed below:
MOSBY-YEAR BOOK, INC.
11830 Westline Industrial Drive
St. Louis, MO 63146

In Canada: TIMES MIRROR PROFESSIONAL PUBLISHING LTD.
130 Flaska Drive • Markham, Ontario
Canada L6G 1B8

Distribution rights for Central and South America: NUEVA EDITORIAL INTERAMERICANA, SA DE CV.

Distribution rights for Japan:
NANKODO CO LTD.

Distribution rights for Indian Subcontinent and South East Asia (except Japan):
TIMES MIRROR INTERNATIONAL PUBLISHERS, LTD.

Arrhythmias: Electrophysiologic Principles/volume editor, Melvin Scheinman.
p. cm. — (Atlas of heart diseases; v. 9)
Includes bibliographical references and index.
ISBN 1-878132-22-9 (hardcover)
1. Arrhythmia—Atlases. I. Scheinman, Melvin M. (Melvin Mayer), 1935-. II. Series.
[DNLM: 1. Arrhythmia—therapy—atlases. 2. Arrhythmia—physiopathology—atlases. 3. Electrophysiology—physiopathology—atlases.
A-524 v.9 / WG 17 A8816 1996 v.9]
RC682.A818 1996 vol. 9
[RC685.A65]
616.1′2 s—dc20
[616.1′28]
DNLM/DLC 95-45708
for Library of Congress CIP

Library of Congress Cataloging-in-Publication Data
ISBN 1-878132-22-9

Printed in Singapore by Imago Productions (FE) Ltd.

10 9 8 7 6 5 4 3 2 1

SERIES PREFACE

Disorders of the cardiovascular system are the most common causes of death and serious morbidity in the industrialized world. In 1991, more than 40% of all deaths in the United States were attributed to cardiac and vascular diseases. These conditions accounted for almost 5 million years of potential life lost.

Despite these sobering statistics, progress in cardiovascular medicine has been immense, and is, in fact, accelerating. Our understanding of the pathobiology of most forms of heart disease has advanced steadily and there have been enormous advances in the diagnosis, treatment, and prevention of cardiovascular disorders. For example, during just one decade, from 1981 to 1991, the overall death rates from cardiovascular disease declined by 26% and death rates from acute myocardial infarction and stroke declined by 32%. Similar progress has been made in other major cardiovascular disorders, including hypertension, valvular and congenital heart disease, congestive heart failure, and the arrhythmias.

The physician responsible for the care of patients with cardiovascular disease now has a number of vehicles available for obtaining up-to-date information, including excellent journals and textbooks of every conceivable size, scope, and depth. In developing new strategies for transmitting information about these conditions, it is important to consider that cardiovascular medicine is the most "visual" of medical specialties. Cardiovascular diagnosis is based on the recognition and understanding of a variety of graphic waveforms, images, decision trees, and microscopic sections. Treatment increasingly involves the intelligent use of algorithms, which are most effectively portrayed visually. Likewise, mechanical correction of cardiovascular disorders, whether catheter-based or surgical, can best be described pictorially. This *Atlas of Heart Diseases* has been designed to provide a detailed and comprehensive visual exposition of all aspects of cardiovascular medicine. Several thousand images, accompanied by detailed captions, have been carefully selected by expert authors and reviewed by the 12 distinguished volume editors. These images are now available separately in print and slide form and also will soon be formatted for CD-ROM use.

Many people deserve credit for the successful completion of this ambitious effort. The expertise and hard work of the authors and the devoted efforts of the volume editors naturally form the foundation of the *Atlas of Heart Diseases*. Great credit is also due to Abe Krieger, President of Current Medicine, who conceived the *Atlas* series; to Maureen McNally, the extremely effective Development Editor, and to Kathryn Saxon, who coordinated the efforts in my office.

All of us who have been engaged in this project hope that each individual volume, and the entire *Atlas*, will be useful to physicians of all specialties who are responsible for the care of patients with cardiovascular disorders, to investigators and teachers of cardiovascular medicine, and ultimately to the millions of patients worldwide with disorders of the heart and circulation.

Eugene Braunwald, MD

PREFACE

The past decade has witnessed an extraordinary growth in both the understanding of basic mechanisms of cardiac arrhythmias as well as in treatment modalities. The contents of this volume are meant to serve as an overview of these areas for the interested internist-cardiologist. Basic advances include our expanded knowledge related to membrane ion channel structure and function, particularly as they relate to the actions of antiarrhythmic agents. Equally spectacular have been the greater understanding of genetic abnormalities as they relate to the problem of sudden cardiac death in the young. It is now appreciated, for example, that patients with the familial long QT syndrome may suffer from genetic abnormalities related to either the delayed rectifier current or to Na^+ channel function. These advances will allow for more precise diagnostic approaches as well as improved genetic counseling. A great deal has been learned about the role of the autonomic nervous system in the genesis of arrhythmias and about the way in which arrhythmias may be triggered by both beta as well as alpha agonists. Moreover, the whole area of arrhythmias related to triggered mechanisms, in particular those that appear to be initiated by early versus late afterdepolarizations, is of great current interest.

Just as profound as the advancements in basic understanding are the advancements in current management strategies. In contrast with the 1980s, which saw great interest and proliferation in the approval and use of antiarrhythmic agents, the 1990s have witnessed a regression in drug use with greater emphasis on ablation or device therapy. The decreased infatuation with drug therapy resulted from limited efficacy of these agents together with substantial adverse effect, particularly in patients with structural heart disease (*ie,* usually those most in need of effective therapy). The great explosion in use of catheter ablation resulted from the fact that this approach provides a definitive cure and is associated with minimal significant adverse effects. Catheter ablative procedures are currently widely used for cure of patients with paroxysmal supraventricular tachycardia and are currently being modified for use in patients with atrial flutter and atrial fibrillation.

The field of clinical cardiac electrophysiology has been greatly impacted by use of device therapy. The types and function of available pacemakers in terms of modes of operation are remarkable. These advances allow our patients to lead more active and full lives. More remarkable is the use of the internal cardioverter-defibrillator, a device that has revolutionized the management of patients with malignant ventricular arrhythmias. This device allows for arrhythmia recognition and delivery of specific therapy, including bursts of antitachycardia pacing or defibrillatory discharges. We hope that this volume presents a clear and complete overview of these impressive advances.

Melvin Scheinman, MD

CONTRIBUTORS

JAMES L. COCKRELL, MD
Director, Cardiac Electrophysiology
Washington Adventist Hospital
Takoma Park, Maryland

TODD J. COHEN, MD
Director of Electrophysiology
Cardiology Section
North Shore Hospital
Manhasset, New York

LAURENCE M. EPSTEIN, MD
Assistant Professor of Medicine
Harvard Medical School
Director, Electrophysiology and Pacing Laboratory
Beth Israel Hospital
Boston, Massachusetts

G. THOMAS EVANS JR, MD
Assistant Clinical Professor of Medicine
Department of Medicine
University of California, San Francisco
San Francisco, California

ADAM FITZPATRICK, MD, MRCP
Consultant Cardiologist
Manchester Heart Center
Manchester Royal Infirmary
Manchester, England

HARLAN R. GROGIN, MD, FACC
Clinical Instructor
Department of Medicine
University of California, San Francisco, Medical Center
Electrophysiologist
Salinas Valley Memorial Hospital
Salinas, California

GERARD GUIRAUDON, MD, FRCS(C), FACC
Professor of Surgery
Department of Surgery
The University of Western Ontario
Staff Surgeon
University Hospital
London, Ontario, Canada

EDMUND C. KEUNG, MD
Assistant Professor of Medicine
University of California, San Francisco
Director, Western Regional Pacemaker Surveillance Program
Director, Arrhythmia Clinic
Director, Electrophysiology
Veterans Affairs Medical Center
San Francisco, California

RANDALL J. LEE, MD, PhD
Assistant Professor of Medicine in Residence
Division of Cardiology
University of California, San Francisco
San Francisco, California

MICHAEL D. LESH, MD
Assistant Professor of Medicine
Department of Medicine
University of California, San Francisco
San Francisco, California

ANDREANA SIU, RN
University of California, San Francisco, School of Nursing
San Francisco, California

CONTENTS

CHAPTER 1

Basic Electrophysiology and Mechanisms of Cardiac Arrhythmias

Randall J. Lee and Edmund C. Keung

CHAPTER 2

Pharmacology/Pharmacokinetics and Clinical Use of Antiarrhythmic Agents

Randall J. Lee

CHAPTER 3

Electrocardiographic Predictors of Cardiac Rhythm Disturbances

G. Thomas Evans Jr

CHAPTER 4

Sinus Node Disorders

Laurence M. Epstein

CHAPTER 5

Supraventricular Tachycardia

Harlan R. Grogin

CHAPTER 6

Ventricular Tachycardia: Mechanisms, Diagnosis, and Treatment

Michael D. Lesh

CHAPTER 7

The Long QT Syndrome

Harlan R. Grogin

CHAPTER 8

Implantable Pacemakers for the Management of Cardiac Rhythm Disorders

James L. Cockrell and Andreana Siu

CHAPTER 9

Implantable Defibrillators for the Management of Cardiac Rhythm Disorders

James L. Cockrell and Andreana Siu

CHAPTER 10

Surgical Treatment of Cardiac Arrhythmias

Gerard M. Guiraudon

CHAPTER 11

Catheter Ablation

Harlan R. Grogin

CHAPTER 12

Syncope and Sudden Cardiac Death

Adam Fitzpatrick

CHAPTER 13

Cardiopulmonary Resuscitation

Todd J. Cohen

Basic Electrophysiology and Mechanisms of Cardiac Arrhythmias

1

CHAPTER

Randall J. Lee and Edmund C. Keung

An understanding of the atrioventricular conduction system and the basic cellular electrophysiologic properties of that system is essential to the understanding of the mechanisms that occur in the generation of cardiac arrhythmias. The tissues involved in the conduction system are responsible for the initiation and conduction of the electrical activity that results in myocardial contraction. The conduction system comprises specialized myocardial tissue that can be distinguished histologically from the "working" atrial and ventricular myocardium.

The structures composing the atrioventricular conduction tissue are the sinoatrial (SA) node, the atrioventricular (AV) node, the atrioventricular bundle (the His bundle), the right and left bundles, and the ventricular conduction system, predominantly consisting of the Purkinje fibers. Each of these specialized tissues has different electrophysiologic properties that determine their excitability and conduction properties. The SA node synchronizes the heart and is called the pacemaker of the heart because of its ability to spontaneously depolarize and initiate conduction at a faster rate than any other specialized tissue within the conduction system. The atrioventricular junction, the AV node, and the His bundle compose the specialized conduction tissue that connects and synchronizes the atrial and ventricular working muscles. The right and left bundles of the heart channel the electrical signals from the atrioventricular junction throughout the Purkinje fibers, which excite the ventricular working muscles and initiate contraction. Differences in excitability and conduction contribute to the different mechanisms that can generate an arrhythmia. This chapter highlights the structures involved in the conduction system and the various electrophysiologic properties of the specialized conduction tissue, and introduces readers to the proposed mechanisms that generate arrhythmias.

Normal Pathway of Electrical Conduction

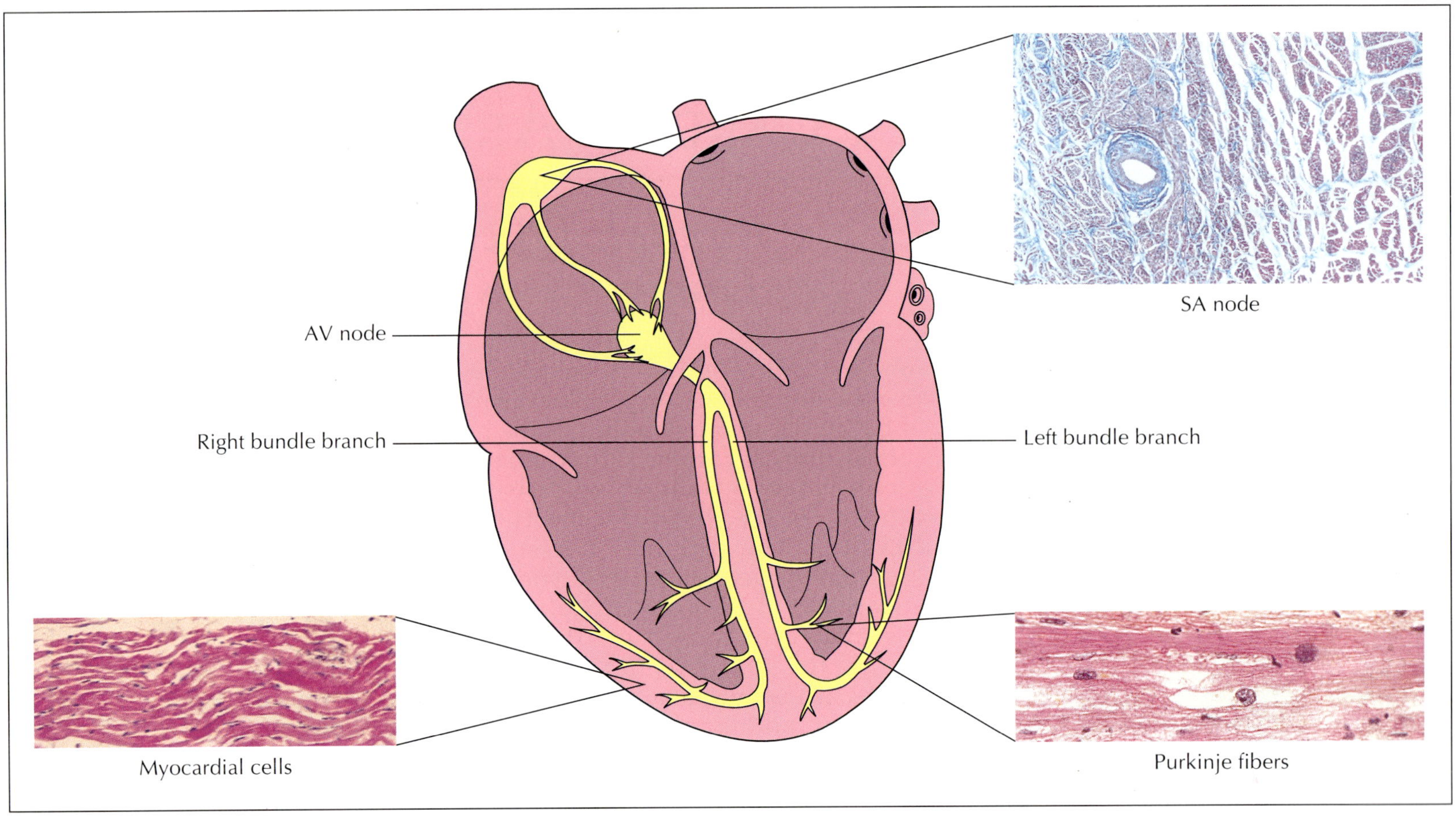

Figure 1-1. Normal pathway of electrical conduction in the heart. Note the differences between the conductive and the contractile tissue of the heart (*insets*). The sinus nodal cells are smaller and interwoven so as to form a network of cells grouped together by the surrounding fibrous matrix. They contain relatively few myofilaments compared with "working" myocardial cells. The Purkinje fibers are comprised of short, cylindrical cells that are irregularly shaped. The ultrastructure of an irregularly shaped cell, which increases cell-to-cell contact, and the large gap junctions at both the ends and sides of the cells provide the membrane properties of rapid impulse conduction. AV—atrioventricular; SA—sinoatrial.

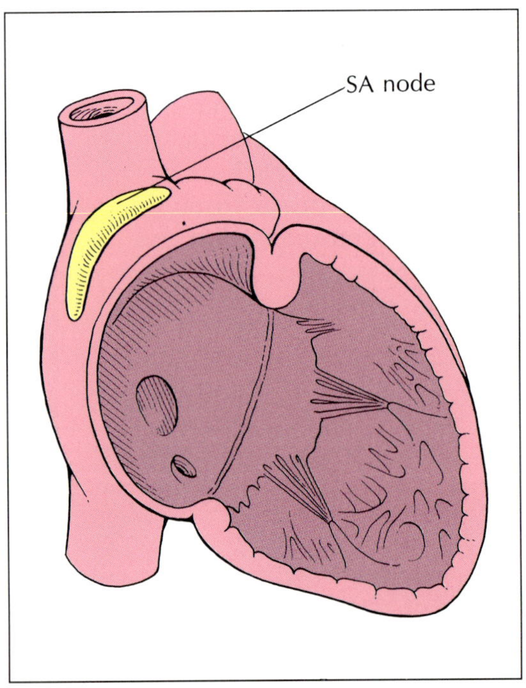

Figure 1-2. Electrical activity of the heart begins with the pacemaker cells of the SA node. The SA node is a crescent-shaped area of specialized muscle lying in the cristae terminalis, which begins high in the right atrium at the border of the superior vena cava and atrial appendage and extends along the lateral aspect of the right atrium. The pacemaker cells of the SA node spontaneously initiate and propagate electrical activity throughout the atrium, which converges at the AV node via three internodal pathways [1]. These pathways appear to reflect the atrial myocardial input into the AV node.

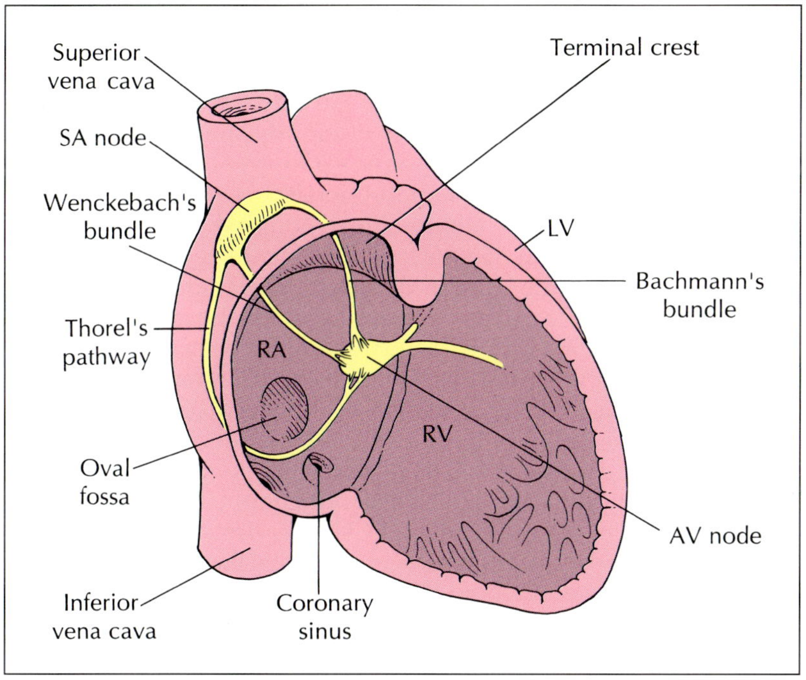

FIGURE 1-3. The internodal pathways are designated as the anterior internodal tract (Bachmann's bundle), the middle internodal tract (Wenckebach's bundle), and the posterior internodal tract (Thorel's pathway). Evidence for specialized internodal tissue is controversial. Becker and Anderson [2] could not find discrete atrial pathways. Furthermore, preferential conduction via an anatomic "pathway" may be explained as a functional pathway existing as muscle bundles forming the entirety of the atrial septum and the terminal crest [3]. LV—left ventricle; RA—right atrium; RV—right ventricle.

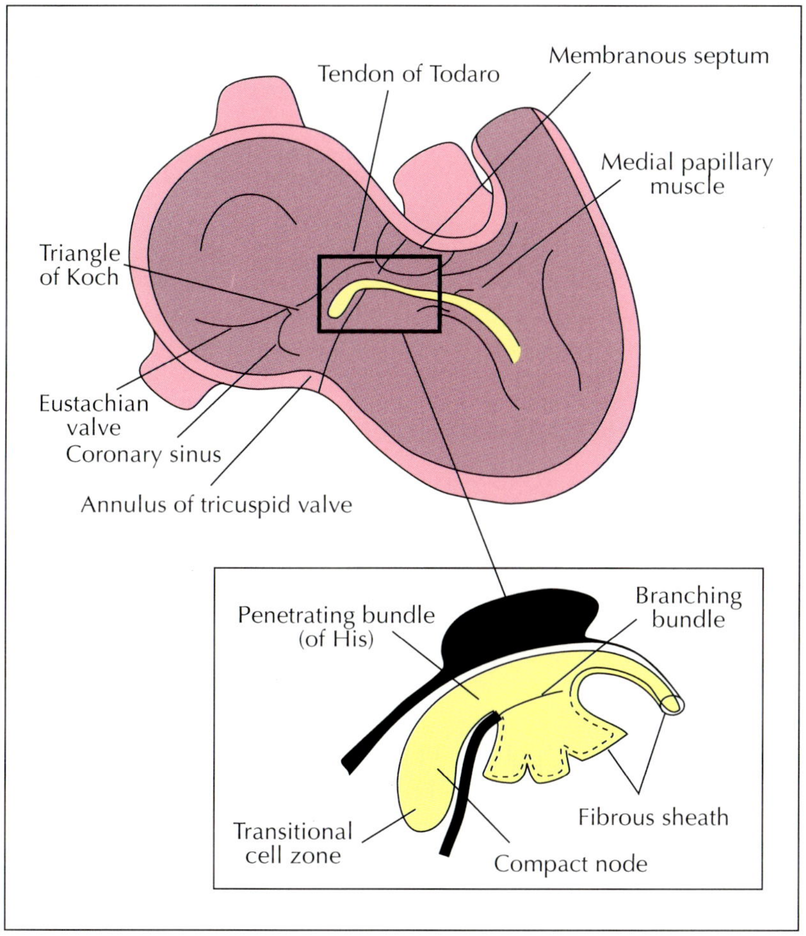

FIGURE 1-4. The AV node is located at the apex of the triangle of Koch, whose borders consist of the tendon of Todaro, the septal tricuspid valve annulus, and the os of the coronary sinus. The AV junction is the area of specialized conduction tissue that provides the electrical links between atrium and ventricle. It is subdivided into anatomic zones: (1) compact AV node and its transitional zone, (2) the penetrating bundle (His bundle), and (3) the branching atrioventricular bundle (*inset*). The speed of conduction of the electrical activity is modulated at the AV node in a decremental fashion before it travels down the His bundle and activates the ventricles via the Purkinje fibers. RA—right atrium. (*Adapted from* Mandel [4]; with permission.)

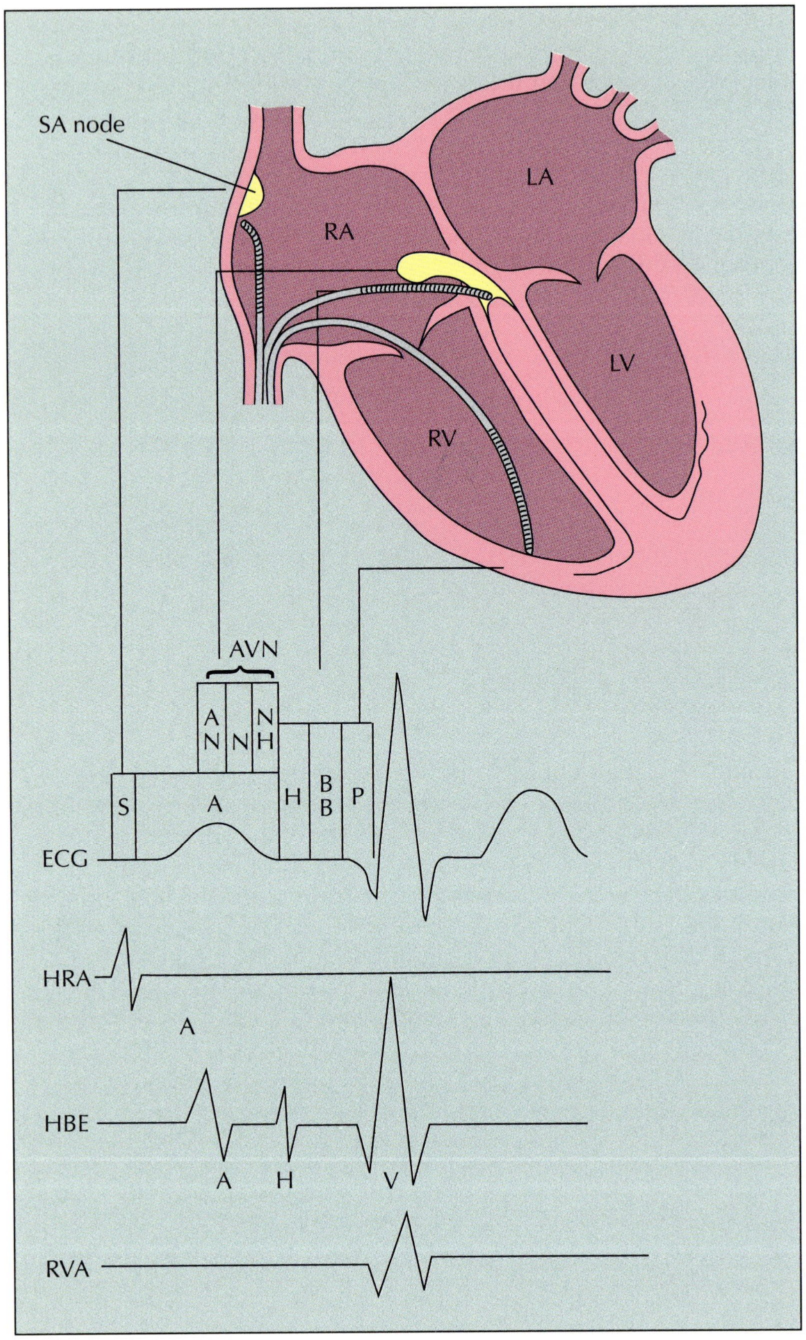

FIGURE 1-5. Sequence of activation through the conduction system relative to surface electrocardiogram (ECG) events and intracardiac electrograms. The intracardiac catheters are positioned in the high right atrium (to record atrial intracardiac ECGs), the low atrioseptal right atrium (RA; to record the His bundle ECG), and the right ventricular (RV) apex (to record the ventricular intracardiac ECG). Note the activation of the sinoatrial (SA) node prior to the onset of the P wave. Conduction through the AV node begins well before atrial depolarization is completed, while conduction through the His-Purkinje system precedes contraction of the ventricles (reflected as the QRS complex). Intracardiac ECGs confirm the activation sequence and timing of the conduction system. Note that the atrial activity in the atrial intracardiac ECG precedes the atrial activity in the His bundle recording, as atrial conduction begins high in the SA node. A—atrial conduction; AN—nodal conduction; AVN—AV nodal conduction; BB—bundle branch conduction; H—His bundle conduction; HBE—His-bundle ECG; HRA—high RA intracardiac ECG; LA—left atrium; LV—left ventricle; N—nodal conduction; NH—nodal–His conduction; P—Purkinje fiber conduction; RVA—RV apex ECG; S—SA node conduction; V—ventricular conduction. (*Adapted from* Marriot and Conover [5]; with permission.)

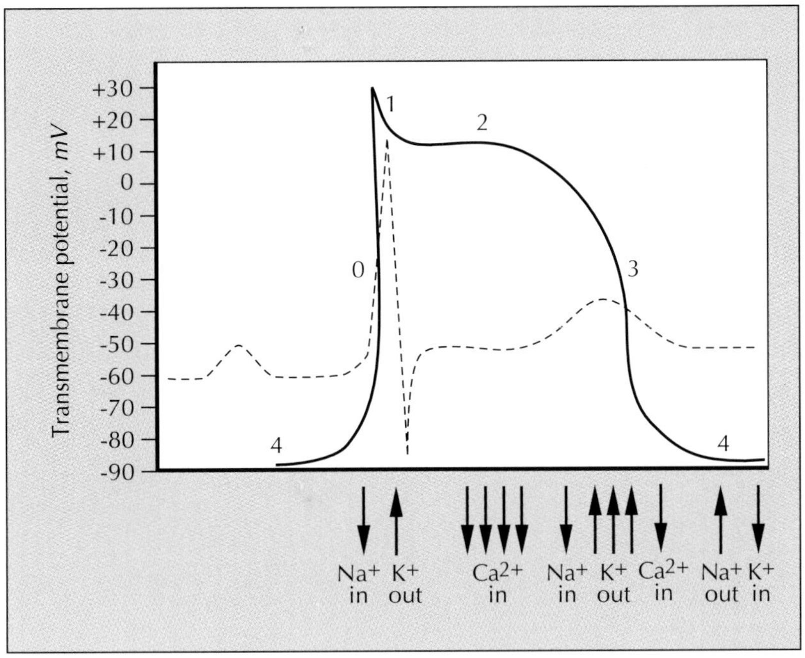

FIGURE 1-6. Relationship of the transmembrane resting and action potential to the surface electrocardiogram (ECG). The action potential of a Purkinje fiber is classically divided into five phases (0,1,2,3, and 4). The depolarization phase (phase 0) occurs when a rapid influx of sodium ions enters the cell, causing a rapid, positively charged change in the transmembrane potential (-90 mV to +30 mV). The resulting positive spike is called depolarization and corresponds to the QRS complex of the surface ECG. The positive depolarization of one cell causes adjacent cardiac cells to depolarize, thus propagating the electrical impulse throughout the heart. The velocity of depolarization, Vmax (reflected by the slope of phase 0), determines the speed of conduction of the electrical impulse throughout the heart.

Repolarization begins with phase 1, which represents the early and rapid repolarization due to the transient potassium outward current. Phase 2 of the action potential, the plateau phase, is mediated by the slow calcium channels, which allow the positively charged calcium ions to enter the cell. The inward calcium current interrupts repolarization, thus increasing the duration of the action potential and prolonging the refractory period. The plateau phase is the absolute refractory period and is the main component of the QT interval of the surface ECG. Repolarization ends with phase 3, which is a period of rapid repolarization predominantly mediated by the outward flow of potassium ions and to a lesser extent by the inward flow of calcium and sodium ions. Phase 3 corresponds to the relative refractory period and is reflected in the surface ECG as the T wave.

The resting phase (phase 4) is the interval from the end of repolarization to the beginning of the next action potential. In most cardiac cells, there is no net change in ion movement across the cell membrane. However, in certain "pacemaker" cells, there is a slow gradual inward flow of positive ions during phase 4, which causes a gradual depolarization in the membrane potential. Once the membrane potential threshold is reached, sodium channels are activated, allowing depolarization to occur. This phase 4 activity leads to spontaneous depolarization and propagation of electrical impulse across the heart (automaticity). The shape of the action potential reflects the conduction velocity, refractory period, and automaticity of the cardiac cells. Ca^{2+}—calcium ions; K^{+}—potassium ions; Na^{+}—sodium ions.

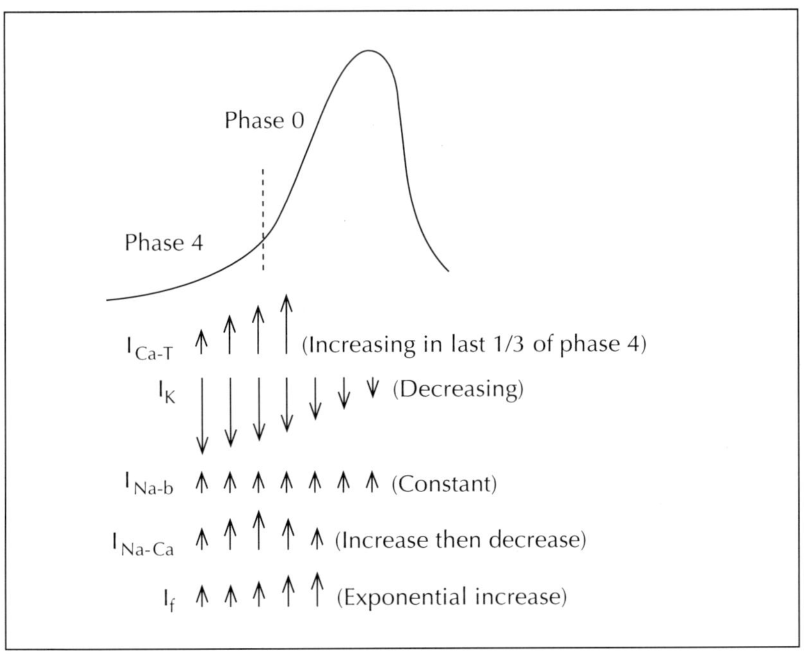

FIGURE 1-7. In the normal heart, cells in the sinoatrial node have the fastest phase 4 activity, hence controlling the sinus rate and rhythm. The ionic currents involved during the phase 4 depolarization are believed to be the combination of a decrease in the outward potassium current (I_K), a continued background inward sodium current ($I_{Na\text{-}b}$), an increasing calcium current ($I_{Ca\text{-}T}$) during the later third of phase 4 depolarization, and probably, a small contribution from the inward sodium current generated from the sodium-calcium exchange current ($I_{Na\text{-}Ca}$). The contribution of an increasing inward sodium current activated by hyperpolarization of the membrane potential (I_f) is unclear. The I_f current has the potential to be a major contributor to diastolic depolarization if the membrane potential becomes hyperpolarized. If the membrane potential does not reach threshold for I_f, then the inward sodium current does not contribute to phase 4 depolarization.

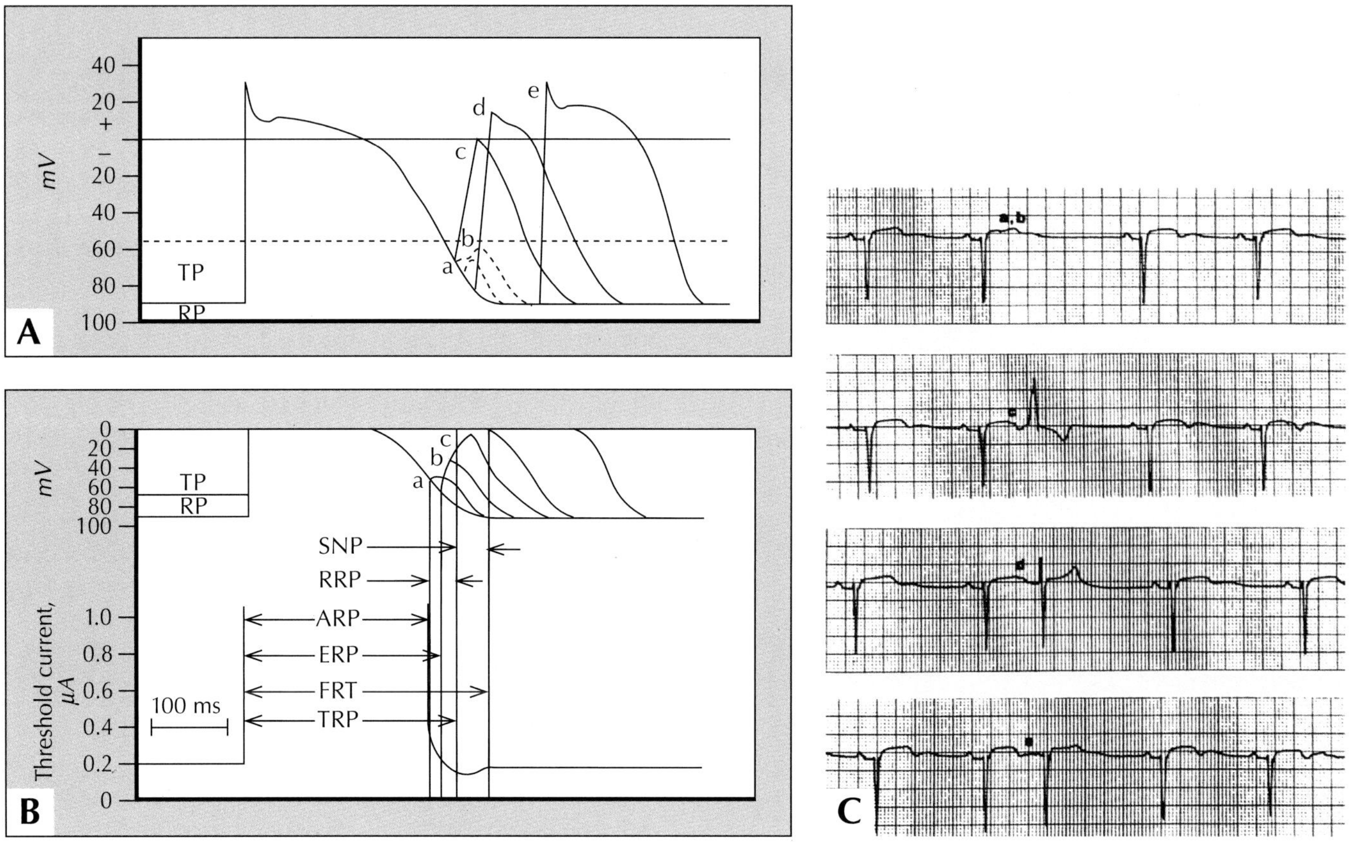

FIGURE 1-8. A, A normal action potential and its relative refractory period. This diagram represents a normal action potential and the responses elicited by stimuli applied at different stages of repolarization. The amplitude and upstroke velocity of the elicited responses are directly related to the membrane potential stimuli applied early during repolarization. As *a* and *b* arise from such a low level of membrane potential, they are too small to propagate graded or local responses. The earliest propagated action potential is response *c*, which defines the end of the effective refractory period (ERP). However, response *c* propagates slowly due to its low amplitude and low upstroke velocity. Response *d* is elicited during the supernormal period (SNP) of excitability and its rates of rise and amplitude are greater than those of *c* because it arises from a higher membrane potential. However, it still propagates more slowly than the normal response *e,* which occurs after complete repolarization and therefore has a normal rate of depolarization and amplitude. Response *e* propagates rapidly [6].

B, The refractory periods in respect to the action potential. The fiber becomes inexcitable beginning with the inscription of phase 0 of the action potential. Recovery of excitability progresses slowly during phase 3 of repolarization. A period of supernormal excitability, in which a submaximal stimulus can elicit a propagated action potential, occurs at the terminal portion of phase 3. The diagram also illustrates the absolute refractory period (ARP), ERP, relative refractory period (RRP), total refractory period (TRP), full recovery time (FRT), and the SNP of excitability. The threshold currents are indicated in microamperes (μA). Vertical lines demonstrate the relationship of the refractory period to the elicited responses during repolarization. This diagram demonstrates the time course relationships among repolarization, refractoriness, and excitability.

C, The electrocardiographic strips of atrial premature beats are examples of stimuli during the different periods of repolarization. Beats *a* and *b* occur during the total refractory period and are either not conducted or result in a nonconducted atrial premature beat. Beats *c* and *d* occur with aberration, since recovery is incomplete. Beat c, being earlier, is conducted more aberrantly. Beat *e* occurs after full recovery and is conducted normally. (Part A *adapted from* Singer and Ten Eick [6]; part B *adapted from* Mandel [4]; with permission.)

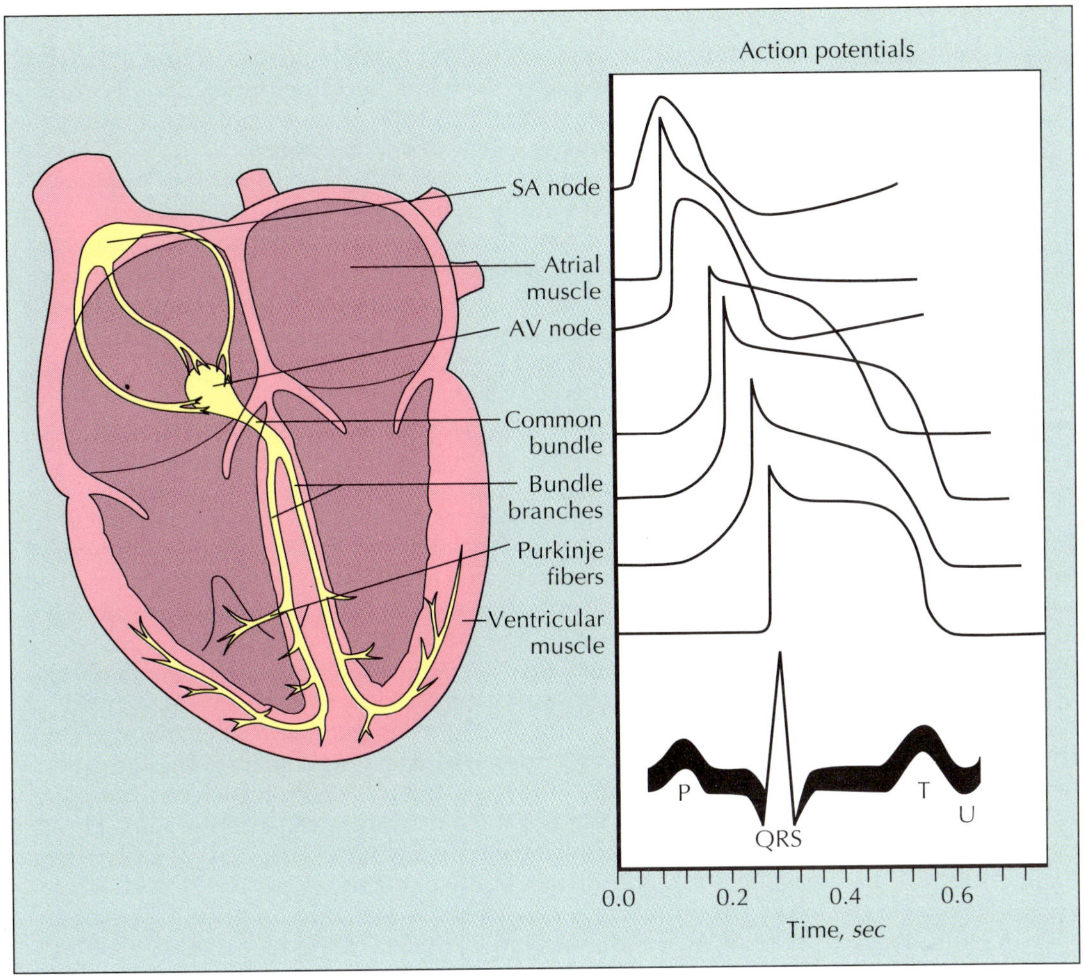

FIGURE 1-9. Localized variations in the action potential of the heart's electrical system. Cardiac action potentials from different locations in the heart have different shapes, leading to different electrophysiologic properties. The SA node and AV node depolarize in response to the slow inward current of calcium and sodium. The two nodes differ in that the SA node possesses the property of automaticity and the AV node does not. All other cardiac cells depolarize in response to the rapid inward current of sodium ions. Note the progressive increase in the action potential duration beginning at the AV node and reaching its maximum in the Purkinje fiber. This results in the functional refractory period of the ventricular tissue being dependent on the effective refractory period of the Purkinje cell. Furthermore, specialized cells depolarize during phase 4, whereas atrial and ventricular muscle does not. (*Adapted from* CIBA Pharmaceutical Company Division of CIBA-GEIGY Corporation [7]; with permission.)

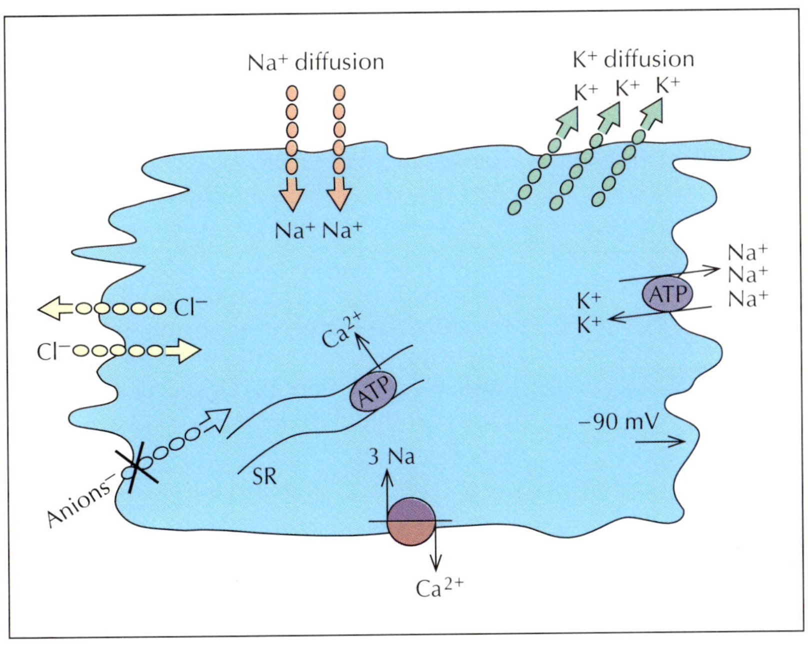

FIGURE 1-10. The resting membrane potential (-90 mV) of a cardiac cell is determined by the net sum of the inward and outward currents. Inward ionic currents are caused by the movement of cations into the cell or anions moving out of the cell, resulting in a more positive membrane potential. Outward ionic currents are caused by cations moving out of the cell or anions moving into the cell, resulting in a more negative membrane potential. At rest, the membrane is highly permeable to potassium ions (K^+), only minimally permeable to chloride (Cl^-) and sodium (Na^+) ions, and impermeable to anions (anions$^-$). Maintenance of the resting membrane potential is aided by both active pumps (*ie*, Na^+/K^+ pump) and passive carriers (*ie*, Ca^{2+}/Na^- carrier). Furthermore, the release of calcium from the sarcoplasmic reticulum (SR) is dependent on intracellular calcium and ATP.

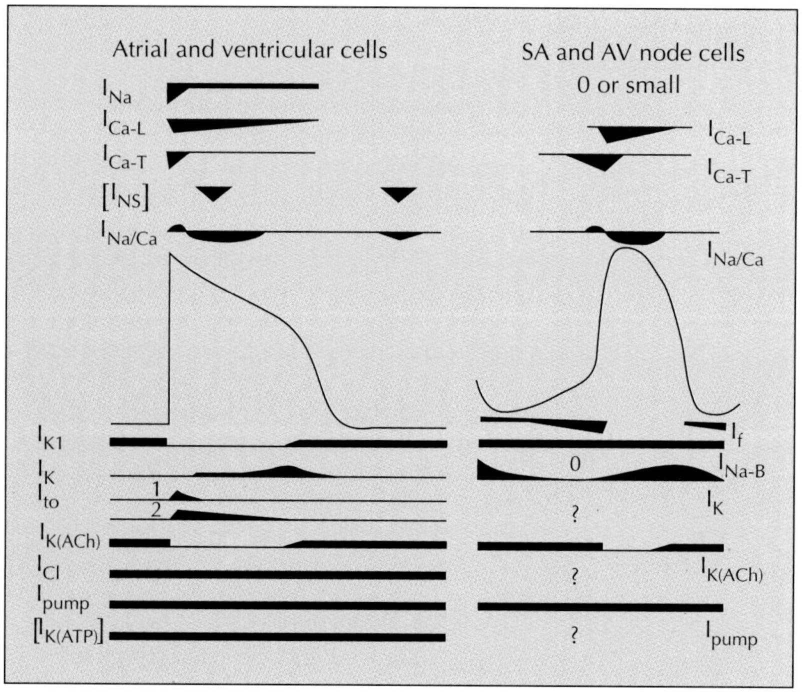

FIGURE 1-11. Currents and channels involved in generating the resting and action potential. Above and below the respective action potentials are the various channels and pumps that contribute to the currents underlying the electrical events. Approximate time courses of the currents associated with the channels or pumps are shown symbolically without effort to represent their magnitudes relative to each other. The heavy bars for I_{Cl}, I_{pump}, and $I_{K(ATP)}$ do not correspond to the magnitude of currents. They only indicate the presence of these channels or pumps. Channels identified by brackets, I_{NS} and $I_{K(ATP)}$, imply they are active only during pathologic conditions. I_{Na} and I_{K1} are small or absent in the SA node cells. Question marks indicate that experimental evidence is not yet available to determine the presence of these channels in the SA node. Other ionic currents are likely to exist. However, at this time, they are not sufficiently well defined and are not included in the figure.

I_{Na} is the inward excitatory current carried by sodium through a voltage-activated sodium channel. I_{Na-B} is the proposed background sodium current through a voltage-independent channel in the SA nodal cells. I_{Ca-L} is the inward calcium current that utilizes a calcium channel blocked by verapamil, diltiazem, and the dihydropyridines. I_{Ca-T}, the inward calcium current, has been identified in pacemaker tissues and is mediated through a different voltage-gated channel that is activated at a potential intermediate between thresholds for I_{Na} and I_{Ca-L}. I_f is an inward current carried by sodium through a relatively nonspecific cationic channel that is activated by polarization to high membrane potentials in the SA and AV nodal cells and the His-purkinje cells. I_{NS} is a channel that is gated by intracellular concentration of calcium. It is a cationic nonselective channel that is activated at the resting potential and produces an inward current carried by sodium [8]. I_{K1} is potassium current responsible for maintaining the resting potential near the potassium equilibrium potential in atrial, AV nodal, His-purkinje, and ventricular cells [9]. I_K is the potassium carried through a voltage-gated channel with slow activation kinetics and delayed rectifier current. I_{to} is a potassium current that turns on rapidly after depolarization and then inactivates [10]. $I_{K(ACh)}$ is a potassium current whose channels are activated by the muscarinic (M2) receptor via GTP regulatory G protein signal transduction [11]. $I_{K(ATP)}$ is a current carried through a metabolically regulated channel [12]. I_{Cl} is a chloride current that is generally quite small but can greatly increase by adrenergic receptor activation, thus favoring repolarization [13]. $I_{Na/Ca}$ is the current generated by the sodium-calcium counter transport system, which exchanges one calcium for three sodium [14]. (*Adapted from* The Sicilian Gambit [15]; with permission.)

MECHANISMS OF ARRHYTHMIAS

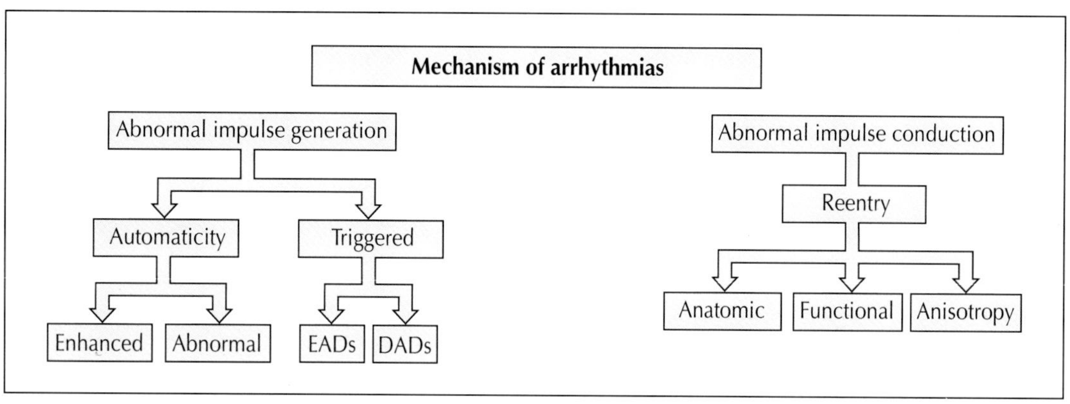

FIGURE 1-12. Mechanism of arrhythmias. Mechanistically, arrhythmias can be separated into those due to abnormal impulse generation and those due to abnormal impulse conduction. EAD—early afterdepolarization; DAD—delayed afterdepolarization.

A. RHYTHMS RESULTING FROM ABNORMALITIES IN IMPULSE FORMATION

Sinus bradycardia or sinus tachycardia
Atrial, junctional, or ventricular escape
Atrial tachycardias (*ie*, digitalis toxicity)
Accelerated junctional (nonparoxysmal junctional tachycardia), accelerated ventricular (accelerated idioventricular)
Atrial or ventricular parasystole

B. RHYTHMS RESULTING FROM ABNORMALITIES IN IMPULSE CONDUCTION

Atrial flutter
Atrial fibrillation
Sinoatrial or atrial reentry
AV nodal reentry
Reciprocating tachycardia associated with accessory pathway
Ventricular tachycardia
Ventricular fibrillation
Ventricular flutter

Figure 1-13. A, Rhythms resulting from abnormalities in impulse generation. **B,** Rhythms resulting from abnormalities in impulse conduction.

Automaticity

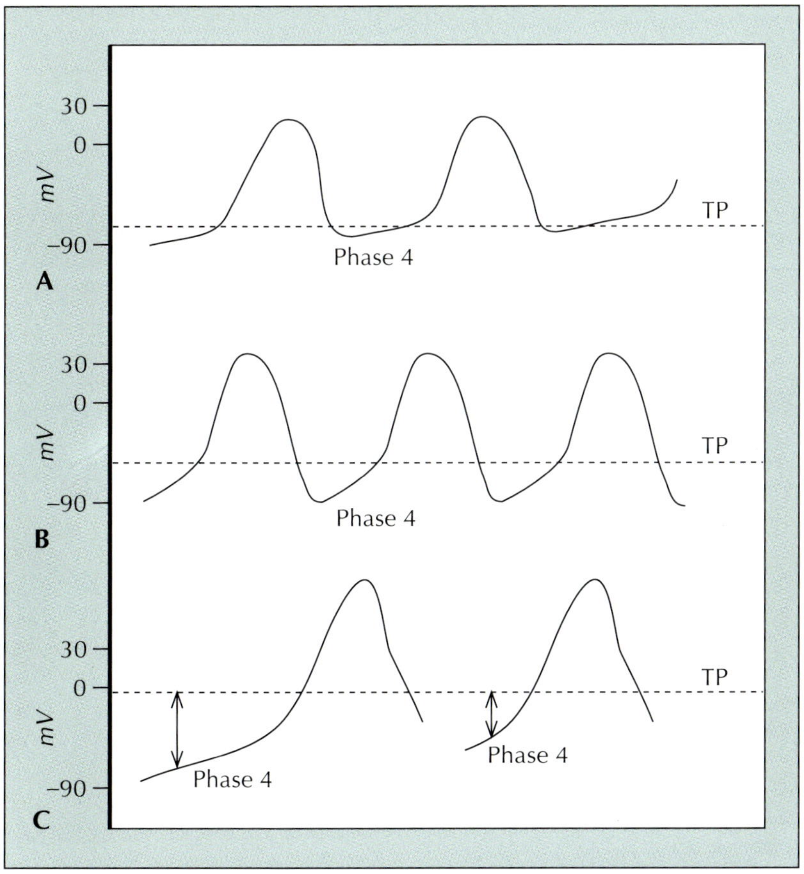

Figure 1-14. A, Normal automaticity of the SA node during sinus rhythm. **B,** Enhanced automaticity with an increase in the slope of phase 4, resulting in an increase in heart rate (shown as an increased number of action potentials. **C,** The effect of hyperpolarization (action potential on the left), which makes it more difficult for the SA nodal cell to reach threshold potential (TP), thus leading to slower heart rates. Depolarization (action potential shown on the right) would allow phase 4 depolarization to reach the threshold potential earlier, thus leading to a potentially increased heart rate.

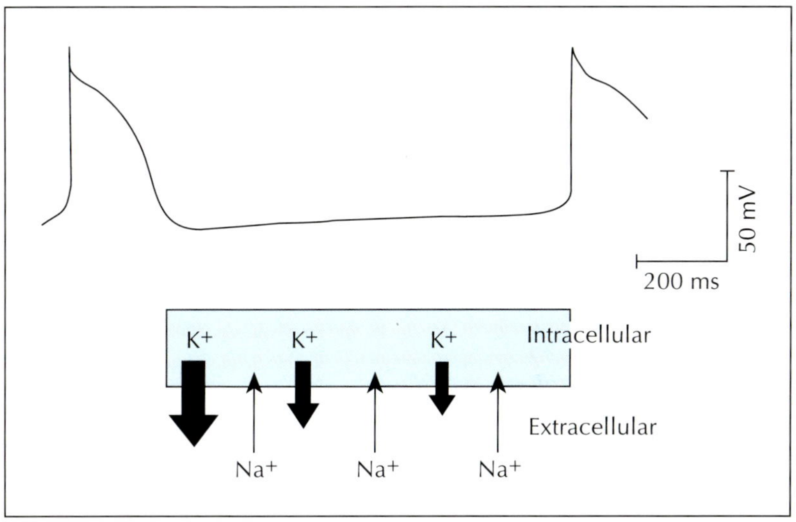

Figure 1-15. A schematic diagram demonstrating the ionic currents responsible for propagating one cycle of an automatic rhythm. Under the recording are the transmembrane potassium (outward) and sodium (inward) ionic currents. The slowly declining potassium (pacemaker) current allows a steady sodium current to cause gradual depolarization until threshold potential is reached (*Adapted from* Rosen and coworkers [16]; with permission.)

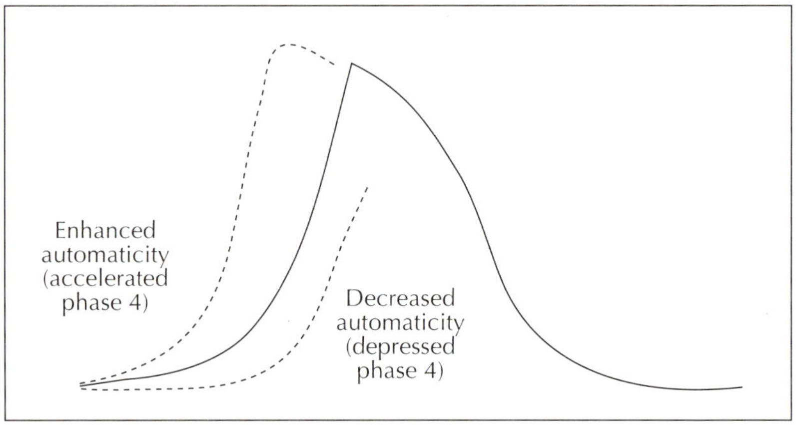

FIGURE 1-16. Increased sympathetic stimulation or decreased parasympathetic stimulation leads to enhanced automaticity of either the sinoatrial node or a latent subsidiary pacemaker. Conversely, decreased sympathetic stimulation or increased parasympathetic stimulation leads to decreased automaticity.

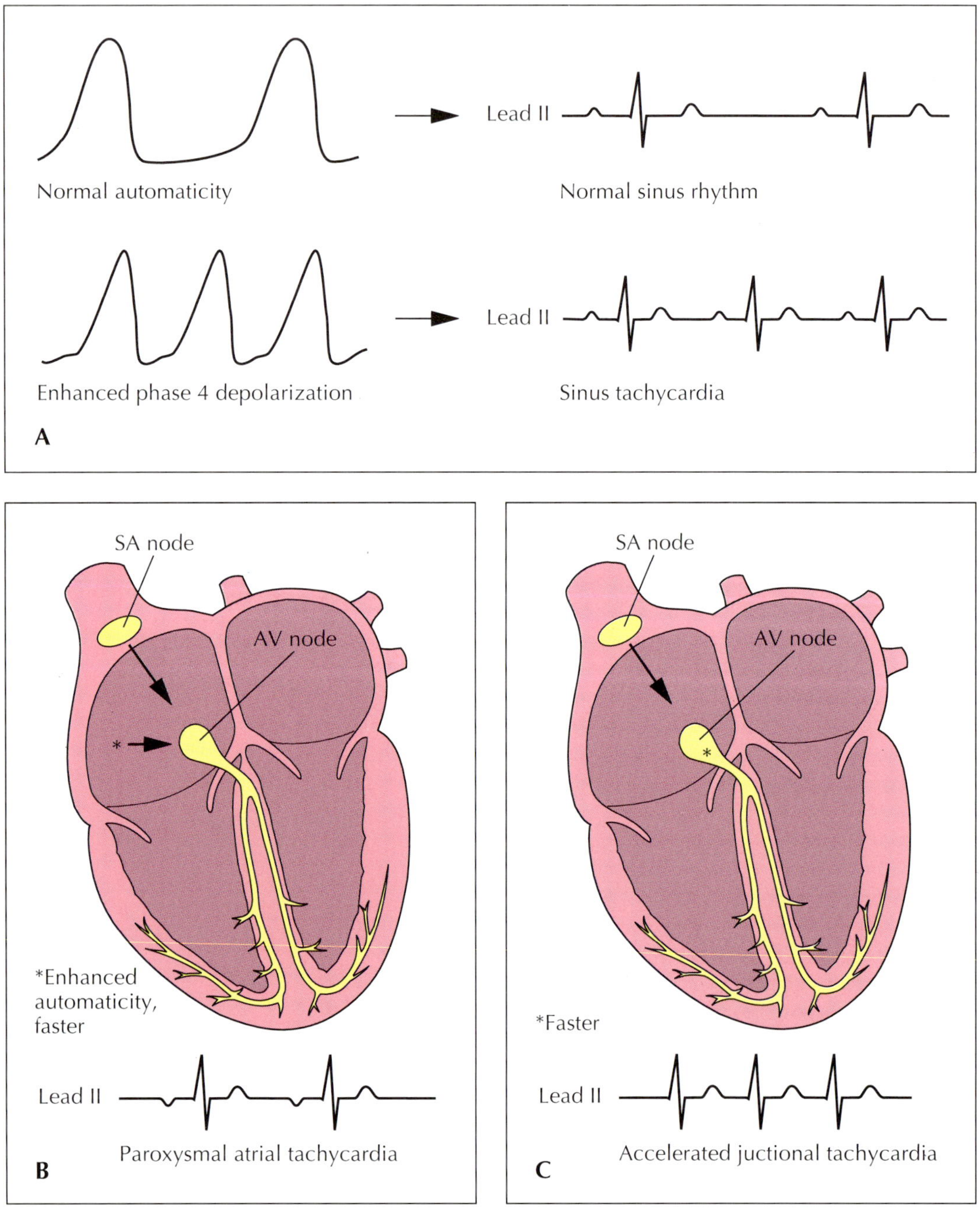

FIGURE 1-17. A, The resting sinus heart rate (note the positive P waves in lead II) is predominantly under the control of parasympathetic stimulation. Normal physiologic responses to exercise or psychologic stresses result in increased sympathetic tone, which produces enhanced normal automaticity and sinus tachycardia. Alternately, sinus tachycardia may result from automaticity caused by abnormally enhanced sympathetic tone resulting in arrhythmias such as inappropriate sinus tachycardia. **B,** There are certain types of atrial tachycardias that arise because of abnormal enhanced automaticity within atrial cells other than the sinus node. The atrial cells with abnormal automaticity compete with the sinus node, producing paroxysmal atrial tachycardia. Atrial tachycardias originating away from the sinus node region will produce an abnormal P wave axis (illustrated as a negative P wave in lead II). **C,** Some types of accelerated junctional tachycardias arise from abnormal enhanced automaticity.

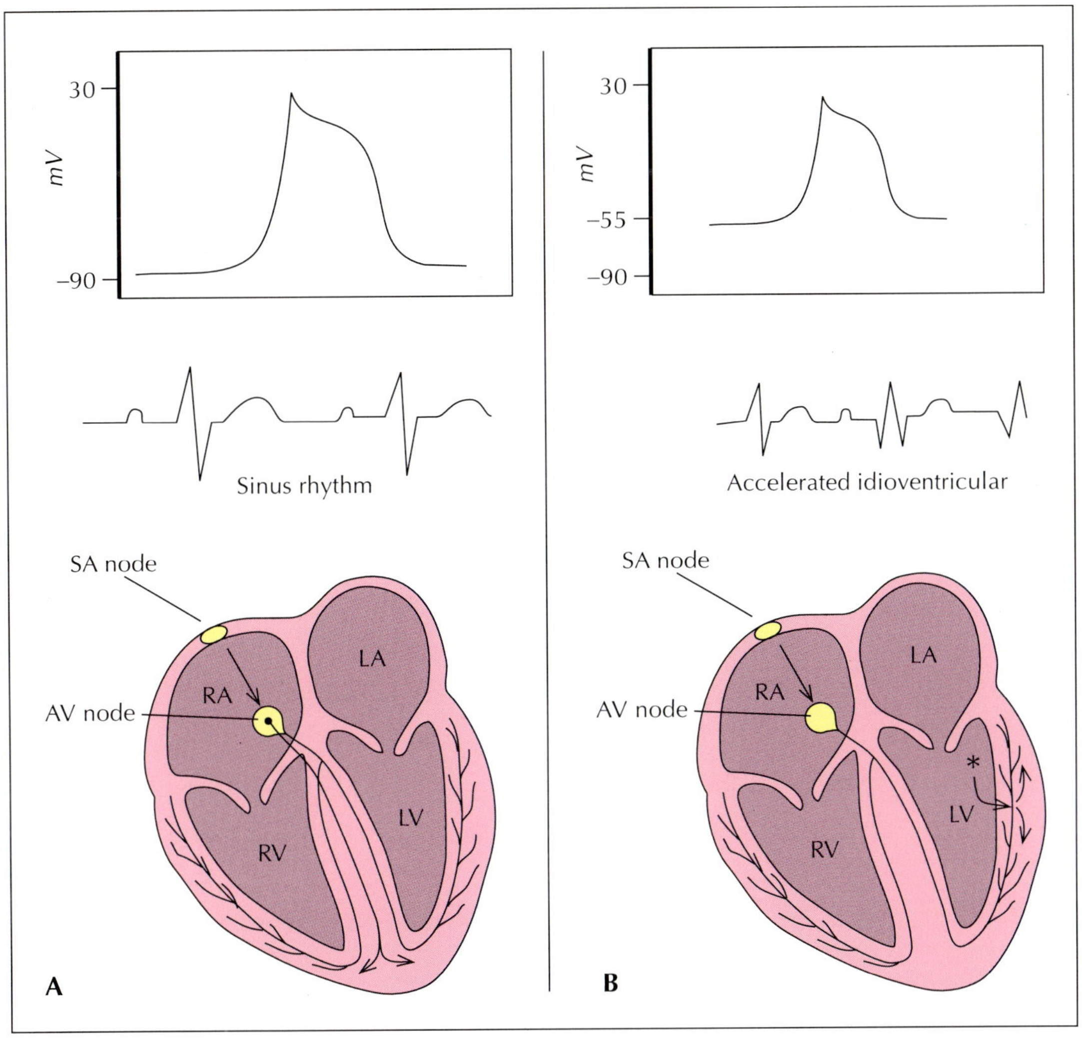

FIGURE 1-18. Abnormal automaticity occurs when spontaneous depolarizations are generated in partially depolarized tissue (reduced maximum diastolic potential or resting membrane potential) as a result of some pathologic process such as ischemia. Arrhythmias that may arise because of abnormal automaticity are certain types of ectopic atrial tachycardias, accelerated idioventricular rhythms, and ventricular tachycardias (especially within the first 72 hours after a myocardial infarction). Compared are normal ventricular tissue (**A**) and ischemic ventricular tissue (asterisk in **B**). Shown are the action potentials along with a schematic drawing of the possible conduction throughout the heart and the resultant rhythms. LA—left atrium; LV—left ventricle; RA—right atrium; RV—right ventricle.

TRIGGERED ARRHYTHMIAS

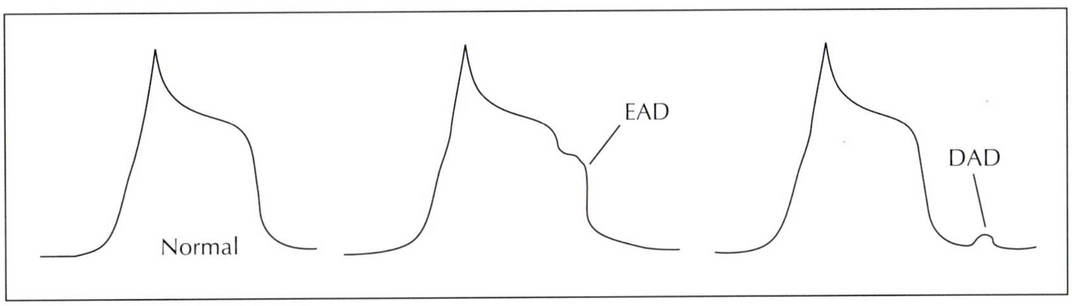

FIGURE 1-19. Triggered activity arises as a consequence of increased positive ions within the cardiac cell, leading to distortion of the action potential (after-depolarization). After-depolarizations can occur in the late phase 3 (early after-depolarization [EAD]) or early phase 4 (delayed after-depolarization [DAD]).

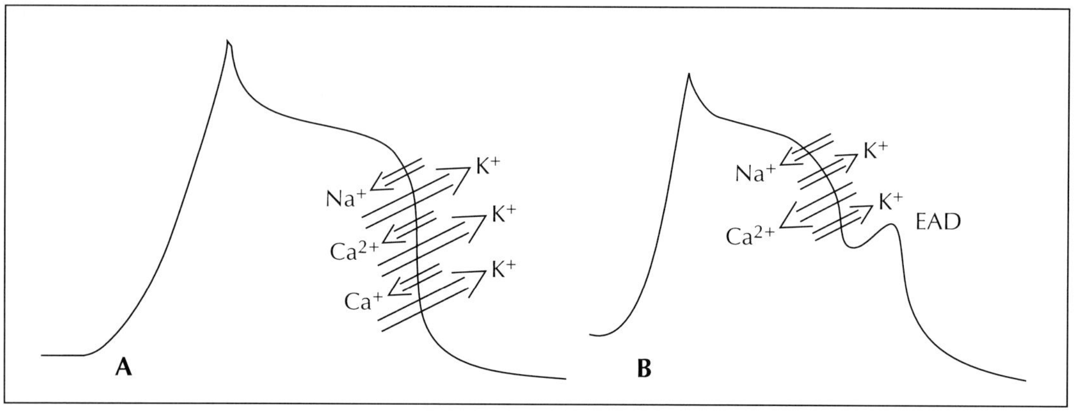

FIGURE 1-20. **A**, During repolarization of the action potential, the outward potassium current is the major ion responsible for the rapid repolarization phase of the action potential. Inward calcium and sodium ions have minor roles during phase 3. **B**, Early after-depolarizations (EADs) arise when there is a reduction of the outward potassium current, a prolongation of the inward calcium or sodium current, or a combination of reduced outward current and enhanced inward current. They are associated with a prolonged action potential duration.

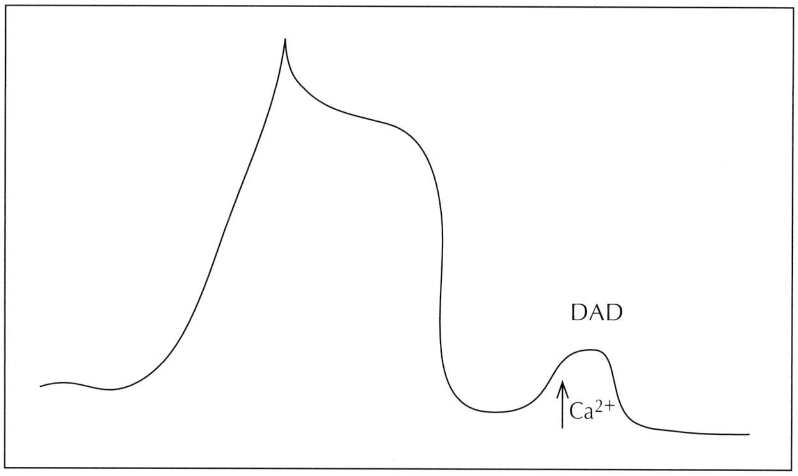

FIGURE 1-21. Delayed after-depolarizations (DADs) occur when there is intracellular calcium overload. The repetitive release of calcium from the sarcoplasmic reticulum results in an inward, depolarizing current that leads to the generation of DADs.

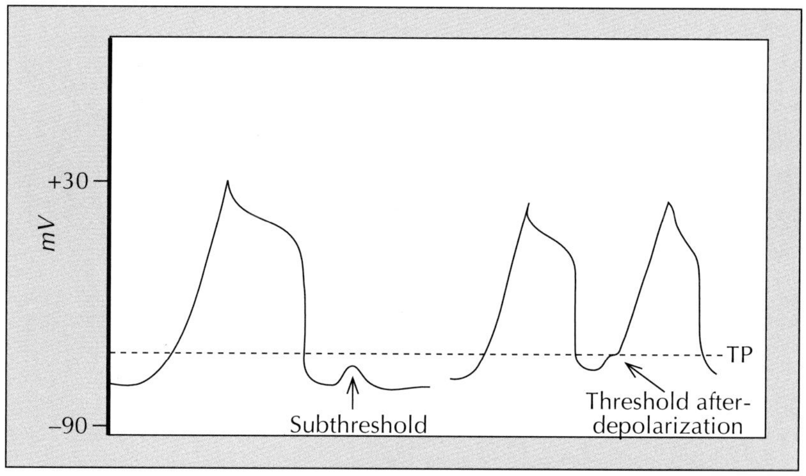

FIGURE 1-22. Delayed after-depolarizations of sufficient magnitude will activate the rapid sodium channels, leading to the generation of another action potential. TP—threshold potential.

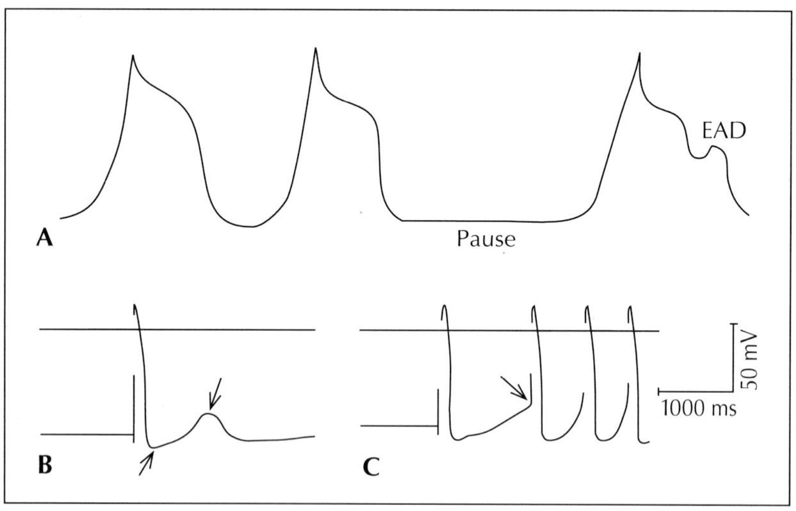

FIGURE 1-23. Triggered activity is not spontaneous but depends on the "preconditioning" of prior impulses. **A,** Early after-depolarizations (EADs) most commonly occur at slow heart rates or following a pause. They are thought to be the mechanism underlying torsade de pointes [17,18] and certain reperfusion arrhythmias [19]. **B,** Delayed after-depolarizations (DADs) (*arrow to the right*) are often preceded by an after-hyperpolarization (*arrow to the left*). **C,** If the DAD reaches threshold potential (*arrow*), it will produce a premature action potential called a triggered impulse [20], because it was dependent upon the preceding beat. Arrhythmias associated with DADs include digitalis intoxication and catecholamine-sensitive ventricular tachycardia. (Parts B and C *adapted from* Wit and coworkers [21]; with permission.)

Reentry as a Mechanism for Arrhythmias

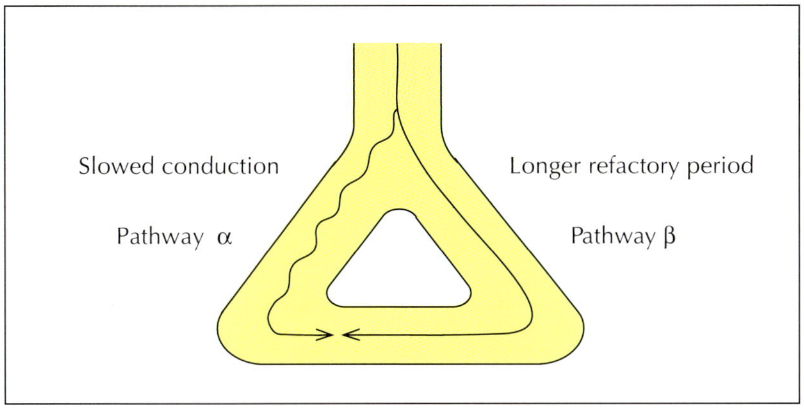

Figure 1-24. Prerequisites for reentry arrhythmias include: (1) an anatomic circuit with two pathways eventually joined by a common tissue, (2) the two pathways have different electrophysiologic properties, and (3) a section within the circuit (pathway β) has a longer refractory period than the pathway α, thus permitting unidirectional block.

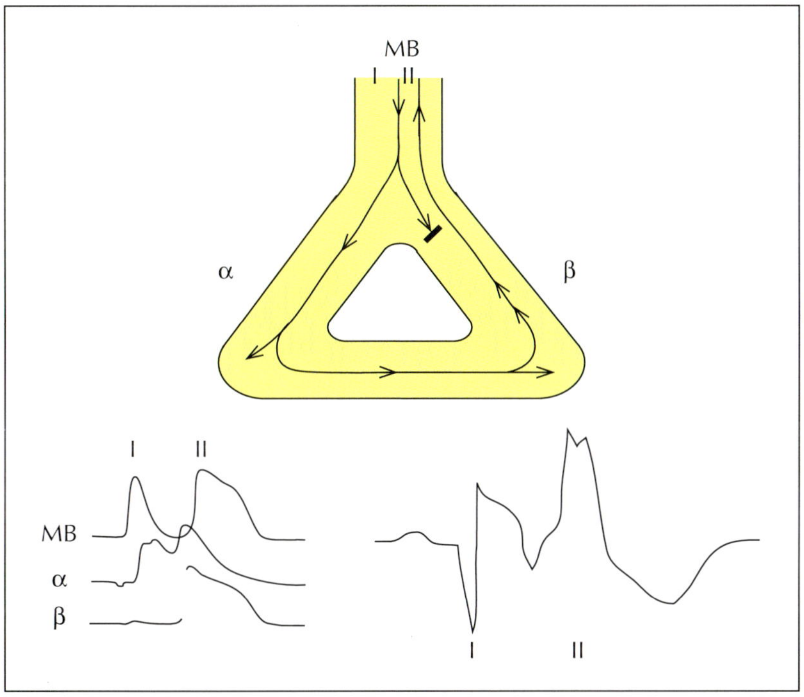

Figure 1-25. The sequence of activation within the reentry circuit, indicated by arrows I and II. Arrow I indicates an impulse of sinus origin entering the circuit. Arrow II is the reentry impulse leaving the loop. Under the reentry circuit are action potentials recorded from myocardial branches (MB) α and β together with an example of how an electrocardiogram might appear. Impulse I would cause ventricular depolarization and impulse II would cause a ventricular extrasystole. (*Adapted from* Wit and Bigger [22]; with permission.)

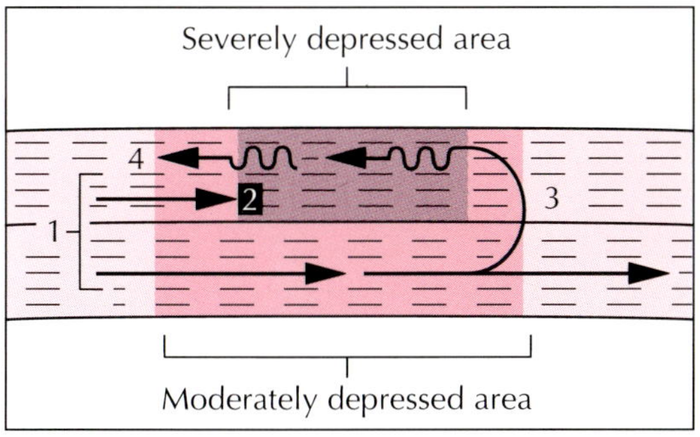

Figure 1-26. Another type of reentry is produced through longitudinal dissociation or reflection. An impulse may turn around within a depressed segment of tissue. The impulse (1) is blocked in the severely depressed fiber (2), but conduction of the impulse proceeds slowly in the less depressed fiber and eventually returns in the retrograde direction (3) through the depressed tissue (4).

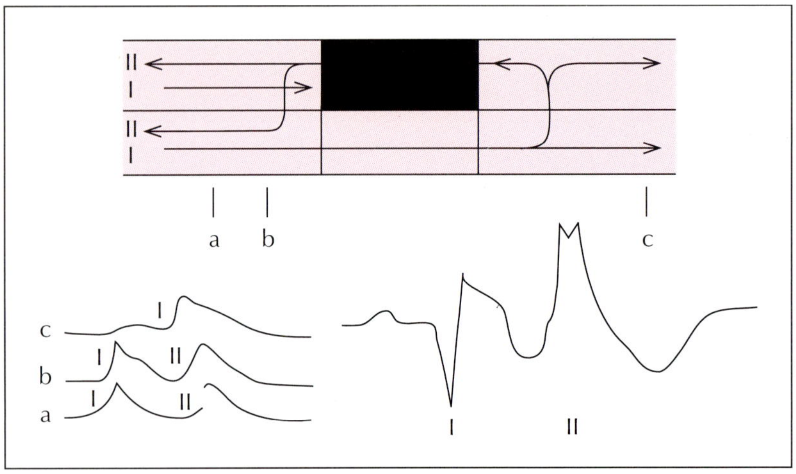

FIGURE 1-27. Reentry due to reflection. The *top panel* demonstrates how reentry can occur even in a single bundle of muscle or Purkinje fibers. The entire shaded area is depressed, but depression in the darkest area of the upper fiber is so severe that unidirectional conduction block occurs. Arrows indicate the sequence of activation, then the bundles. The arrow labeled I indicates the impulse entering the bundle, and the arrow labeled II shows the reentry impulse returning to its origin. The *lower panel* represents action potential measured at sites a, b, and c, with an example of how an electrocardiogram may appear, I being the normal conducted beat and II being the ventricular extrasystole. (*Adapted from* Wit and Bigger [22]; with permission.)

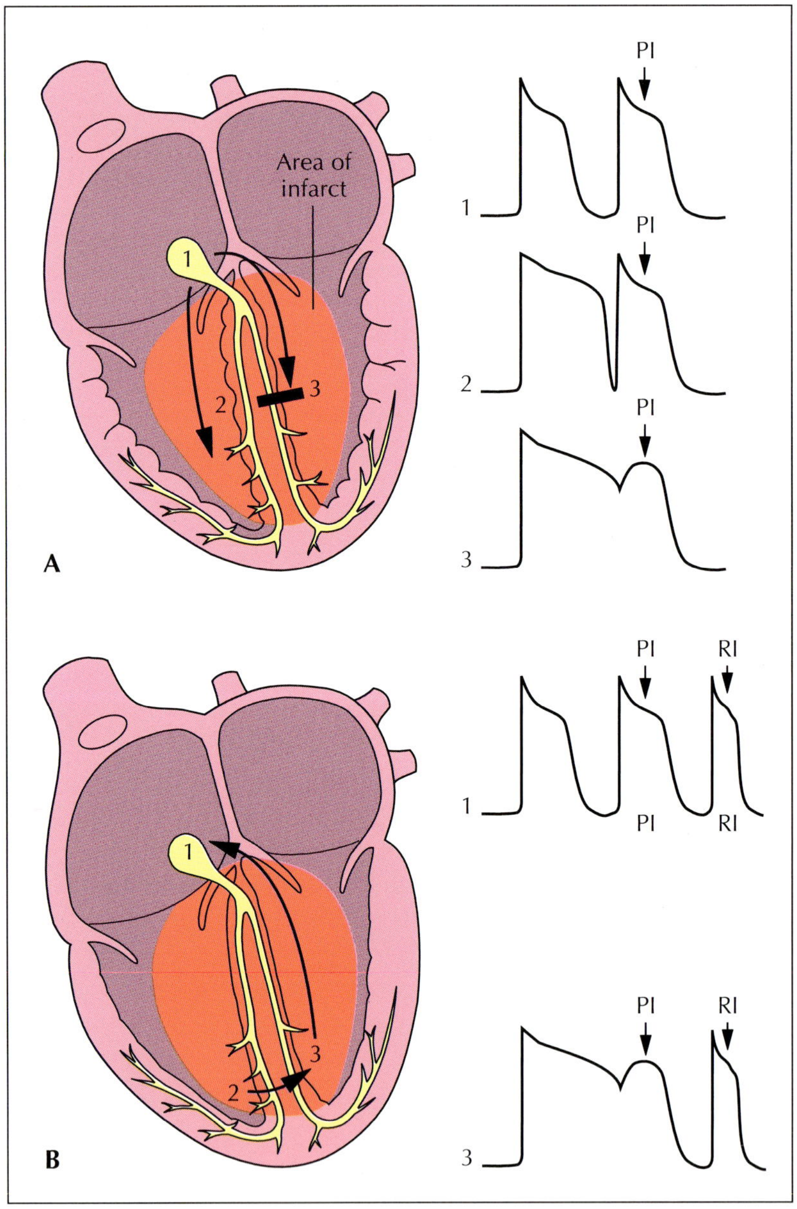

FIGURE 1-28. Mechanism for reentry resulting from dispersion of refractoriness in the subendocardial Purkinje fiber network over an area of extensive myocardial infarction. This figure shows the endocardial surface of the left ventricular anterior papillary muscle. The color area in each diagram is the scar resulting from the myocardial infarct that is covered by a blanket of the surviving Purkinje fibers. As depicted, Purkinje fibers in different regions have markedly different action potentials with respect to duration and refractory periods. Action potentials are recorded from normal tissue (site 1) and from subendocardial Purkinje fibers with prolonged repolarization phases (sites 2 and 3), surviving in the infarct. In **A,** premature impulse (PI) occurs at the infarct border (site 1) and conducts into the infarcted regions as indicated by the large arrows. Note that the action potentials are prolonged. The action potential at site 3 is longer than at site 2 in the infarcted area. Consequently, premature impulses can excite cells at site 2, but conduction blocks at site 3. **B,** The continuation of these events after the premature impulse conducts through site 2 and activates the cells at site 3. As a reentering impulse (RI), it then proceeds to its site of origin (site 1), which also re-excites as a reentry impulse (RI). (*Adapted from* Wit and coworkers. [23]; with permission.)

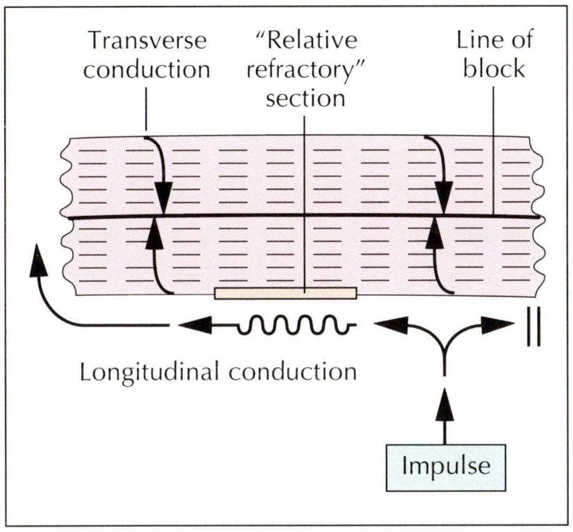

FIGURE 1-29. Another type of functional reentry is anisotropic reentry. Anisotropic reentry differs from a purely functional reentry in that reentry is not based on differences in transmembrane currents causing the action potential but on differences in the physical properties of muscle orientation. As shown in the schematic representation of an anisotropic reentry circuit, conduction parallel to the fiber orientation (longitudinal conduction) is fast, whereas conduction perpendicular to the fiber axis (transverse conduction) is slow. These differences in the conduction properties of the fiber orientation allow an anatomic line of block to form. Furthermore, differences in their conduction allow differences in refractoriness of the tissue. The portion of the circuit that is absolutely refractory is depicted in black and the part of the circuit that is relatively refractory is striped. Excitable gaps can only form in the longitudinal direction. Therefore, an impulse originating outside of the circuit can only enter the circuit through the excitable gap in the longitudinal limbs. Depending on the refractoriness of the tissue in both the antegrade and retrograde directions, penetrating impulse may block retrograde as a result of the collision of the oncoming wavefronts and conduct antegrade, thus initiating a reentry pattern.

References

1. James TN: Morphology of the human atrioventricular node, with remarks pertinent to its electrophysiology. *Am Heart J* 1961, 62:756.
2. Becker AE, Anderson RH: Morphology of the human atrioventricular junctional area. In *The Conduction System of the Heart. Structure, Function and Clinical Implications*. Edited by Wellens HJJ, Lie KI, Janse MJ. Leiden: Stenfert Kroese; 1976:263.
3. Spach MS, Lieberman M, Scott JG, *et al.*: Excitation sequences of the atrial septum and AV node in isolated hearts of the dog and rabbit. *Circ Res* 1971, 29:156.
4. Mandel WJ: *Cardiac Arrhythmias*. Philadelphia: JB Lippincott, 1980:21, 214.
5. Marriot HJC, Conover MH (eds): *Advanced Concepts in Arrhythmias*. St. Louis: CV Mosby; 1983:13–15.
6. Singer DH, Ten Eick RE: Pharmacology of cardiac arrhythmias. *Prog Cardiovasc Dis* 1969, 11(6):488–514.
7. CIBA Pharmaceutical Company Division of CIBA-GEIGY Corporation: The CIBA Collection of Medical Illustrations by Frank H. Netter, MD, 1969.
8. Ehara T, Noma A, Ono K: Calcium activated nonselective cation channel in ventricular cells isolated from adult guinea pig heart. *J Physiol (Lond)* 1988, 403:117–133.
9. Giles WR, Imaizumi Y: Comparison of potassium currents in rabbit atrial and ventricular cells. *J Physiol (Lond)* 1988, 405:123–145.
10. Coraboeuf E, Carmeliet E: Existence of two transient outward currents in sheep cardiac Purkinje fibers. *Pflugers Arch* 1982, 392:352–359.
11. Sakmann B, Noma A, Trautwein W: Acetycholine activation of single muscarinic K channels in isolated pacemaker cells of the mammalian heart. *Nature* 1983, 303:250–253.
12. Carmeliet E, Storms L, Vereecke J: The ATP-dependent K channel and metabolic inhibition. In *Cardiac Electrophysiology: From Cell to Bedside*. Edited by Zipes DP, Jalife J. Philadelphia: WB Saunders; 1990:103–108.
13. Harvey RD, Clark CD, Hume JR: Chloride current in mammalian cardiac myocytes. *J Gen Physiol* 1990, 95:1077–1102.
14. Gadsby DC: The Na/K pump of cardiac cells. *Ann Rev Biophys Bioeng* 1984, 13:373–378.
15. Task Force of the Working Group on Arrhythmias of the European Society of Cardiology: The Sicilian Gambit: A new approach to the classification of antiarrhythmic drugs based on their actions on arrhythmogenic mechanisms. *Circulation* 1991, 84:1831–1851.
16. Rosen MR, Hordof AJ, Roberts NK, Gelband H: *Cardiac Arrhythmias in the Neonate, Infant and Child*. New York: Appleton Century Crofts; 1977:116.
17. Brachman J, Scherlag BJ, Rosenshtraukh LV, Lazzara R: Bradycardia-dependent triggered activity: relevance to drug-induced multiform ventricular tachycardia. *Circulation* 1983, 68:846–856.
18. Krikler DM, Curry PVL: Torsade de pointes: an atypical ventricular tachycardia. *Br Heart J* 1976, 38:117–120.
19. Priori SG, Mantica M, Napolitano C, Schwartz PJ: Early afterdepolarizations induced in vivo by reperfusion of ischemic myocardium: a possible mechanism for reperfusion arrhythmias. *Circulation* 1990, 81:1911–1920.
20. Cranefield PF, Aronson RS: *Cardiac Arrhythmias: The Role of Triggered Activity and Other Mechanisms*. Mt. Kisco, NY: Futura Publishing Co; 1988.
21. Wit AL, Boyden PA, Gadsby DC, Cranefield PF: In *Cardiac Arrhythmias: Electrophysiology, Diagnosis, and Management*. Edited by Narala OS. Baltmore: Williams & Wilkins; 1979:459.
22. Wit AL, Bigger JT: Possible electrophysiologic mechanism for lethal arrhythmias accompanying myocardial ischemia and infarction. *Circulation* 1975, 3(Suppl 51, 52):96.
23. Wit AL, Rosen MR, Hoffman BF: Electrophysiology and pharmacology of cardiac arrhythmias. II: Relationship of normal and abnormal electrical activity of cardiac fibers to the genesis of arrhythmias. B. Reentry. *Am Heart J* 1974, 88:799.

Pharmacology/Pharmacokinetics and Clinical Use of Antiarrhythmic Agents

2

CHAPTER

Randall J. Lee

The concept that drugs bring about their effects by interacting with specific receptors in or on cells was postulated almost 100 years ago and has been confirmed by the isolation and characterization of many receptors during the past two decades. The hypothesis has been extremely effective in explaining drug effects and is fully applicable to the action of antiarrhythmic drugs.

The goal of pharmacologic therapy in the treatment of cardiac arrhythmias is to utilize drug interactions with appropriate receptors to correct pathologic membrane excitability caused by the abnormal electrophysiology of the heart. Abnormalities of impulse generation and impulse conduction that lead to cardiac arrhythmias are believed to result from abnormal membrane channel action or from imbalances in the ionic milieu. The initial management of arrhythmias includes the correction of reversible causes of cardiac arrhythmias (*eg*, revascularization for ischemic heart disease, correction of electrolyte imbalances, and removal of any drug that is causing proarrhythmic effects). If these initial therapies do not correct the arrhythmias, then specific pharmacologic intervention is warranted.

Pharmacologic therapy should be directed toward altering the primary mechanism initiating or maintaining the arrhythmia. For example, in an ischemic reentry ventricular tachycardia, therapy could be directed toward slowing conduction through, or increasing refractoriness in, the circuit by using drugs with type I effects or by increasing refractoriness within the circuit by using drugs with class III effects. Since all antiarrhythmic agents have adverse effects, benefits versus risks must always be considered. Furthermore, dosing of the antiarrhythmic drug should be aimed at producing therapeutic effects with minimal toxicity.

This chapter reviews the putative receptors for antiarrhythmic drugs, the basic pharmacologic principles in achieving the desired therapeutic effect, and the classification of antiarrhythmic drugs.

Ion Channel Concepts

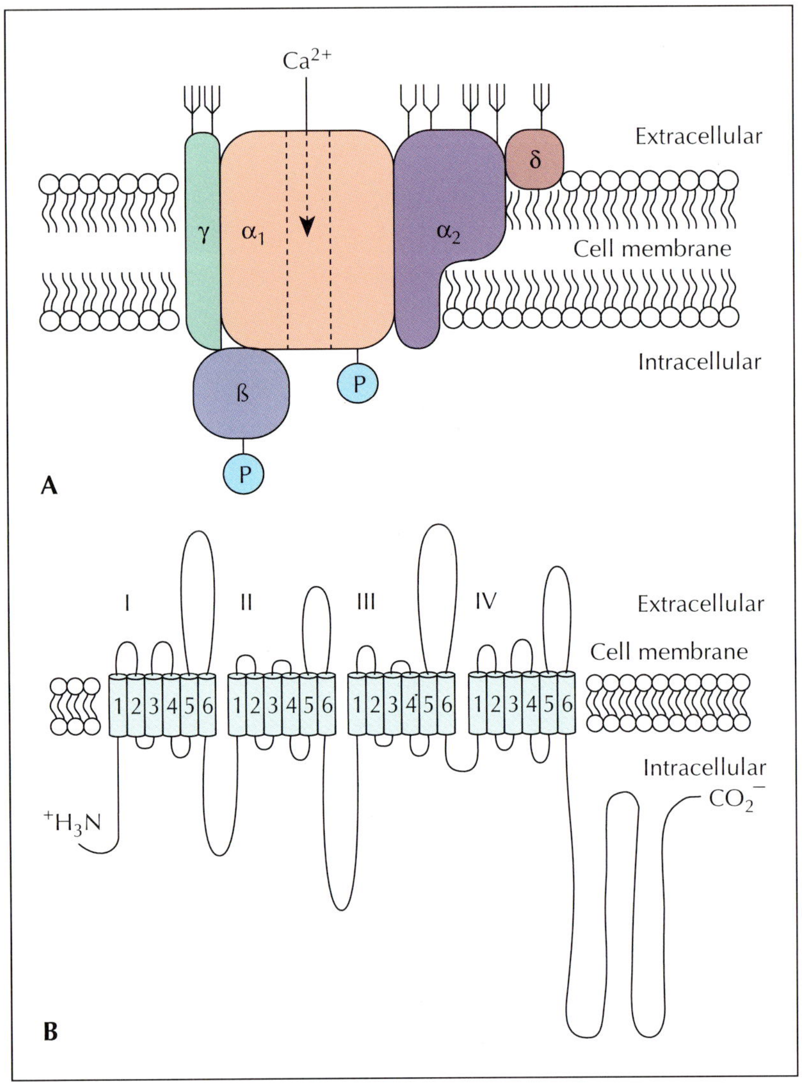

FIGURE 2-1. Cardiac channels and receptors. The receptors for most antiarrhythmic drugs are ion channels that maintain the resting membrane potential and generate the currents involved in the action potential. Advances in molecular biology have recently led to the cloning of sodium, calcium, and potassium channels. Each of these membrane portals represents a family of channels that contain several subtypes with varying cellular electrophysiologic properties. **A** depicts the structure of the calcium channel of rabbit skeletal muscle. There are four subunits: (α_1, α_2/δ, β, and γ), each subunit being coded by a different gene. Note that the channel pore is contained within the alpha subunit. **B**, shows more detailed representation of the α_1 receptor site subunit of the putative transmembrane structure. This subunit is composed of four repeating motifs, each motif containing six membrane-spanning helices. CO_2^-—carboxyl terminus; ^+H_3N—amino terminus; P—putative phosphorylation sites. (*Adapted from* Catterall [1]; with permission.)

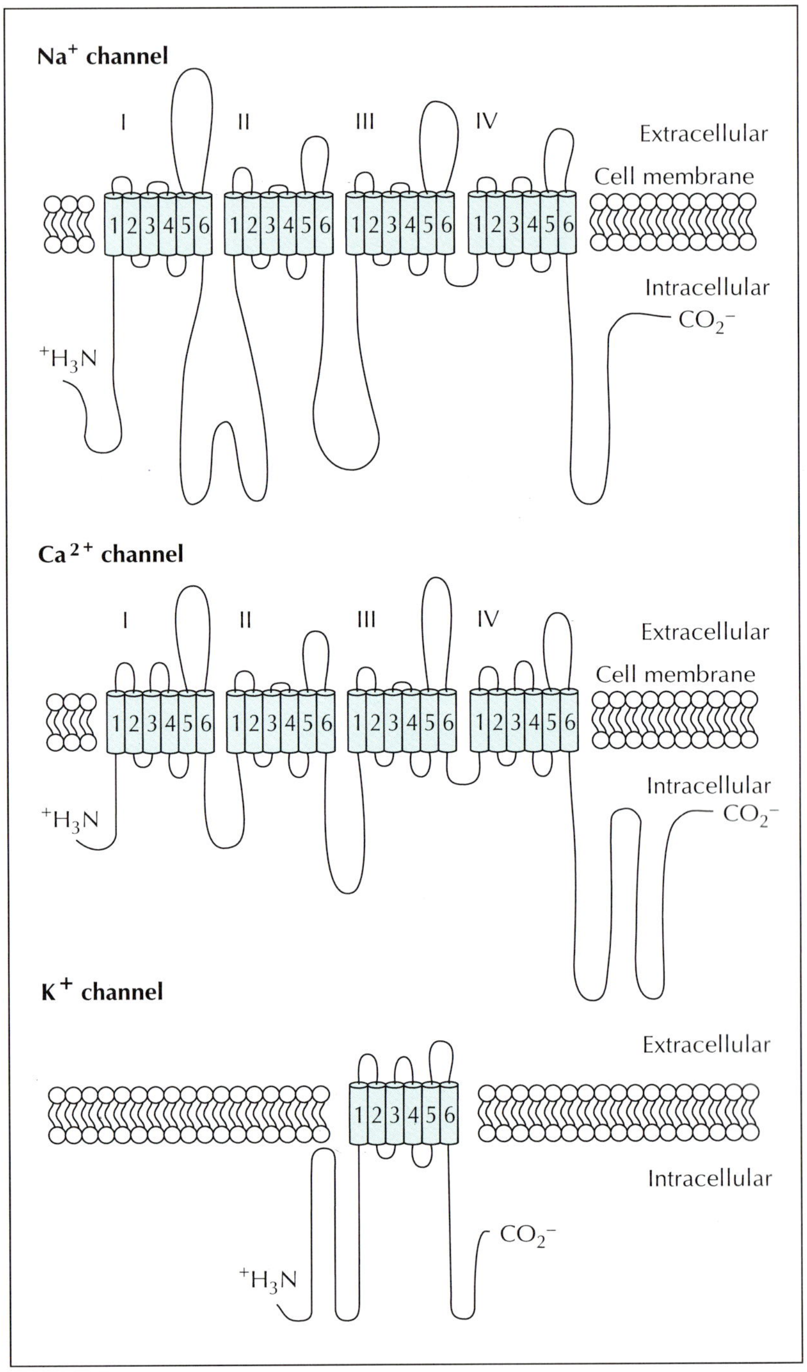

FIGURE 2-2. Cardiac ion channels: proposed configurations of sodium, calcium, and potassium subunit structures. Note the similar folding pattern of the subunits of the sodium and potassium voltage-gated ion channels. CO_2^-—carboxyl terminus; ^+H_3N—amino terminus. (*Adapted from* Catterall [1]; with permission.)

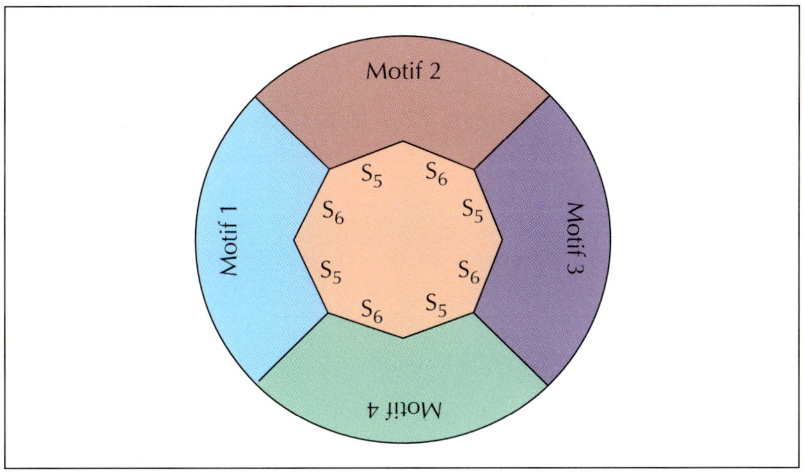

FIGURE 2-3. Cardiac ion channels. A view of the channel pore structure from above. The portion of the molecule forming the surface lining the pore of the α_1 subunit of the calcium channel is believed to involve the S5 and S6 transmembrane helices of each of the four motifs. A ring of negatively charged glutamine residues (not shown) lines the pore. This ring of negative charges has been postulated to be the major determinant of ion selectivity [2]. Similar configurations for the sodium and potassium channels are plausible. (*Adapted from* Catterall and Striessnig [3]; with permission.)

PHARMACOKINETIC PRINCIPLES

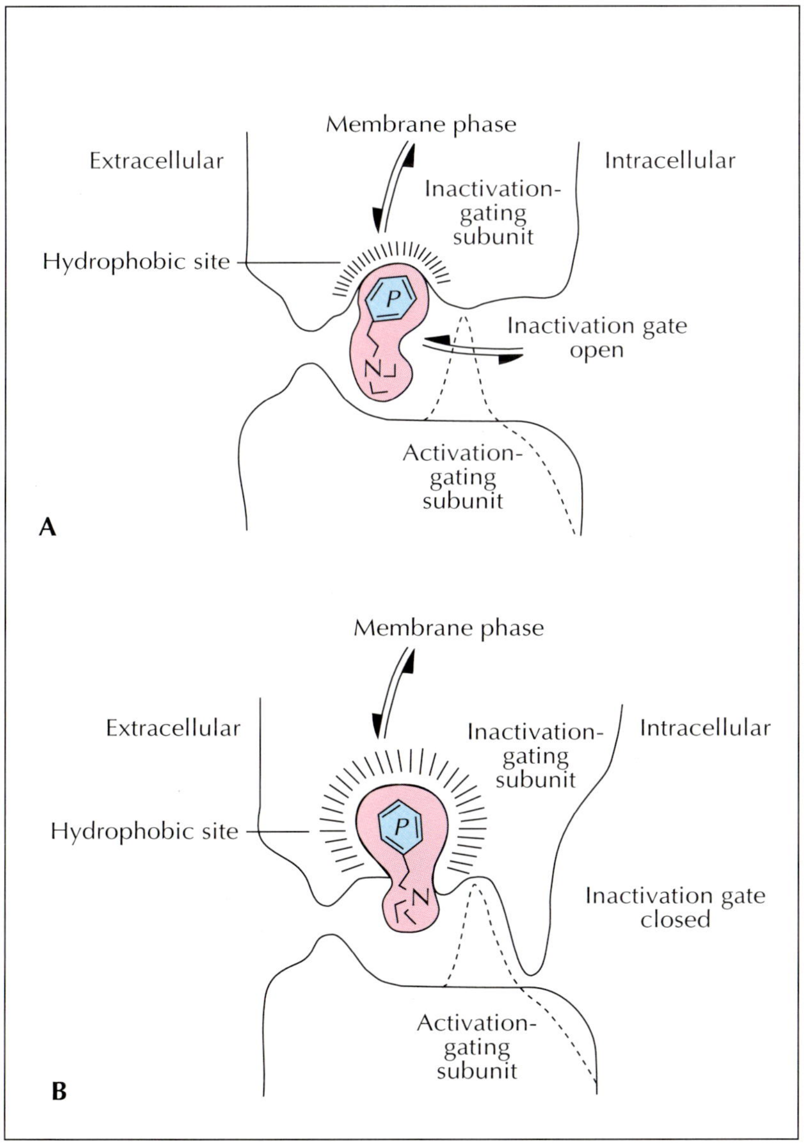

FIGURE 2-4. Drug binding in a sodium channel. The advances in molecular biology and cellular electrophysiology allow investigators to study structural and functional relationships of ion channels and test current hypotheses for antiarrhythmic drug modulation of ion channels. **A**, Procainamide *(P)*, an antiarrhythmic drug with local anesthetic properties, binds to a hydrophobic site within the pore of the sodium channel; this binding promotes inactivation of the channel. The procainamide receptor is in the channel near the inactivation-gating subunit. Intracellular procainamide can reach its binding site if activation (m-gating subunit) and inactivation (h-gating subunit) gates are open; however, the binding is not very firm. If one or both gates are closed, only procainamide located within the membrane phase can interact with its binding site. **B**, Closure of the inactivation gate modifies the binding site. The conformational change in the channel increases its affinity for procainamide. Studies in progress—to define the precise characteristics of the drug-binding site—may lead to more selective and less toxic drugs. N—amino group. (*Adapted from* Hille [4]; with permission.)

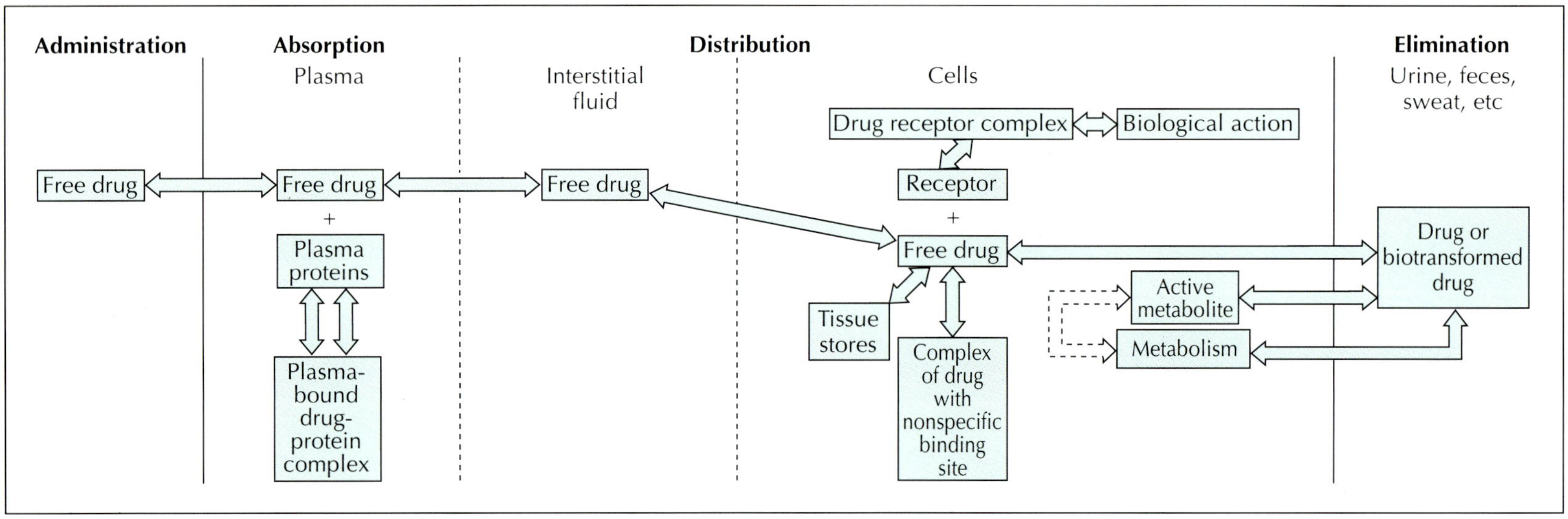

FIGURE 2-5. Flow chart of pharmacokinetics of antiarrhythmic drugs. A drug must be present in a specific concentration at its site of action to produce the desired biologic effect. Entry of the drug into the body is initially dependent on absorption from the site of administration. Once the drug is in the central circulation, it may bind to plasma proteins, thus decreasing the free concentration of the drug. Most antiarrhythmic drugs are basic compounds and tend to bind to alpha-acid glycoprotein. The free drug distributes into the interstitial fluid, which accounts for approximately 11% of total body water. As the drug distributes through the interstitial fluid, it perfuses and enters cells. Free drug can then be stored in tissue reservoirs, can nonspecifically bind to intracellular components, and can be metabolized into active or inactive metabolites. The free or biotransformed drug can then be excreted in urine, feces, or sweat. The drug can also bind to its site of action and form a drug-receptor complex, thus initiating its desired biologic action.

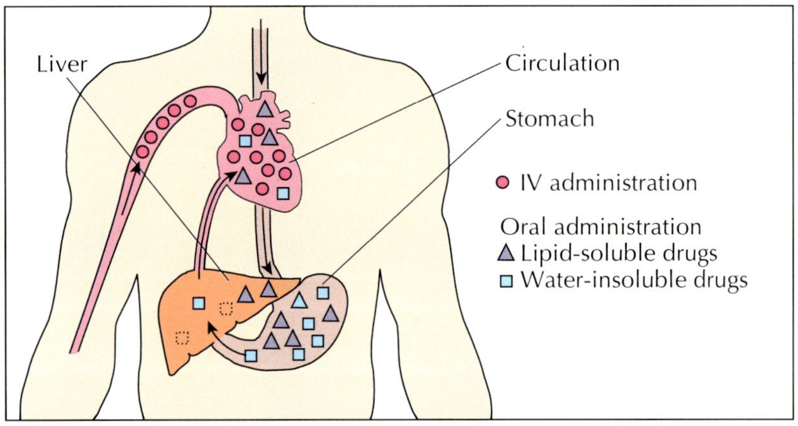

FIGURE 2-6. Drug absorption. Absorption is the process whereby a drug leaves its site of administration. Absorption of a drug depends on the route of administration and on the properties of the drug itself, such as lipid solubility and molecular size. Bioavailability is a measure of the efficiency of absorption. It may be defined as the fraction of a dose that reaches the systemic circulation when compared with the same dose administered intravenously (IV). Smaller lipid-soluble drugs can be readily absorbed into the systemic circulation and direct IV injection of a drug provides greater bioavailability than oral administration of the same drug. The lower bioavailability after oral administration results from incomplete absorption, metabolism, or elimination by the liver before it reaches the systemic circulation. If the drug is metabolized in the gut or liver or excreted in the bile, a fraction of the active drug is inactivated or diverted from the systemic circulation (the first-pass effect).

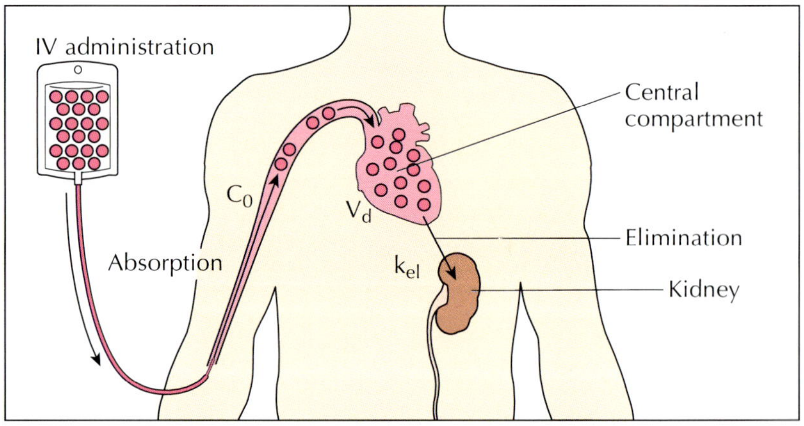

FIGURE 2-7. Drug distribution. Following absorption or infusion of the drug, the concentration of the drug is dependent upon its distribution within and elimination from the body. Distribution of a drug within the body depends on the ability of the drug to diffuse through membranes. In a single-compartment model, the drug distributes throughout its total volume of distribution. Plasma concentration immediately after an intravenous bolus and corrected for distribution delay (C_o) is a function of the intravenous (IV) dose and the volume of distribution (Vd). Volume of distribution is the volume that would be needed to account for all of the drug within the body at the drug concentration in the plasma (Cp). It is a mathematically abstract term that need not equate to any of the physical volumes within the body at the drug concentration in the plasma. The Vd can be calculated from Vd = amount in the body $\div C_o$. An example of a single-compartment drug is one that is completely confined to the vascular compartment. Drug elimination (elimination constant [k_{el}]) is determined by the clearance of the drug (Cl). Clearance is defined as the volume of blood from which the drug is removed per unit of time. Drug elimination generally proceeds as a first-order process, *ie*, it is proportionate to the concentration of drug remaining: rate of elimination = Cl × Cp.

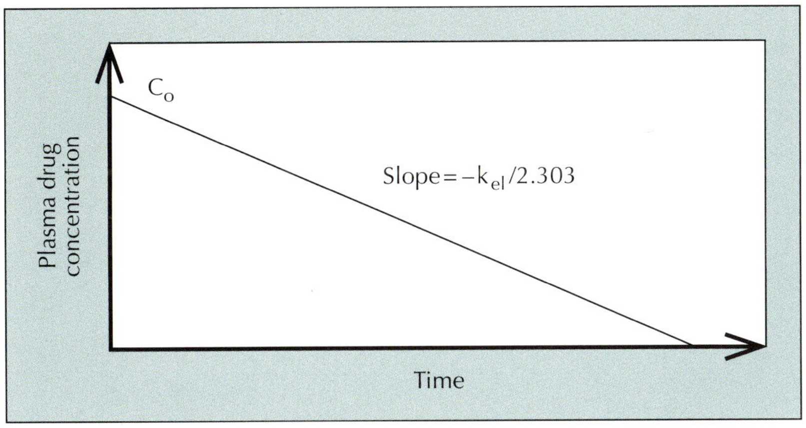

FIGURE 2-8. Pharmacokinetic calculations. For drugs that can be described by the single-compartment model and are rapidly distributed, the plasma level at any time (C_t) can be determined from the equation: $C_t = C_o \times e^{-k_{el} \times t}$, where C_o = plasma concentration immediately after the intravenous bolus, k_{el} = elimination constant, and t = time. In practice, C_o is determined by extrapolating the concentration–time curve back to zero time on the y axis.

At steady-state, the rate of elimination is equal to the rate of administration. Thus, if the clearance and the target concentration (*ie,* the concentration required to produce a therapeutic effect) of a drug are known, the steady-state infusion rate can be calculated by the equation: $K_o = Cl \times C_{ss}$, where K_o = infusion rate, Cl = clearance, and C_{ss} = plasma drug concentration at steady-state.

Similarly, the loading dose (LD) can be calculated from LD = $C_{ss} \times$ Vd, where Vd = volume of distribution. By substituting Cl for K_{el} x Vd, drug concentration at steady-state after constant infusion of a drug can be estimated by the equation: $C_{ss} = K_o \div Cl$. Furthermore, the elimination half-life of a drug ($t_{1/2}$) can be estimated from the equation $t_{1/2} = 0.693 \times Vd \div Cl$, where $t_{1/2}$= half-life.

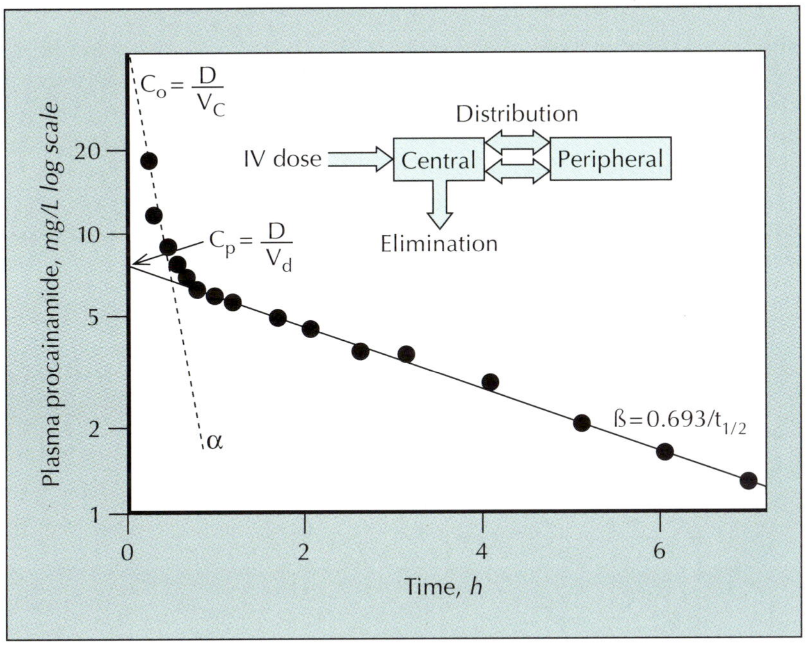

FIGURE 2-9. Plasma concentration decay curve. The concentration of procainamide (*closed circles*) following an intravenous bolus of procainamide hydrochloride shows the biphasic curve, indicating a two-compartment distribution pattern for their drug [5]. This illustrates the following principles: in a two compartment model, the drug distributes throughout the central volume of distribution, which includes blood volume plus the volume of highly perfused body tissues. From the central compartment, the drug then distributres into a second peripheral compartment. The straight lines are fitted to the points, using the model shown in the inset, in which the first phase of decay of plasma concentration represents distribution into the second compartment and declines with a half-life $T_{1/2}\alpha$ and the second phase represents elimination, which declines with a half-life $T_{1/2}\beta$. The volumes of distribution can be calculated from the curves shown in the inset. The volume of distribution for the central compartment (V_c) is determined by: V_c+D/V_c or C_o initial drug concentration, where D=intravenous dose and V_c=central volume of distribution. The total apparent volume of distribution (VD) is the sum of the volumes of the central and peripheral compartments. It can be calculated by extrapolating the peripheral compartment curve back to the Y axis to obtain C_p. The total apparent volume of distribution can then be calculated as: V_d=D/C_p.

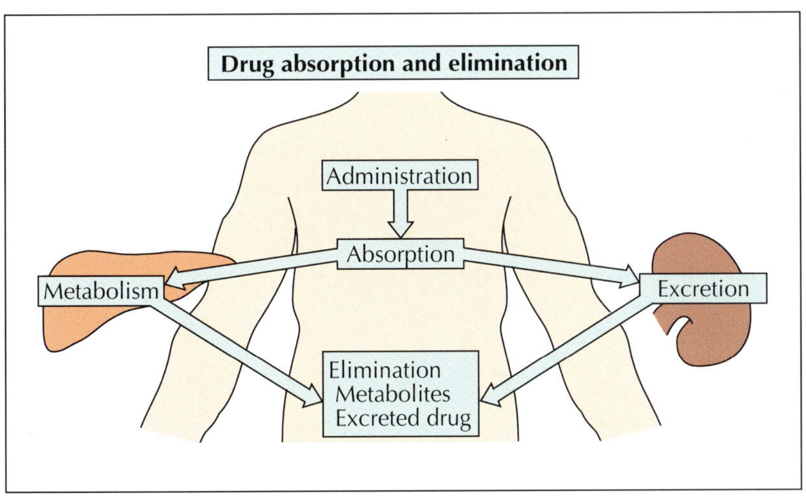

FIGURE 2-10. Elimination. Concentration of a drug depends on the balance of the drug's absorption into and rate of elimination from the body. Drugs may be eliminated by metabolism or by excretion of the unchanged molecule. Excretion of the drug and its metabolites may be via the urine, feces, sweat, or other routes. Renal elimination may be affected by alterations in renal blood flow, glomerular filtration rate, tubular secretion, and tubular resorption. Protein-bound drugs are eliminated slowly by this route. Bound as well as unbound drugs can also undergo hepatic elimination, which is affected by the flow of blood to the liver and the hepatic extraction ratio (efficiency of the hepatic drug-metabolizing enzymes). Reductions in hepatic blood flow can be caused by cardiac diseases such as congestive heart failure, by agents commonly used to treat cardiac diseases such as β-adrenergic antagonists, and by other drugs such as H_2 histamine receptor antagonists.

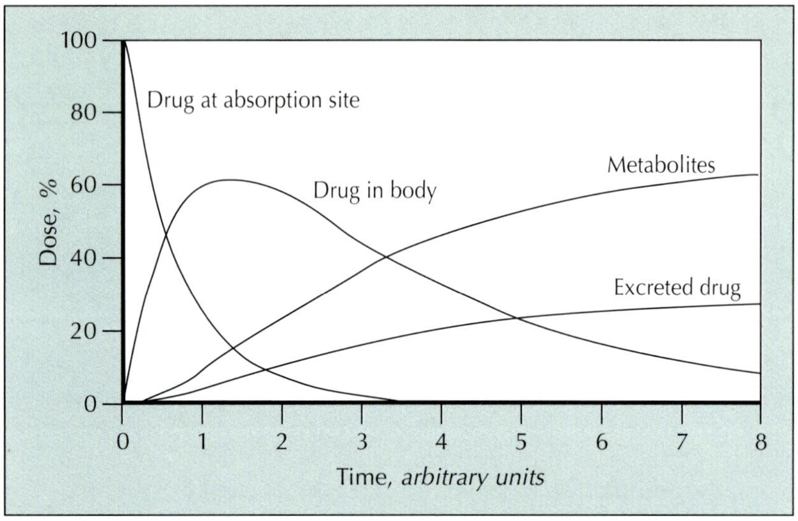

FIGURE 2-11. The fate of a drug after a single administration. Time course and relationship between drug at the site of administration (absorption), drug within the body, and elimination of the drug (excretion and metabolism) are shown. (*Adapted from* Rowland and Tozer [6]; with permission.)

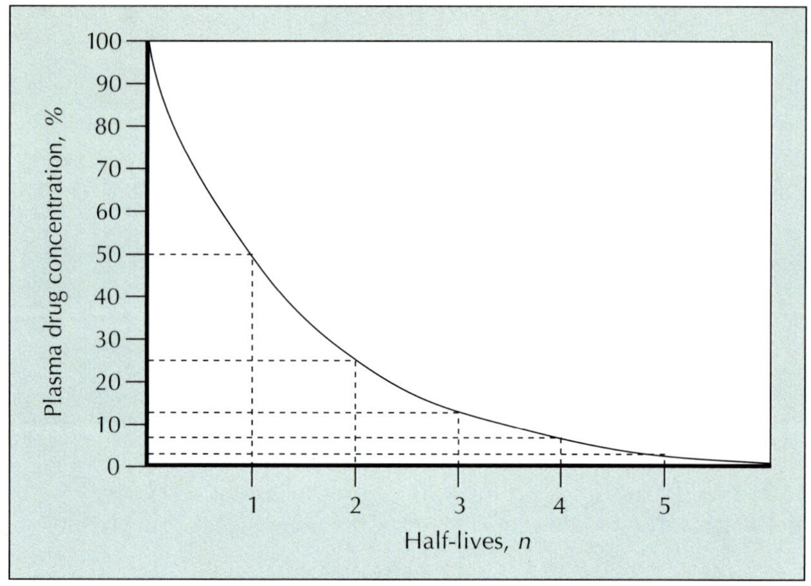

FIGURE 2-12. Time course after stopping drug administration. The time course of the concentration of a drug in the body after stopping administration can be predicted if the elimination half-life is known. As shown in the graph of plasma concentration of drug versus number of half-lives, greater than 90% of the drug will be eliminated after four half-lives and greater than 95% will be eliminated after five half-lives. To assure plasma levels whose peaks and troughs differ by 50% or less, a dose should be administered at each half-life.

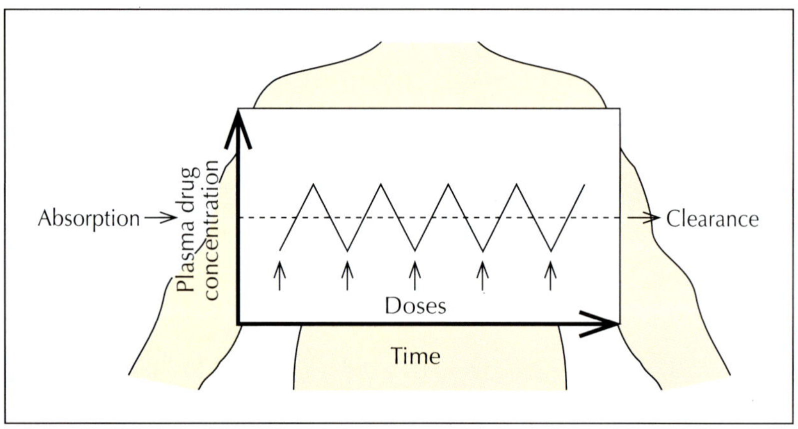

FIGURE 2-13. Intermittent dosing regimen. To maintain a relatively constant steady-state plasma drug concentration, various parameters depicted in the figure, such as fraction of the drug absorbed (F), elimination rate constant of the drug (k_{el}), and apparent volume of distribution (Vd), must be taken into consideration. These factors are related by the following equation: $C_{ss} = F \times dose/Cl \times Di$, where C_{ss} = plasma drug concentration at steady-state (remember that Cl [clearance] = $k_{el} \times Vd$). To assure plasma levels whose peaks and troughs differ by 50% or less, a dose should be given at intervals of one half-life or less. Slow-release preparations are available for some antiarrhythmic agents (*eg*, procainamide) to reduce the variation in plasma concentration. Such preparations can be given at intervals longer than fast-release preparations. Di—interval between doses.

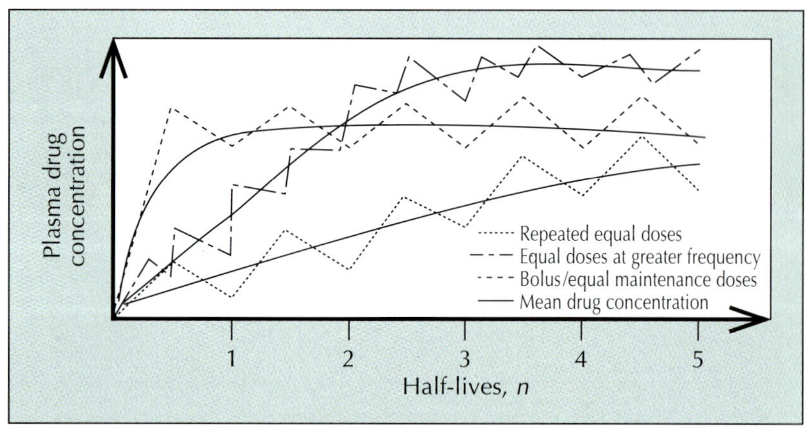

FIGURE 2-14. Time course of drug concentrations after repeated equal doses, after a bolus loading dose followed by equal maintenance doses, and following equal doses administered at a higher dosing frequency. Note that the dosing frequency is related to accumulation of the drug. An important difference between a loading dose and the maintenance dose is that the loading dose is not determined by the rate of clearance of a drug, whereas the drug clearance is a major determinant of the steady-state concentration of a drug.

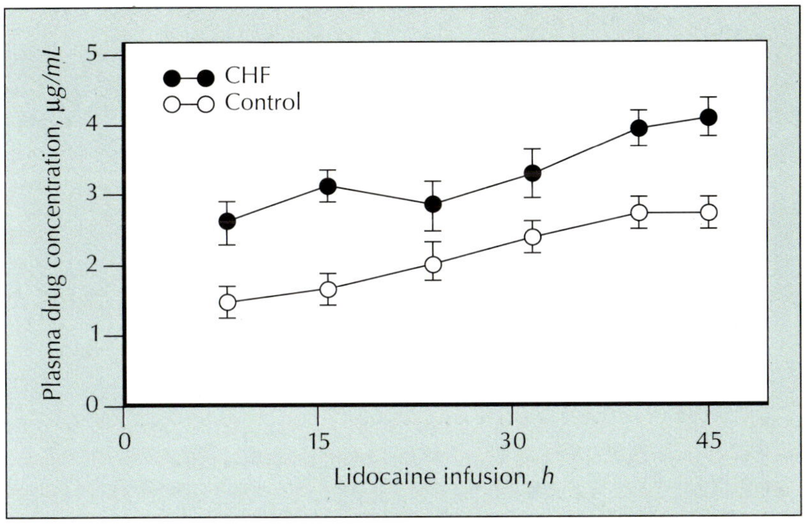

FIGURE 2-15. Effects of congestive heart failure (CHF). The pharmacokinetic changes caused by CHF include delayed and incomplete oral and intramuscular absorption; increased volume of distribution of water-soluble drugs (due to the increase in extracellular volume); decreased volume of distribution for lidocaine [7], quinidine [8], procainamide [5], and disopyramide [9]; and decreased clearance resulting from hepatocellular damage and decreased liver and renal perfusion. The graphs demonstrate the effects of CHF on plasma lidocaine concentration. Displayed are the mean (± SD) plasma concentrations of lidocaine during a constant infusion of lidocaine, 1.4 mg/min. (*Adapted from* Prescott and coworkers [10]; with permission.)

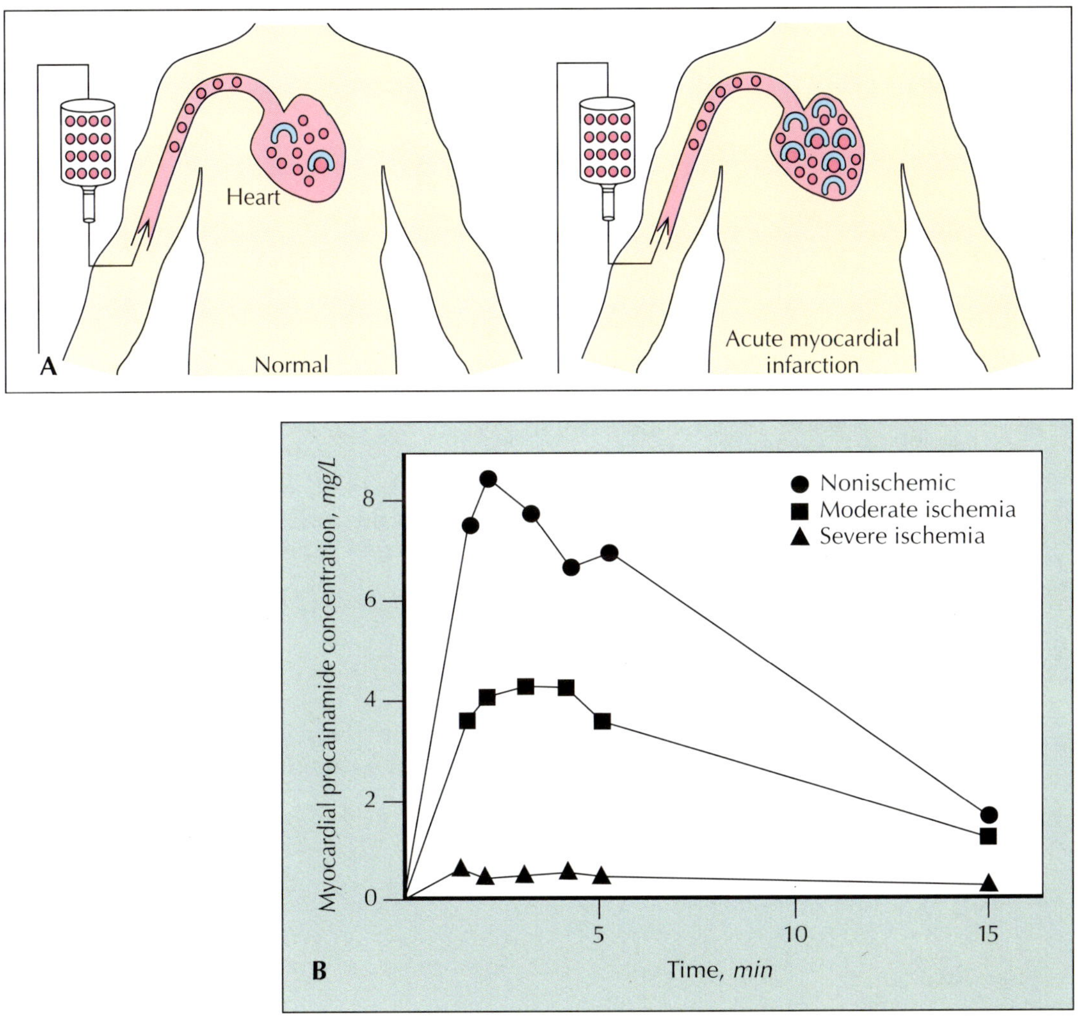

FIGURE 2-16. Effects of myocardial infarction on pharmacokinetics. Patients with acute myocardial infarction can have altered hemodynamics and increased levels of alpha$_1$-acid glycoprotein. During the acute phase of infarction, the total lidocaine plasma level becomes elevated because of the increased plasma protein binding resulting from increased levels of alpha$_1$-acid glycoproteins [11] (**A**). However, the unbound free lidocaine concentration remains relatively constant. Therefore, patients with acute myocardial infarction may tolerate higher plasma levels of antiarrhythmic drugs as observed with lidocaine, quinidine [12], and disopyramide [13]. Furthermore, experimental data suggest that areas of myocardial ischemia accumulate drugs more slowly, thus acting as a peripheral compartment rather than a central compartment. This alteration of myocardial drug disposition is demonstrated in **B**, which shows procainamide concentration in nonischemic regions versus regions of moderate and severe ischemia. (*Adapted from* Wenger and coworkers [14]; with permission.)

Classification of Antiarrhythmic Drugs

A. CLASSIFICATION OF ANTIARRHYTHMIC DRUGS ACCORDING TO THEIR MECHANISM OF ACTION

CLASS	ACTION	REPRESENTATIVE DRUGS
I	Sodium channel blockers, mechanism defined	
	Moderate phase 0 depression; moderate conduction slowing; prolongs repolarization	Quinidine*, Procainamide, Disopyramide
	Minimal phase 0 depression; shortens repolarization	Lidocaine (IV), Tocainide, Mexiletine
	Marked phase 0 depression; marked conduction slowing; slight effect on repolarization	Flecainide, Encainide, Propafenone
	Sodium channel blockers, mechanism not clearly defined	Moricizine, Recainam
II	β-blockers	Propranolol, Metoprolol , Atenolol, Esmolol
III	Prolong repolarization	Bretylium, Amiodarone†, Sotalol
IV	Calcium channel blockers	Verapamil, Diltiazem
Miscellaneous		
Purine		Adenosine
Digitalis glycosides		Digoxin, Digitoxin

*Quinidine also prolongs repolarization (class III effects).
†Amiodarone also blocks sodium channels (class I effects).

DRUG	CHANNELS: Na Fast	Na Med	Na Slow	Ca	K	I_f	RECEPTORS:	ß	M_2	P	PUMPS: Na/k ATPase
Lidocaine	Low										
Mexiletine	Low										
Tocainide	High (I)										
Moricizine		High (A)									
Procainamide		High (A)			Moderate						
Disopyramide		High (A)			Moderate				Low		
Quinidine		High (A)			Moderate		Low		Low		
Propafenone		High (A)						High			
Flecainide			High (A)		Low						
Encainide											
Bepridil	Low			High	Moderate						
Verapamil	Low			High			Moderate				
Diltiazem				Moderate							
Bretylium					High		Agonist/antagonist	Agonist/antagonist			
Sotalol					High			High			
Amiodarone	Low			Low	High		Moderate	High			
Alinidine				Moderate	High						
Nadolol								Moderate			
Propranolol	Low							Moderate			
Atropine									High		
Adenosine										Agonist	
Digoxin									Agonist		Moderate

Relative blocking potency: Low, Moderate, High; Agonist; Agonist/antagonist; A-Activated state blocker; I-Inactivated state blocker

B

Figure 2-17. Methods of antiarrhythmic drug classification. Two schemes have been used to classify antiarrhythmic drugs. **A**, The modified Vaughan Williams–Harrison system classifies antiarrhythmic drugs according to their cellular electrophysiologic effects on the cell. This classification is a listing of drug *actions* rather than of *drugs* themselves because most antiarrhythmic drugs have effects on more than one type of channel or autonomic receptor. **B**, The Task Force of the Working Group on Arrhythmias of the European Society of Cardiology classifies antiarrhythmic drugs on the basis of their pharmacologic site of action [15]. This is a better system because it recognizes the multiple effects of many of these drugs. It fails, however, to predict the types of arrhythmias likely to respond to any particular drug. (*Adapted from* The Sicilian Gambit [15]; with permission)

PHARMACOKINETIC SUMMARY OF ANTIARRHYTHMIC DRUGS

A. CLASS I. SODIUM CHANNEL BLOCKADE

DRUG	ROUTE OF ADMINIS-TRATION	ORAL BIOAVAIL-ABILITY, %	PROTEIN BINDING, %	HALF-LIFE OF PARENT COMPOUND, *h*	PRINCIPAL ROUTE OF ELIMINATION	ACTIVE METABOLITES	THERAPEUTIC RANGE, *μg/mL*	USUAL ORAL MAINTENANCE DOSE, *mg, FREQUENCY*
A.								
Quinidine	PO, IM, IV	80	75–95	6	Hepatic	3-Hydroxy-quinidine	2–7	200–400 qid
Procainamide	PO, IV	85	15	3	Hepatic, renal	*N*-acetyl-procainamide	4–10	500–1500 qid
Disopyramide	PO	80	40–81	7	Renal, hepatic	mono-N-dealkylated disopyramide	2–8	100–200 qid
B.								
Lidocaine	IV	35	70	1.7	Hepatic	MEGX	1.5–6.0	1.4 mg/min
Phenytoin	PO, IV	90	—	22	Hepatic	No	10–20	200–600 qd
Tocainide	PO	95	15	13–15	Hepatic, renal	No	4–10	300–600 tid
Mexiletine	PO	85	70	10–12	Hepatic	No	0.5–2	150–300 tid
C.								
Moricizine	PO	38	95	2–5 (9 chronic)	Hepatic	No	?	200–300 tid
Flecainide	PO	90	40	20	Hepatic, renal	No	0.4–1	100–150 bid
Encainide	PO	30 (85)*	70	2–3 (EM)	Hepatic	ODE 3-mode	?	25–50 tid
Propafenone	PO	<25	95	4–6 (EM)	Hepatic	OH-propafenone	?	150–300 tid
Recainam	PO	80	15	6–10	Renal, hepatic	No	?	200–600 tid

B. CLASS II. β-ADRENERGIC BLOCKADE

DRUG	ROUTE OF ADMINIS-TRATION	ORAL BIOAVAIL-ABILITY, %	PROTEIN BINDING, %	HALF-LIFE OF PARENT COMPOUND, *h*	PRINCIPAL ROUTE OF ELIMINATION	ACTIVE METABOLITES	THERAPEUTIC RANGE, *μg/mL*	USUAL ORAL MAINTENANCE DOSE, *mg, FREQUENCY*
Propranolol	PO, IV	10	—	3–6 (PO)	Hepatic	No	100–190	10–40 qid
Acebutolol	PO	40	25	3–4	Hepatic, renal	Diacetolol	?	200–400 qd
Esmolol	IV	NA	56	9 min	Hepatic	No	?	500μg/kg, load

FIGURE 2-18. Major pharmacokinetic properties of the antiarrhythmic drugs. **A**, Class I drugs are sodium channel blockers. **B**, Class II drugs provide β-adrenergic blockade. (*continued*)

C. CLASS III. PROLONGED REPOLARIZATION

DRUG	ROUTE OF ADMINIS-TRATION	ORAL BIOAVAIL-ABILITY, %	PROTEIN BINDING, %	HALF-LIFE OF PARENT COMPOUND, *h*	PRINCIPAL ROUTE OF ELIMINATION	ACTIVE METABOLITES	THERAPEUTIC RANGE, *µg/mL*	USUAL ORAL MAINTENANCE DOSE, *mg, FREQUENCY*
Bretylium	IV	NA	—	8	Renal	No	?	1–4 mg/min
Amiodarone	PO, IV	50	90	53 d	Hepatic	Desethyl-amiodarone	1.5–2.5	200–400 qd
Sotalol	PO, IV	90	50	7–15	Renal	No	?	80–320 bid

D. CLASS IV. CALCIUM CHANNEL BLOCKADE

DRUG	ROUTE OF ADMINIS-TRATION	ORAL BIOAVAIL-ABILITY, %	PROTEIN BINDING, %	HALF-LIFE OF PARENT COMPOUND, *h*	PRINCIPAL ROUTE OF ELIMINATION	ACTIVE METABOLITES	THERAPEUTIC RANGE, *µg/mL*	USUAL ORAL MAINTENANCE DOSE, *mg, FREQUENCY*
Verapamil	PO, IV	16	90	5 (PO)	Hepatic	No	0.1–0.4	0.1 g/kg IV; 80–160 PO, tid
Diltiazem	PO, IV	40	75	3.5	Hepatic	No	?	30–90 PO tid
Miscellaneous								
Adenosine	IV	NA	—	10 s	Cellular	No	?	6–12 mg IV
Digoxin	PO, IV	70	25	36–48	Renal	No	0.1–2.0	0.25 mg qd
Digitoxin	PO	95	90	7–9 d	Hepatic	No	10–20	0.15 mg qd

FIGURE 2-18. (*continued*) **C**, Class III agents prolong repolarization. **D**, Class IV drugs provide calcium channel blockade. A *question mark* indicates that a therapeutic range has not been established; an *asterisk* indicates that active metabolites have been taken into account. bid—twice a day; EM—extensive metabolizers; IM—intramuscularly; IV—intravenously; PO—orally; qid—four times a day; qd—once per day; tid—three times a day.

ANTIARRHYTHMIC DRUG INTERACTIONS

DRUG	INTERACTING DRUG	RESULT
Quinidine	Digoxin	Doubled digoxin levels
Propafenone	Digoxin	Doubled digoxin levels
Amiodarone	Digoxin	Doubled digoxin levels
	Quinidine, procainamide, disopyramide, flecainide	15%–35% increase in Na^+ channel blocker levels
	Warfarin	Double–triple increase in prothrombin times
Disopyramide	Phenytoin	Decreased disopyramide levels
Verapamil	Digoxin	Increased digoxin levels
Moricizine	Theophylline	Decreased theophylline levels

FIGURE 2-19. Important antiarrhythmic drug interactions.

MECHANISMS OF ACTION OF ANTIARRHYTHMIC DRUGS AND EFFECTS ON THE INTACT HEART

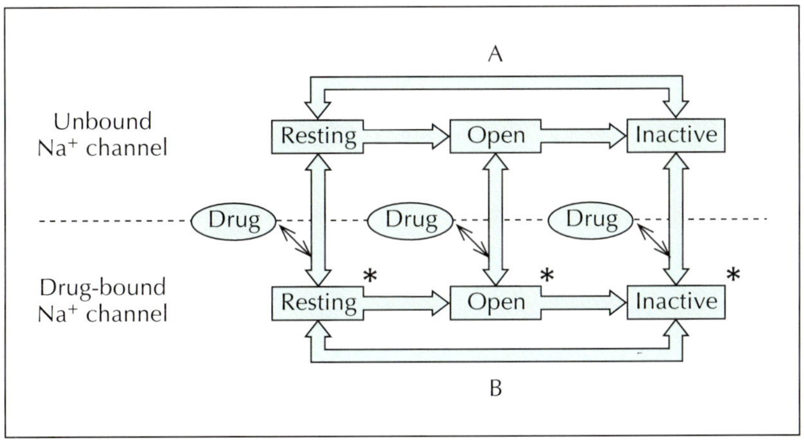

FIGURE 2-20. Modulated receptor hypothesis. Antiarrhythmic drugs (especially agents with class I effects) are known to have greater depressant effects on diseased cardiac tissue compared with healthy tissue. The modulated receptor hypothesis has been developed to describe the mechanism of action of the class I antiarrhythmic drugs and explain the selectivity of these agents for arrhythmic tissue. This hypothesis proposes that the class I antiarrhythmic drugs block the function of the sodium channel in a state-dependent fashion. Drug interaction with the sodium channel receptor is represented in this figure. The channel molecule is assumed to cycle through the resting, open, and inactivated states, as proposed by Hodgkin and Huxley [16]. Asterisks (*) indicate the nonconducting resting, open, and inactive states of the drug-bound sodium channel. As long as the drug is bound to the sodium channel, sodium conductance is zero [4,17,18]. Path A represents the time- and voltage-dependent recovery of the sodium channel, while path B is the recovery path of the sodium channels altered by the drug. A drug may bind to any of the three states of the channel but may have preferential affinity for a particular channel state.

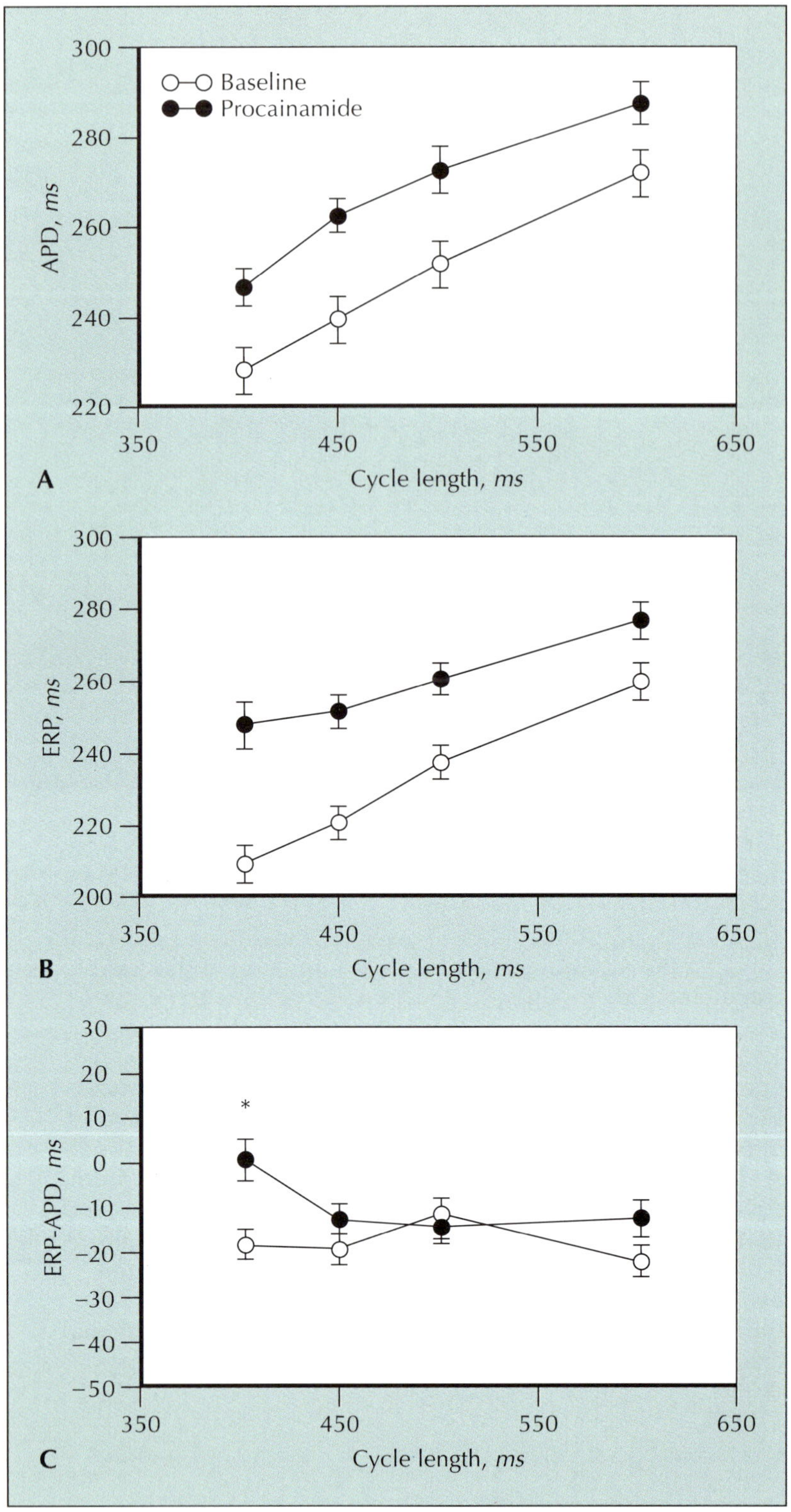

FIGURE 2-21. Frequency-dependent action. The modulated receptor model has been used to develop the concept of use-dependent or frequency-dependent action of antiarrhythmic drugs. It is hypothesized that antiarrhythmic agents have a greater affinity for the channel in its open or inactivated state and that recovery is slowed or incomplete at resting transmembrane voltages. The model predicts that there will be a greater opportunity for, and intensity of, drug binding to the ion channels at faster heart rates, leading to an incremental increase in antiarrhythmic drug action. This use-dependence of blockade, *ie,* greater block at higher rates, is what is actually observed *in vitro* and *in vivo*. The antiarrhythmic drug effects of procainamide (Class I) *in vivo* on action potential duration (APD), effective refractory period (ERP), and the difference between effective refractory period and action potential duration (ERP - APD) over several cycle lengths in human patients are shown in this figure. Procainamide prolongs APD at each cycle length by a near constant amount (**A**). However, procainamide causes a greater prolongation of ERP at shorter cycle lengths (**B**), which is clearly shown by the significant difference (*, $P < 0.01$) of ERP - APD at a cycle length of 375 ms versus 600 ms (**C**). These findings are consistent with the use-dependent blockade of sodium channels by procainamide, as predicted by the modulated receptor hypothesis. (*Adapted from* Lee and coworkers [19], with permission.)

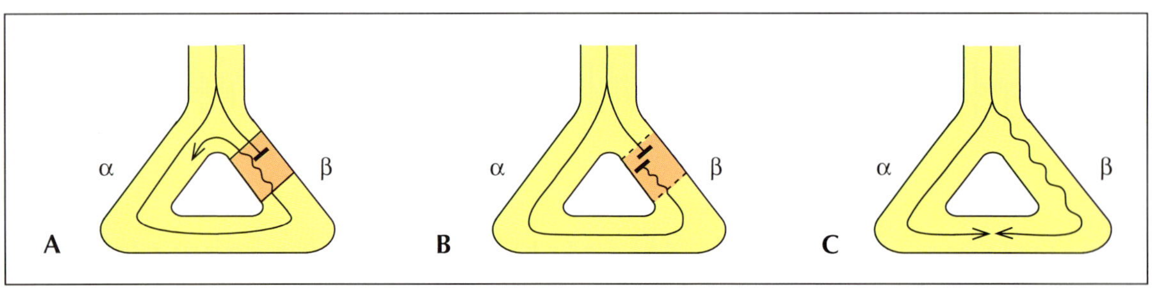

FIGURE 2-22. Effect of antiarrhythmic drugs on reentry. The question of how antiarrhythmic drugs suppress arrhythmias must be addressed by considering arrhythmia mechanisms. Most arrhythmias based on abnormal conduction involve reentry circuits, as illustrated in **A** (described in Chapter 1, Figs. 24 and 25). The *shaded area* represents the depolarized tissue in which conduction block occurs, and retrograde conduction is slow enough to allow the cells in limb α to recover and propagate the reentrant impulse. Antiarrhythmic drugs can eliminate reentry tachyarrhythmias by impairing conduction sufficiently to cause interruption of conduction through the circuit (**B**) or by improving conduction in limb β, which prevents the development of conduction block (**C**). Class I drugs prevent reentry by causing a greater amount of slow conduction in depolarized tissue, thus producing conduction block in both the forward and reverse directions in limb β.

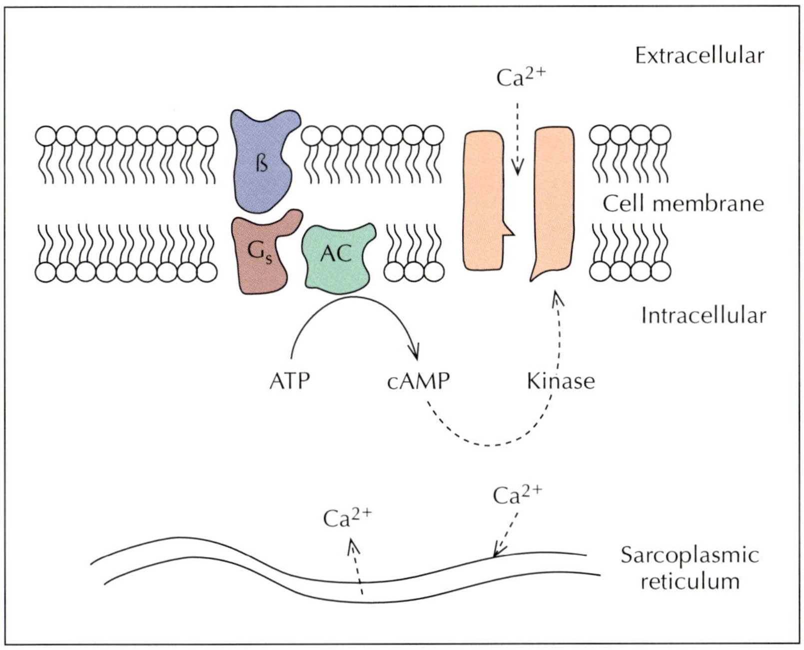

Figure 2-23. Class II antiarrhythmics. Class II antiarrhythmic action consists of sympatholytic effects on the heart; the most common drugs with this action are the β-adrenoceptor blockers. β adrenoceptor (denoted β) blockade results in a decrease of cAMP by preventing the stimulatory effects of β agonists (usually norepinephrine) on the cardiac receptors. These receptors are coupled by the G-protein (G_s) to the production of cyclic adenosine monophosplate (cAMP) by adenylyl cyclase (*AC*). The decreased cAMP level leads to a decrease in the activation of a protein kinase and thus inhibition of phosphorylation of the calcium channel. This results in inhibition of calcium current through the voltage-gated calcium channel and a reduction in calcium-dependent electrical activity. Furthermore, intracellular calcium concentration is reduced, which decreases the calcium-induced release of calcium from the sarcoplasmic reticulum. ATP—adenosine triphosphate, Ca^{++}—calcium ions.

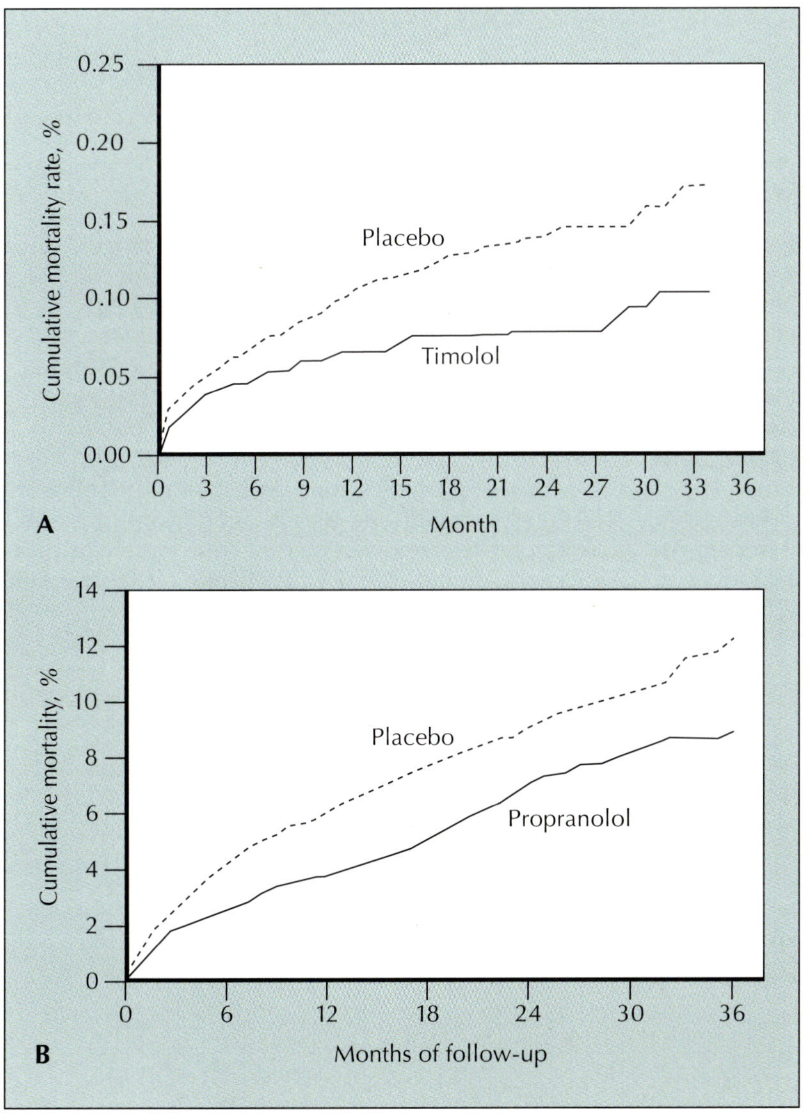

Figure 2-24. Therapeutic use of Class II drugs. Blockade of the sympathetic nervous system (especially β blockade) leads to a decrease in the slope of phase 4 of the sinoatrial and atrioventricular (AV) nodal cell action potentials, resulting in a decreased heart rate and slower conduction through the AV node (seen as prolongation of the PR interval). In addition to its use for controlling heart rate, the beneficial effect of prophylactic use of β-blocker therapy on the cumulative death rate in patients following myocardial infarction is well recognized (reviewed by Yusuf and coworkers [21]). Shown in **A** and **B** are two of the early multicenter, randomized, double-blind, and placebo-controlled trials of β-adrenergic blockade of patients with myocardial infarction.

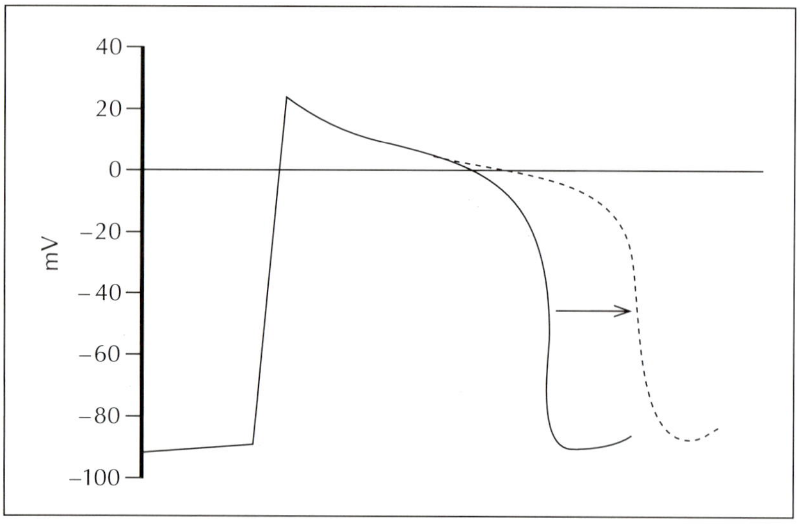

FIGURE 2-25. Class III Antiarrhythmics. Class III action consists of prolongation of the action potential duration, which leads to a prolongation of refractoriness. The diagram represents a normal action potential of a Purkinje cell (*solid line*) and the effects of d-sotalol (*dotted line*) on the action potential duration.

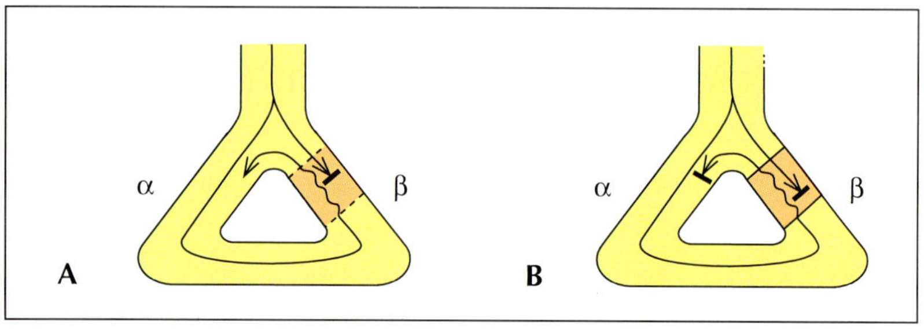

FIGURE 2-26. The probable effect of a drug with Class III antiarrhythmic action on a reentry circuit. Class III drugs can affect a prototypic reentry circuit (**A**; described in Chapter 1, Figs. 24 and 25) by sufficiently prolonging the refractory period of path α, thus preventing reentry from occurring (**B**).

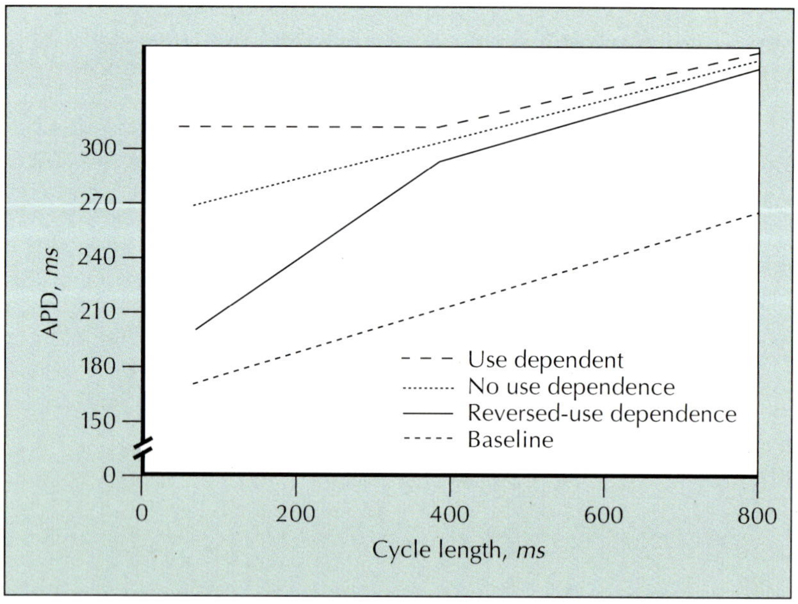

FIGURE 2-27. Class III reversed use dependence. A property seen with some drugs with class III antiarrhythmic action (but not amiodarone) is reversed-use dependence. The effect of such class III drugs increases as the rate of the arrhythmia slows (Hondeghem and Snyders [22]). This is depicted in the schematic illustration as an increasing prolongation of the action potential duration (APD) at longer cycle lengths. Unfortunately, maximal prolongation of refractoriness is most beneficial during rapid heart rates. The class III action of quinidine and the active metabolite of procainamide (NAPA) along with the class II agent, sotalol, exhibit reversed use dependence of potassium channel blockade. However, newer investigational class III agents appear to prolong APD in a use dependent manner [20, 23].

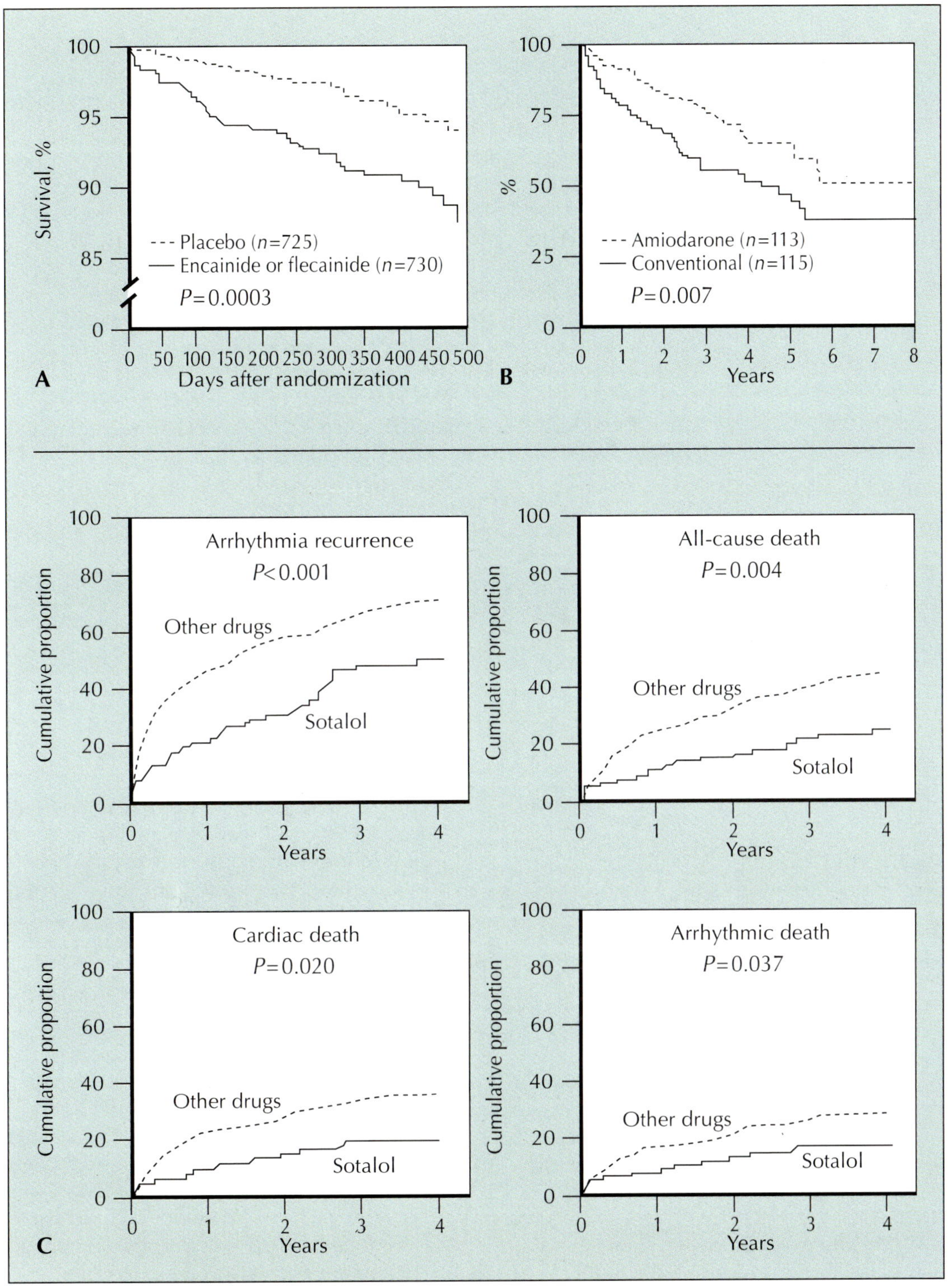

Figure 2-28. Comparison of Antiarrhythmic Drugs. The surprising results of CAST I (**A**), which demonstrated an increase in mortality in post–myocardial infarction patients treated with the class Ic antiarrythmic agents, encainide and flecainide, compared with placebo (CAST) [24]. These results were corroborated by CAST II [25] (comparison of moricizine, also a Class I agent, versus placebo for post–myocardial infarction survival) and provided a strong incentive for the development of alternatives to the use of class I drugs. The recent findings of the CASCADE study [26] (**B**) and the ESVEM trial [27] (**C**), demonstrating improved survival in patients with life-threatening ventricular arrhythmias, confirmed the usefulness of the class III agents and has led to their use as first line agents in ventricular arrhythmias. B compares the cumulative cardiac survival of patients with aborted cardiac arrest treated with empiric amiodarone with that of conventional antiarrhythmic therapy, Class I agents. C compares the cumulative effect of sotalol therapy on arrhythmia recurrence, all-cause death, cardiac death, and arrhythmic death as compared with class I agents. The popularity of class III agents has led to the development of a multitude of refractory period-prolonging drugs as shown in **D**. CAST, CAST II—Cardiac arrhythmic suppression trial; CASCADE—cardiac arrest in Seattle, conventional versus amiodarone drug evaluation; ESVEM—electrophysiologic study versus electrocardiographic monitoring. (Part A *adapted from* CAST I [24] and CAST II [25]; with permission; Part B *adapted from* The CASCADE Investigators [26]; with permission; Part C *adapted from* Mason [27]; with permission.)

D. INVESTIGATIONAL CLASS III ANTIARRHYTHMIC DRUGS

Almokalant	Ambasilide
Dofetilide	Sematilide
MDL-11939	E-4031
Ibutilide	D-sotalol
MS-551	Tedisamil

Effect of Class IV Drugs

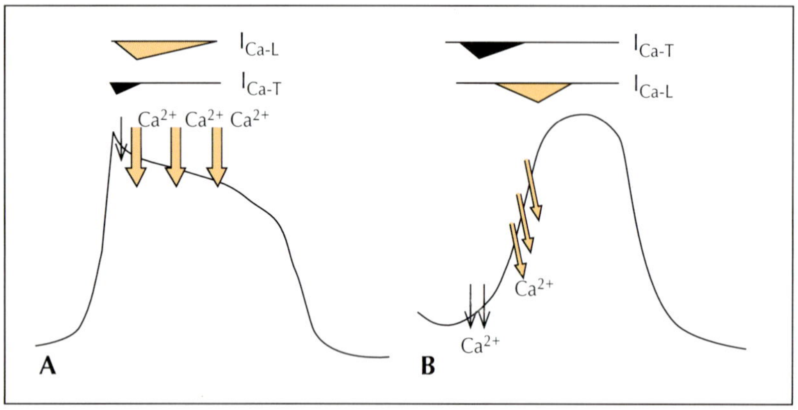

Figure 2-29. Mechanism-Class IV. Class IV antiarrhythmic action consists of blockade of voltage-gated calcium channels. These channels are involved in the plateau phase of the action potential of atrial, Purkinje, and ventricular tissue (**A**) and in the upstroke of the action potential in the sinoatrial and atrioventricular nodes (**B**). They are also involved in some types of triggered automaticity. Currently, the major antiarrythmic uses of the calcium channel blockers are to control ventricular rate during fast atrial rhythms by decreasing conduction through the AV node and to prevent supraventricular tachycardias from arising. Ca^{2+}—calcium ions; I_{Ca-T}—calcium T current; I_{Ca-L}—calcium L current. (*Adapted from* the Sicilian Gambit [15].)

Effects of Miscellaneous Drugs

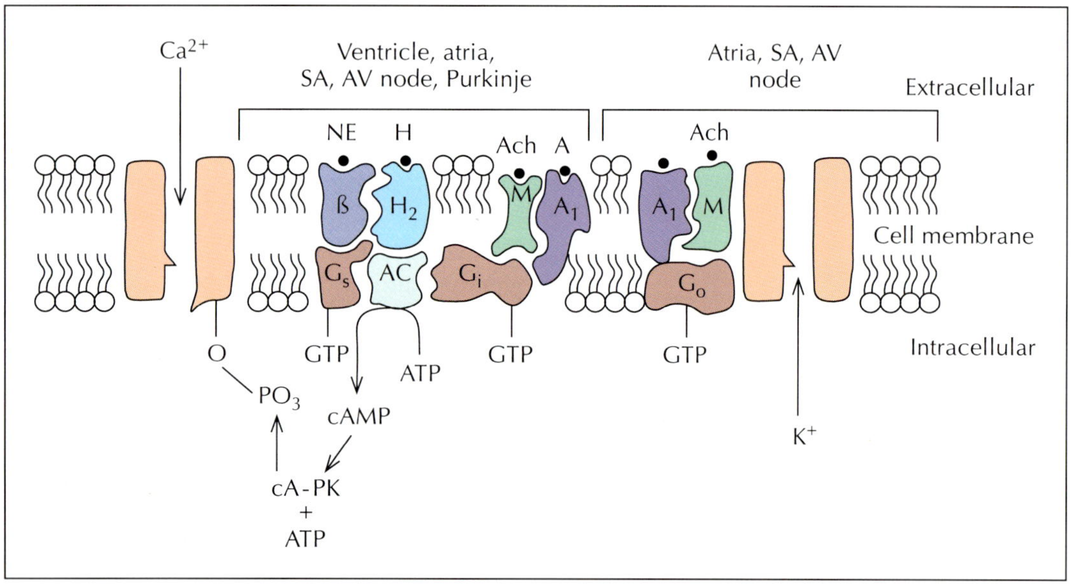

Figure 2-30. Putative site of action of adenosine. A miscellaneous group of agents have effects that are not included in the Vaughan Williams classification. Among the older members of this group are potassium and magnesium. One of the most important of the newer miscellaneous agents is adenosine. Adenosine has several effects. It binds to an adenosine receptor (A_1) linked via an inhibitory GTP-dependent regulator protein (G_1) to adenylyl cyclase. Activation of the A_1 receptor inhibits the enhancement of adenylyl cyclase activity and the associated increase in cyclic adenosine monophosphate (cAMP) caused by norepinephrine (*NE*) and histamine (*H*). In all myocytes, cAMP regulates phosphorylation of the slow calcium channel via a cAMP-dependent protein kinase (*cA-PK*). In atrial and atrioventricular (AV) nodal cells, adenosine activation of the A_1 receptor also enhances K^+ conduction via a different G protein (G_o). This causes hyperpolarization and negative inotropic, chronotropic, and dromotropic effects. The actions of adenosine on the cardiac myocytes are similar to those of the muscarinic receptor (*M*) agonist, acetylcholine (*ACh*). AC—adenylyl cyclase; ATP—adenosine triphosphate; β—β agonist; G_S—regulator protein; GTP—guanosine triphosphates; SA—sinoatrial node. (*Adapted from* Collis [28]; with permission.)

SUMMARY OF EFFECTS OF ANTIARRHYTHMIC DRUGS

EFFECTS OF ANTIARRHYTHMIC DRUGS ON ELECTROPHYSIOLOGIC AND ELECTROCARDIOGRAPHIC INTERVALS

INVERVAL	CLASS I			CLASS II	CLASS III	CLASS IV
	A	B	C			
Sinus rate	0↑	0	0	↓	↓	↓
P-R	0↑	0	↑	↑	↑	↑
A-H	↓0↑	0↓	↑	↑	↑	↑
H-V	0↑	0	↑	0	0↑	0
QRS	↑	0	↑↑	0	0	0
Q-Tc	0↑	0	0	↓0↑*	↑↑↑	0
J-T	↓0↑	↓	↓	↓0↑*	↑↑	0
Ventricular rate in atrial fibrillation	0↑	0	0↑	↓	↓	↓
Sinus node automaticity	0	0	0↓	↓	0	↓
AV node (effective refractory period)	↓0↑	0↓	↑	↑	↓↑	↑
Purkinje fiber automaticity	↓0	↓	↓	↓	↓↑†	0 ↓
Use dependence (kinetics)	Intermediate	Fast	Slow	NA	NA	Intermediate†
dV/dT and conduction velocity	↓↓	↓	↓↓↓	0↓	0↓	0
Action potential duration	↑↑	0	0	↓	↑↑	0
Effective refractory period	↑↑	↓	↑	0↓	↑↑	0
Effective refractory period/ action potential duration	↑	↑	↑	↑	↑	0
Ventricular fibrillation threshold	↑	↑	↑	↑	NA	0
Membrane-stabilizing activity	Yes	Yes	Yes	Yes	0	0

*Depends on the drug (*eg*, propranolol shortens, sotalol lengthens.)

†Calcium channels in the AV node.

FIGURE 2-31. Summary—electrical effects of antiarrhythmic drugs. The effects of the various classes of antiarrhythmics on the electrical properties of the specialized tissue within the conduction systems are listed.

CLASSIFICATION OF DRUG ACTIONS ON ARRHYTHMIA BASED ON MODIFICATION OF VULNERABLE PARAMETER

ARRHYTHMIA	MECHANISMS	VULNERABLE PARAMETER	IONIC CURRENTS MOST LIKELY TO MODULATE VULNERABLE PARAMETER	REPRESENTATIVE DRUGS
Inappropriate sinus tachycardia	Enhanced normal automaticity	Phase 4 depolarization (decrease)	I_f, $I_{Ca\text{-}T}$(block) $I_{K(ACh)}$(activate)	β-blocking agents
Some idiopathic ventricular tachycardias	As above			Sodium channel blocking agents
Ectopic atrial tachycardia	Abnormal automaticity	Maximum diastolic potential (hyperpolarization) or	I_K, $I_{K(ACh)}$(activate)	M_2-agonists
		Phase 4 depolarization (decrease)	$I_{Ca\text{-}L}$, I_{Na}(block)	Calcium or sodium channel blocking agents M_2-agonists
Accelerated idioventricular rhythms	As above	Phase 4 depolarization (decrease)		Calcium or sodium channel blocking agents
Torsade de pointes	Triggered activity: EAD	Action potential duration (shorten) or	I_K(activate)	β-Agonists; vagolytic agents (increase rate)
		EAD (suppress)	$I_{Ca\text{-}L}$, I_{Na}(block)	Calcium channel blocking agents; Mg^{2+}; β- blockers
Digitalis-induced arrhythmias	Triggered activity: DAD	Calcium overload (unload) or	$I_{Ca\text{-}L}$(block)	Calcium channel blocking agents
		DAD (suppress)	$I_{Ca\text{-}L}$, I_{Na}(block)	Sodium channel blocking agents
Certain autonomically mediated ventricular tachycardias	As above	Calcium overload (unload) or		β-blocking agents
		DAD (suppress)		Calcium channel blocking agents, adenosine
Atrial flutter type I	Reentry (sodium channel dependent) Long excitable gap	Conduction and excitability (depress)	I_{Na}(block)	Atrium: sodium channel blocking agents (except lidocaine, mexiletine, tocainide)
Circus movement tachycardia in WPW	As above	Conduction and excitability (depress)		Sodium channel blocking agents (except lidocaine, mexiletine tocainide)
Sustained monomorphic ventricular tachycardia	As above	Conduction and excitability (depress)		Ventricle: sodium channel blocking agents
Atrial flutter type II	Re-entry (sodium channel dependent) Short excitable gap	Refractory period (prolong)	I_K(block)	Potassium, sodium channel blocking agents
Atrial fibrillation	As above	Refractory period (prolong)		Potassium channel blockers
Circus movement tachycardia in WPW	As above	Refractory period (prolong)		Amiodarone, sotalol
Polymorphic and sustained monomorphic ventricular tachycardia	As above	Refractory period (prolong)		Quinidine, procainamide, disopyramide
Bundle branch reentry	As above	Refractory period (prolong)		Quinidine, procainamide, disopyramide
Ventricular fibrillation	As above	Refractory period (prolong)		Bretylium
AV nodal reentrant tachycardia	Reentry (calcium channel dependent)	Conduction and excitability (depress)	$I_{Ca\text{-}L}$(block)	Calcium channel blocking agents
Circus movement tachycardia in WPW	As above	Conduction and excitability (depress)		Calcium channel blocking agents
Verapamil-sensitive ventricular tachycardia	As above	Conduction and excitability (depress)		Calcium channel blocking agents
Other	Reflection	Excitability (decrease)	I_{Na}, $I_{Ca\text{-}L}$(block)	
	Parasystole	Phase 4 depolarization (decrease)	I_f(block) (if maximum diastolic potential high)	

FIGURE 2-32. Choice of antiarrhythmic drug. A different approach in choosing the appropriate antiarrythmic drug utilizes the classification of arrhythmogenic mechanisms at the cellular level to classify antiarrhythmic drugs based on their actions on modifying the vulnerable parameter [15]. DAD—delayed after-depolarization; EAD—early after-depolarization; WPW—Wolff-Parkinson-White syndrome.

COMPARATIVE EFFICACY OF ORAL ANTIARRHYTHMIC DRUGS

DRUG	PREMATURE ATRIAL CONTRACTIONS	ATRIAL FIBRILLATION	ANTEGRADE SLOWING OF AV NODAL CONDUCTION	AV NODE RE-ENTRANT TACHYCARDIA	EFFECTS ON ACCESSORY PATHWAY CONDUCTION	WPW-PAROXYSMAL SUPRAVENTRICULAR TACHYCARDIA	SUSTAINED VENTRICULAR TACHYCARDIA/VENTRICULAR FIBRILLATION PES, %
Quinidine	++	++	+/-	+	+	+	20–25
Procainamide	++	++	+/-	+	+	+	20–25
Disopyramide	++	++	+/-	+	++	++	20–25
Tocainide	0	0	0	0	+/-	0	10–15
Mexiletine	0	0	0	0	+/-	0	10–20
Moricizine	+	NE	0	NE	+	NE	20
Flecainide	++	++	+	++	+++	+++	20–25
Encainide	++	++	++	++	+++	+++	20–25
Propafenone	++	++	++	++	++	++	20–25
Recainam	+	++	+	++	++	++	20
β blockers	+*	+	++	+	0	+	5
Amiodarone	++	+++	++	++	+	++	20–60
Sotalol	+	++	++	++	+	+	30
Digoxin	0	+*	++	+	+/-	+	NA
Verapamil	0	+*	++	+	+/-	+	NA
Diltiazem	0	+*	++	+	+/-	+	NA

*Rate control data

FIGURE 2-33. Efficacy of antiarrythmic drugs. This table compares the efficacy of a number of antiarrhythmic drugs on some of the more common types of arrhythmias. NA—not applicable; NE—not established; PES—programmed electrical stimulation.

The author would like to thank Bertram G. Katzung for his helpful suggestions and review of this chapter.

REFERENCES

1. Catterall WA: Structure and function of voltage-sensitive ion channels. *Science* 1988, 242:50–61.
2. Tang S, Mikala G, Bahinski A, *et al.*: Molecular localization of ion selectivity sites within the pore of a human L-type cardiac calcium channel. *J Biol Chem* 1993, 268:13026–13029.
3. Catterall WA, Striessnig J: Receptor sites for Ca^{2+} antagonists. *Trends Pharmacol Sci* 1992, 13:256–262.
4. Hille B: Local anesthetics: Hydrophilic and hydrophobic pathways for the drug-receptor reaction. *J Gen Physiol* 1977, 69:497–515.
5. Koch-Weser J: Pharmacokinetics of procainamide in man. *Ann N Y Acad Sci* 1971, 179:370–382.
6. Rowland M, Tozer TN: *Clinical Pharmacokinetics: Concepts and Applications*, ed 2. Philadelphia: Lea & Febiger; 1989.
7. Thomson PD, Melmon KL, Richardson JA, *et al.*: Lidocaine pharmacokinetics in advanced heart failure, liver disease, and renal failure in humans. *Ann Intern Med* 1973, 78:499–508.
8. Ueda CT, Dzindzio BS: Pharmacokinetics of dihydroquinidine in congestive heart failure patients after intravenous quinidine administration. *Eur J Clin Pharmacol* 1979, 16(2):101–105.
9. Ueda CT, Dzindzio BS: Quinidine kinetics in congestive heart failure. *Clin Pharmacol Ther* 1978, 23(2):158–164.
10. Prescott LF, Yamoah-Adjepon KK, Talbot RG: Impaired lidocaine metabolism in patients with myocardial infarction and cardiac failure. *Br Med J* 1976, 1:939–941.
11. Routledge PA, Shand DG, Barchowsky A: Relationship between $alpha_1$-acid glycoprotein and lidocaine disposition in myocardial infarction. *Clin Pharmacol Ther* 1981, 30:154–157.
12. Kessler KM, Kissane B, Cassidy J: Dynamic variability of binding of antiarrhythmic drugs during the evolution of acute myocardial infarction. *Circulation* 1984, 70:472.
13. David BM, Ilett KF, Whitford EG, Stenhouse NS: Prolonged variability in plasma protein binding of disopyramide after acute myocardial infarction. *Br J Clin Pharmacol* 1983, 15(4):435–441.

14. Wenger TL, Browning DJ, Masterton CE, *et al.*: Procainamide delivery to ischemic canine myocardium following rapid intravenous administration. *Circ Res* 1980, 46:789.

15. The Sicilian Gambit: A new approach to the classification of antiarrhythmic drugs based on their actions on arrhythmogenic mechanisms. *Circulation* 1991, 84:1831–1851.

16. Hodgkin AL, Huxley AF: The components of membrane conductance in the giant axon of Loligo. J Physiol (London) 1952, 116:473–496.

17. Hondeghem L, Katzung B: Time- and voltage-dependent interactions of antiarrhythmic drugs with sodium channels. *Biochim Biophys Acta* 1977, 472:373.

18. Hondeghem LM: Antiarrhythmic agents: modulated receptor applications. *Circulation* 1987, 75(3):514–520.

19. Lee R, Bing Liem L, Cohen T, *et al.*: Relation between repolarization and refractoriness in the human ventricle: cycle length dependence and effect of procainamide. *J Am Coll Cardiol* 1992, 19:614–618.

20. Carmeliet E: Effect of UK-68,798 on delayed rectifier K^+ currents in cardiac myocytes. *Circulation* 1991, 84:II–176.

21. Yusuf S, Peto R, Lewis J, *et al.*: β blockade during and after myocardial infarction: an overview of the randomized trials. *Prog Cardiovasc Dis* 1985, 27(5):335–371.

22. Hondeghem LM, Snyders DJ: Class III antiarrhythmic agents have a lot of potential but a long way to go. Reduced effectiveness and dangers of reverse use dependence. *Circulation* 1990, 81(2):686–690.

23. Spinelli W, Moubarak IF, Parson RW, Colatsky TJ: Cellular electrophysiology of WAY-123,398, a new class III antiarrhythmic agent: Specificity of IK block and lack of reversed-use dependence in cat ventricular myocytes. *Cardiovasc Res* 1993, 27(a):1580–1591.

24. The Cardiac Arrhythmia Suppression Trial (CAST) Investigators: Preliminary report: effect of encainide and flecainide on mortality in a randomized trial of arrhythmia suppression after myocardial infarction. *N Engl J Med* 1989, 321:406–412.

25. The Cardiac Arrhythmia Suppression Trial (CAST) II Investigators: Effect of the antiarrhythmic agent moricizine on survival after myocardial infarction. *N Engl J Med* 1992, 327:227–233.

26. The Cardiac Arrest in Seattle, Conventional Versus Amiodarone Drug Evaluation (CASCADE) investigators: Randomized antiarrhythmic drug therapy in survivors of cardiac arrests (the CASCADE study). *Am J Cardiol* 1993, 72(3):280–287.

27. Mason JW: A comparison of seven antiarrythmic drugs in patients with ventricular tachyarrhythmias. Electrophysiologic study versus electrocardiographic monitoring (ESVEM) investigators. *N Engl J Med* 1993, 329(7):452–458.

28. Collis MG: Influence of adenosine on cardiac activity. In *Adenosine and Adenine Nucleotides as Regulators of Cellular Function*. Edited by Phillis JW. Boca Raton: CRC Press; 1991:249.

ELECTROCARDIOGRAPHIC PREDICTORS OF CARDIAC RHYTHM DISTURBANCES

3

CHAPTER

G. Thomas Evans, Jr.

The electrocardiogram (ECG) is the most cost-effective method of determining the cardiac rhythm. Although the precise mechanism of any cardiac rhythm may require invasive electrophysiologic studies, the surface ECG may provide important information leading to the diagnosis. This chapter focuses on specific electrocardiographic clues that should alert the physician to the potential for future cardiac rhythm disturbances. The actual arrhythmias for which the ECG signs are predictive are not included, because these may be found in any standard ECG text.

The chapter is divided into four major areas: 1) predictors of supraventricular rhythm disturbances, 2) predictors of ventricular rhythm disturbances, 3) predictors of A-V block, and 4) predictors of miscellaneous disturbances. Readers will find two major categories among the various subsections: 1) findings on the resting ECG that might predict subsequent arrhythmias and 2) findings during arrhythmias or abnormal conditions that might predict more adverse consequences.

Many of the abnormalities shown in the chapter may be markers for the development of life-threatening ventricular arrhythmias. This has the greatest potential application in patients with electrolyte disturbances, cardiac ischemia and the acquired types of long Q-T syndromes. Therefore, a knowledge of these predictors and alleviation of the underlying problems causing them may enable the clinician to prevent more serious consequences, including death. For example, early recognition and correction of hypokalemia may obviate treatment of potassium-induced ventricular tachycardia.

Predictors of Supraventricular Rhythm Disturbances: Atrial Fibrillation

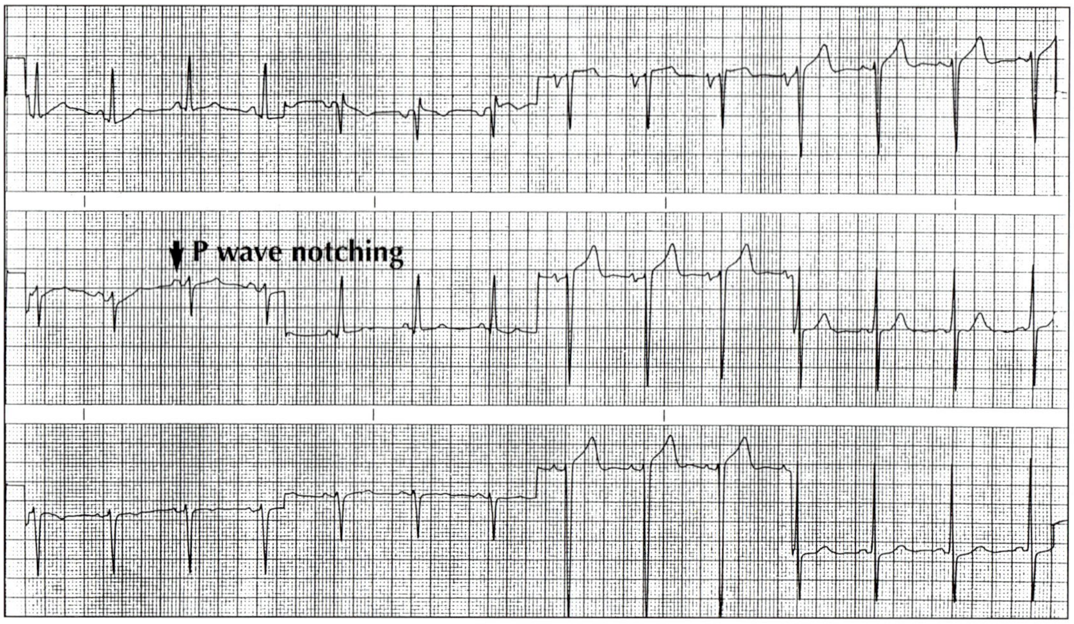

Figure 3-1. Intra-atrial conduction delay, left atrial abnormality, and left ventricular hypertrophy as predictors of atrial fibrillation (AF). A 12-lead electrocardiogram (ECG) from a 45-year-old man with long-standing hypertension and renal failure is shown. There is sinus rhythm, and the P wave duration is prolonged to 0.12 sec, with notching of 0.04 sec in lead II consistent with an intra-atrial conduction delay and the pattern of left enlargement in lead V_1. The ECG precursors of AF are not well understood, but intra-atrial conduction delay has been cited as a possible, although unproved, predictor [1]. There is also left ventricular hypertrophy (LVH) with associated repolarization abnormalities. In the Framingham study, the presence of ECG criteria for LVH doubled or tripled the risk of developing atrial fibrillation [1].

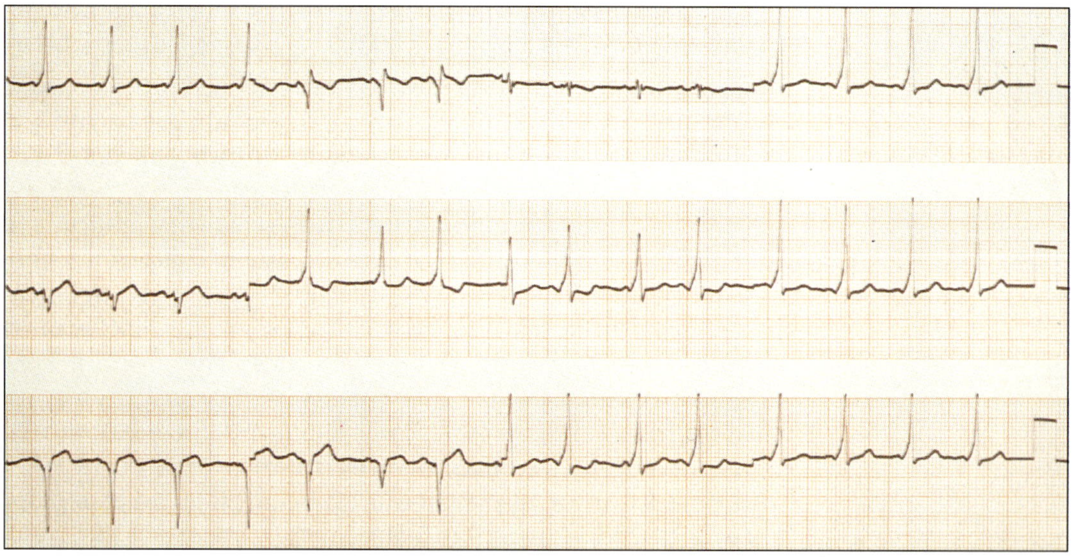

Figure 3-2. Manifest ventricular pre-excitation as a predictor of paroxysmal supraventricular tachycardia or atrial fibrillation (AF). The true incidence of arrhythmias occurring in subjects with the Wolff-Parkinson-White (WPW) pattern is unknown. There were no sudden deaths in over 350 patient-years of follow-up in a prospective natural history study of asymptomatic subjects with the WPW pattern [2]. The two major arrhythmias occurring in patients with WPW syndrome are atrioventricular reentrant tachycardia and AF. Manifest pre-excitation on the surface ECG may be a clue to these arrhythmias in patients with symptoms consistent with recurrent tachycardias. A 12-lead ECG showing the WPW pattern is shown. There is an absent PR segment in leads I, aVL, and V_2 to V_5, and the QRS complex is prolonged to 0.14 sec. There are positive delta waves in leads I, aVL, and V_1 through V_5, and negative delta waves in leads aVF and III, consistent with a pathway located in the posteroseptal space.

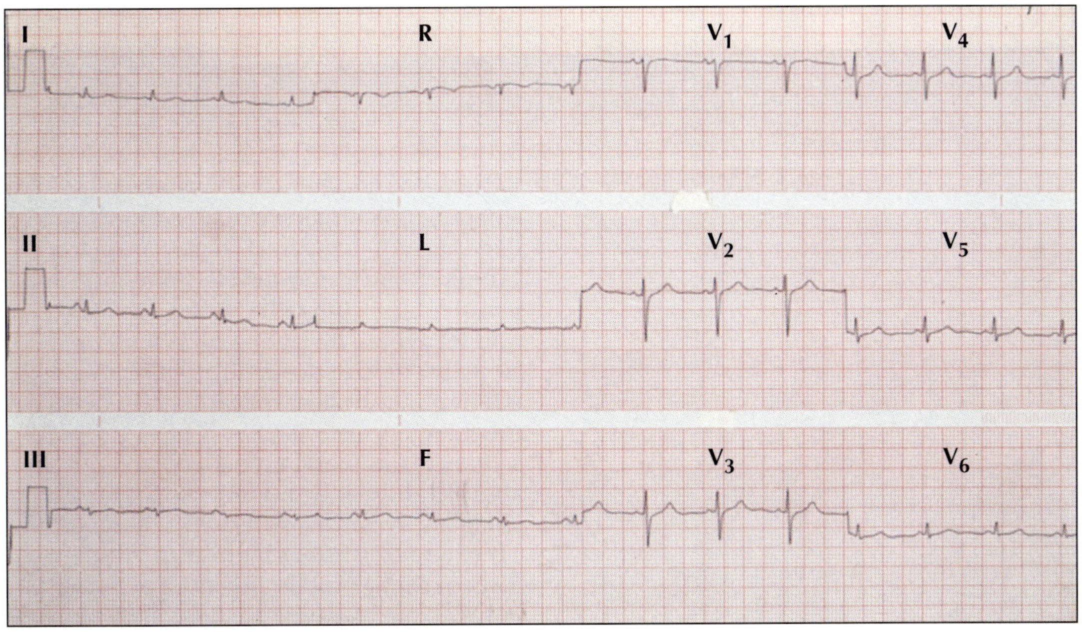

FIGURE 3-3. Short PR syndrome as a predictor of paroxysmal supraventricular tachycardia or atrial fibrillation. In this form of ventricular pre-excitation the PR interval is shortened to less than 0.12 sec (or there is absence of a PR segment), whereas the QRS complex usually is normal, *ie*, showing the same configuration as during a normally conducted sinus rhythm. It should be stressed that not all cases showing a short PR interval on the ECG are examples of ventricular pre-excitation [3]. Most arrhythmias that occur in patients with the short PR syndrome are usually reentrant supraventricular tachycardias. The arrhythmia mechanisms are similar to those seen in patients with normal PR intervals. Therefore, patients with dual atrioventricular (AV) nodal physiology have AV nodal reentrant tachycardia, and patients with concealed bypass tract have atrioventricular reentry tachycardia. Patients with either enhanced AV nodal conduction or atrio-His bypass tracts may exhibit atrial flutter or fibrillation with a rapid ventricular response [4]. A 12-lead ECG showing an absent PR segment without a delta wave or abnormalities of the QRS complex is shown. Although the PR interval in lead II is 0.12 sec, there is an absent PR segment in leads I, II, aVF, and V_4 through V_6.

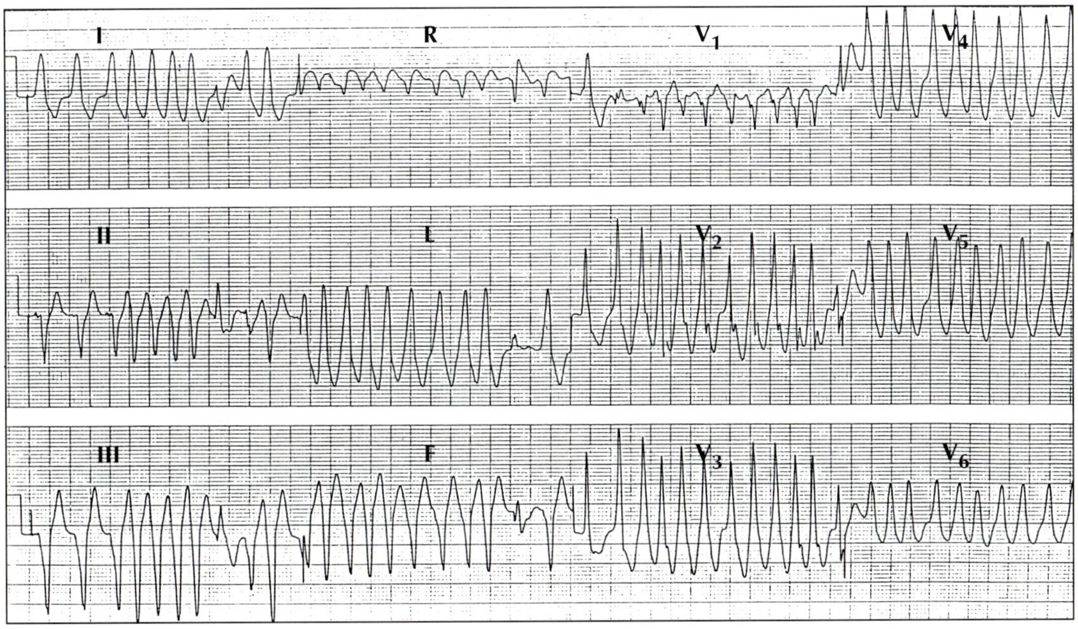

FIGURE 3-4. Atrial fibrillation (AF) with short RR intervals as a predictor of ventricular fibrillation (VF) in the Wolff-Parkinson-White (WPW) syndrome. Atrial fibrillation occurs in up to 40% of patients with the WPW syndrome. Extremely rapid rates can occur over the bypass tract during this rhythm and precipitate VF [4]. Klein *et al.* [5] compared 25 patients with WPW syndrome in whom VF occurred during an episode of AF with a control group of 73 patients. The shortest pre-excited RR interval during AF was less in the group with VF (mean shortest RR interval, 180 ms) than in the control group (mean shortest RR interval, 240 ms). No patient in the VF group had a shortest pre-excited RR interval less than 250 ms. There was some overlap between the groups [5]. This 12-lead ECG is from a 57-year-old man with WPW syndrome who was resuscitated from cardiac arrest, and whose coronary angiography was normal. The tracing shows AF and was obtained during electrophysiologic study that documented a posteroseptal para-Hisian accessory pathway. The shortest RR interval measures 170 ms and is seen in leads V_1 through V_3. (*Courtesy of* Gust H. Bardy, MD, Seattle, WA.)

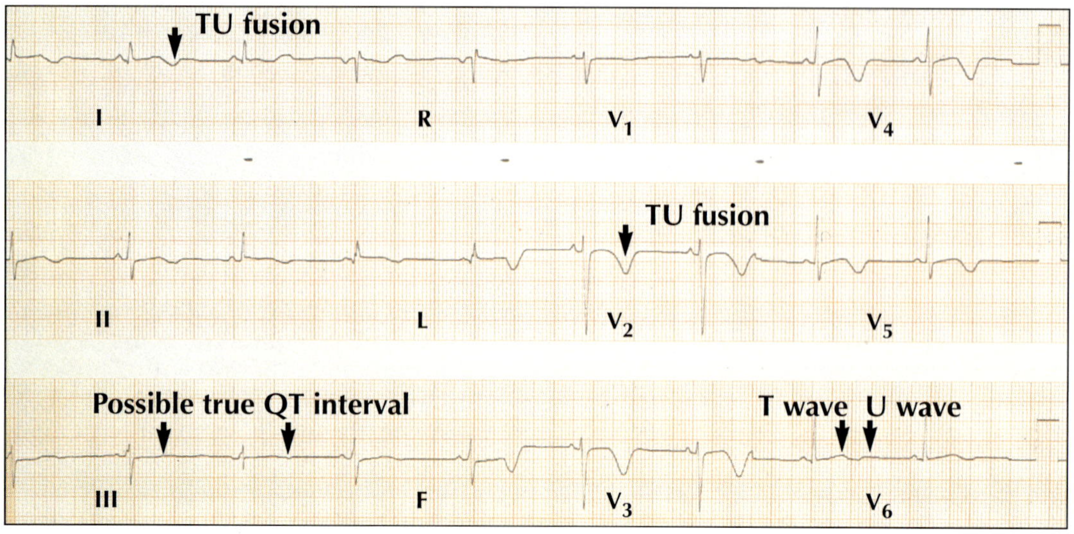

FIGURE 3-5. Prolonged QT syndromes as predictors of ventricular arrhythmias. Patients with congenital or acquired long QT syndromes may develop polymorphic ventricular tachycardia of the torsade de pointes type. The resting ECG may occasionally show abnormalities of repolarization manifested as marked T-wave inversion. A resting 12-lead ECG from a 19-year-old woman who presented with aborted sudden death is shown. There is sinus bradycardia associated with marked TU changes. Although it is difficult to discern the QT interval, it may measure only 0.42 sec, seen best in lead III. The QT-U interval is 0.56 sec. (*Courtesy of* David G. Benditt, MD, Minneapolis, MN.)

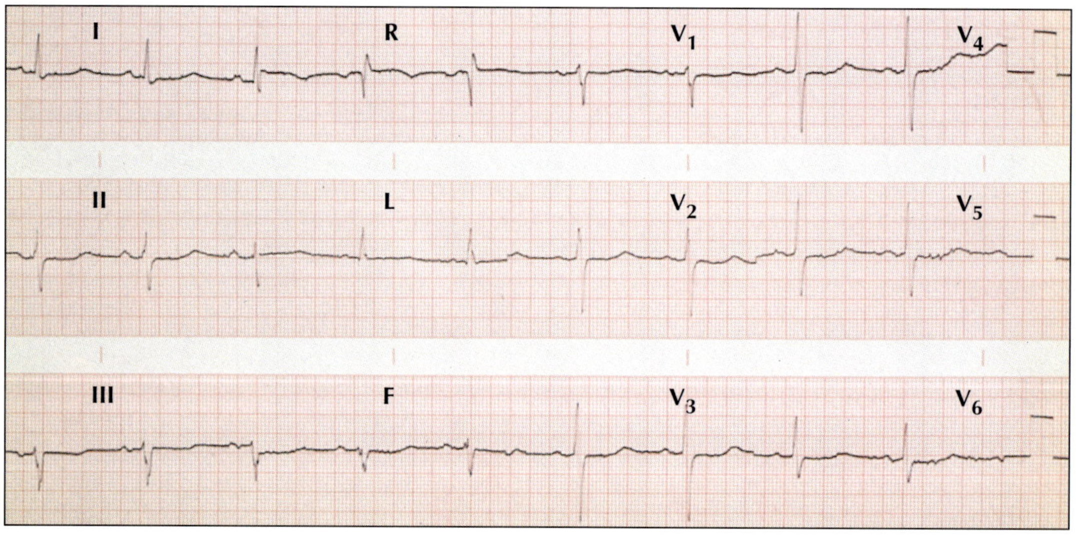

FIGURE 3-6. Prolonged QT interval as a predictor of drug-induced torsade de pointes. A prolonged QT interval is usually required for the diagnosis of the pause-dependent polymorphic ventricular tachycardia of this type. Keren *et al.* [6] reported on 10 patients with this arrhythmia, all of whom had QT interval prolongation longer than 0.60 sec immediately before the onset of torsade de pointes. This 12-lead ECG is from a 65-year-old man who was taking procainamide. There is sinus bradycardia with 1° atrioventricular block (PR interval, 0.26 sec). There is an intraventricular conduction delay with left axis deviation, probably due to left anterior fascicular block. The ST segment is horizontally depressed, with a prolonged ST segment and an apparent QT interval of 0.68 sec.

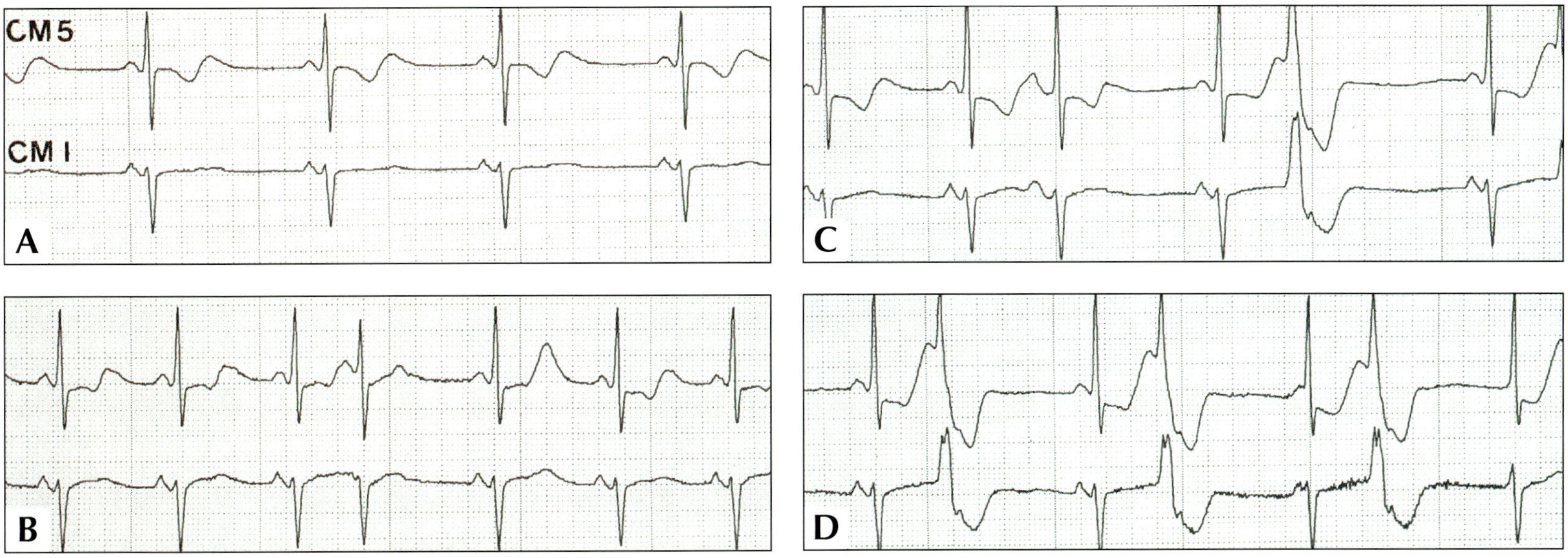

FIGURE 3-7. Marked post-pause accentuation of U wave amplitude or post-pause ventricular bigeminy as a predictor of pause-dependent polymorphic ventricular tachycardia. Jackman *et al.* [7] described two ECG findings that commonly preceded the development of pause-dependent polymorphic ventricular tachycardia of the torsade de pointes type in a series of 46 patients: 1) marked post-pause accentuation of the U wave amplitude, found in 91% of cases, and 2) new post-pause premature ventricular complexes in a bigeminal pattern, found in 93% of cases. Both patterns are shown, taken from leads CM_1 and CM_5 during ambulatory electrocardiographic monitoring in a patient who had recently started oral procainamide therapy. **A,** Sinus rhythm with inverted T waves and prominent U waves. The QT interval is probably 0.44 sec. **B,** a premature atrial complex (PAC) produces a pause, with marked accentuation of the postpause U wave. **C** and **D,** continuous recordings. Another PAC produces a pause that initiates an episode of ventricular bigeminy. The onset of ventricular ectopic activity arises near the apex of the U wave, as discussed by Jackman *et al.* [7]. Although these two signs are very sensitive, postpause accentuation of U wave amplitude is not invariably associated with ventricular arrhythmias.

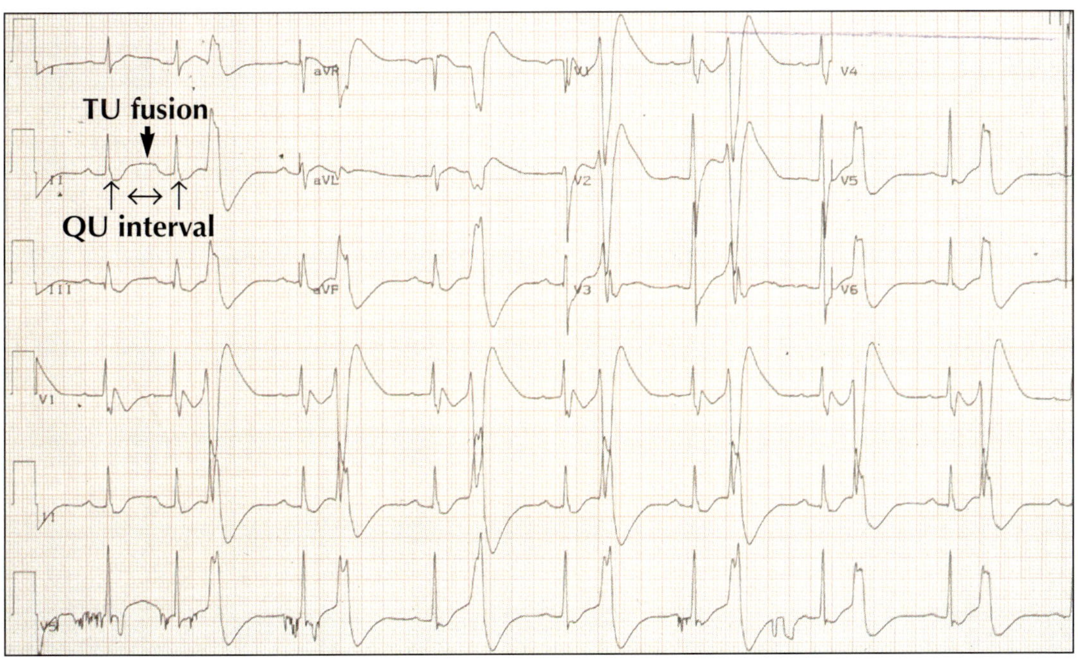

FIGURE 3-8. ECG changes of hypokalemia (TU fusion with an apparent prolonged QT interval) as a predictor of ventricular tachycardia. This 12-lead ECG is from a 30-year-old man with hypokalemic periodic paralysis due to hyperthyroidism. The serum potassium level was 2.0 mEq/L. There is sinus rhythm with 1° atrioventricular block and uniform ventricular bigeminy, with some variability in the coupling intervals. There is a deformity in the J point (best seen in lead V_1) with an altered proximal ST segment. The QU interval is 0.56 sec, but the true QT interval is difficult to discern. This recording preceded an episode of ventricular tachycardia.

Most prior studies of the effects of changing potassium concentrations on the myocardial action potential were performed using rabbit myocytes. More recently, Antzelevitch *et al.* [8] have recorded action potentials from both endocardial and epicardial canine ventricular myocytes and have derived simulated ECG patterns. These experiments more closely simulate the QRS-ST-T waveforms in human ECGs, which can be derived from instantaneous differences in the action potential of the endocardial and epicardial layers of the ventricle. (*Courtesy of* Nora Goldschlager, MD, San Francisco, CA.)

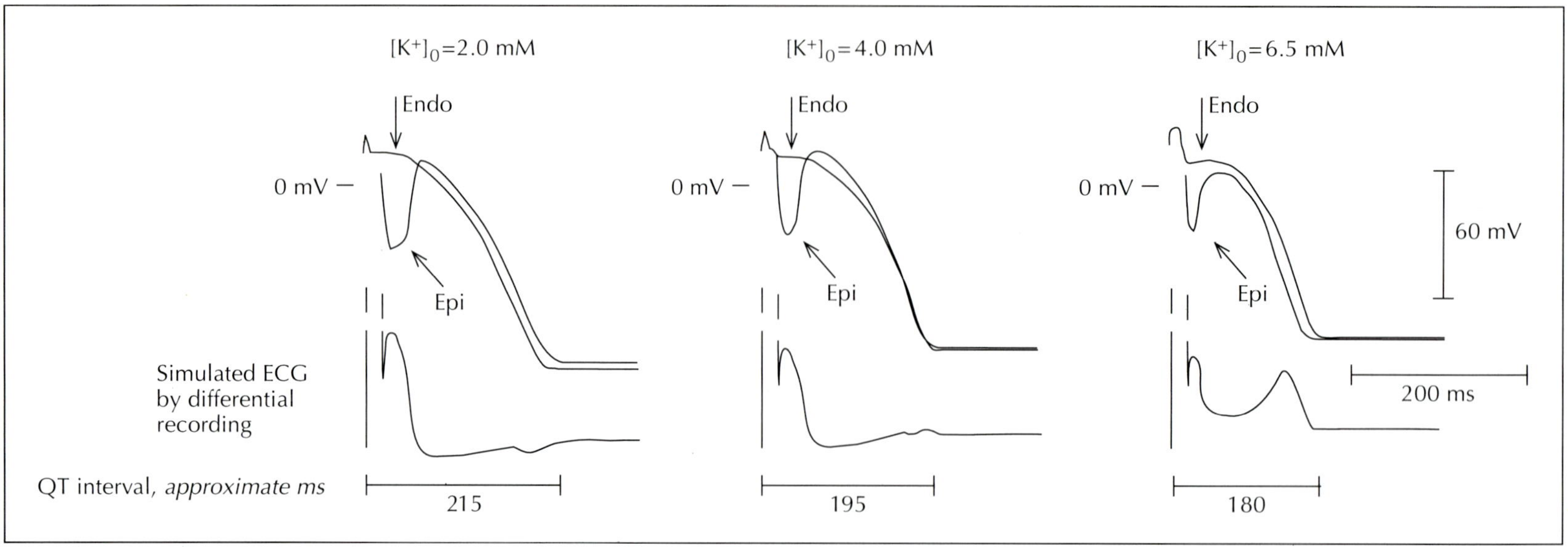

FIGURE 3-9. Effects of changes in extracellular potassium concentration $[K^+]_o$. Each panel shows transmembrane recordings obtained from isolated epicardial (Epi) and endocardial (Endo) canine ventricular preparations and a simulated ECG tracing obtained by differential recording of the same two traces. A slight delay was introduced in the delivery of stimuli to the two tissues to mimic transmural conduction. Note the domed appearance of the J point and prolongation of the QT interval with decreasing levels of potassium. In this experiment, alterations in QRS duration caused by changes in extracellular potassium were not included in the simulation. (*Adapted from* Antzelevitch and coworkers [8]; with permission.)

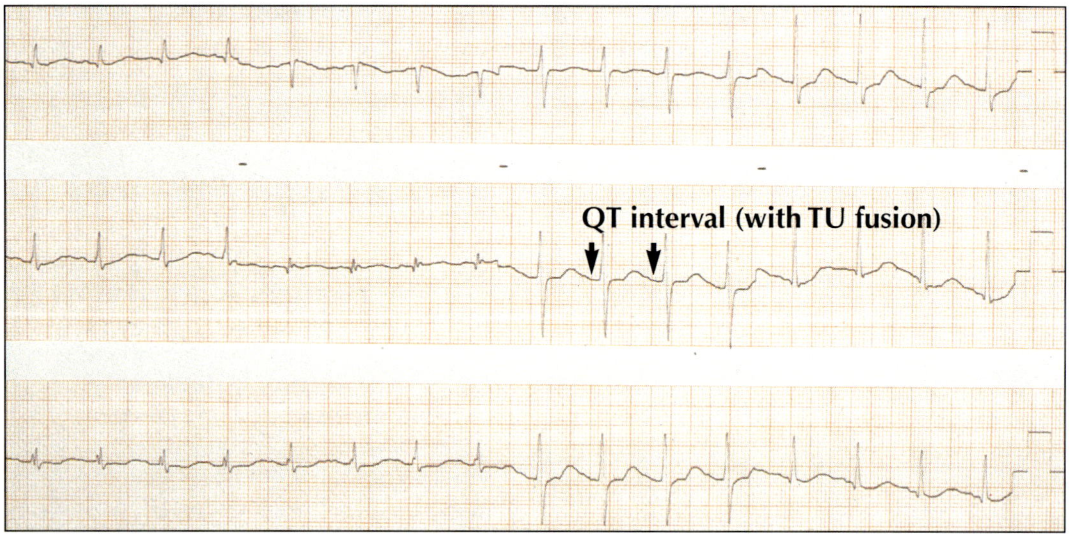

FIGURE 3-10. TU fusion with apparent prolonged QT interval as a predictor of hypokalemia. This 12-lead ECG is from a 41-year-old man who presented with recurrent inability to walk because of familial periodic paralysis. The serum potassium level was 2.2 mEq/L at the time the ECG was obtained. There is sinus rhythm. The ECG shows diffuse ST segment lowering and straightening, with broad-based T waves. The apparent QT interval is 0.48 seconds because of TU fusion.

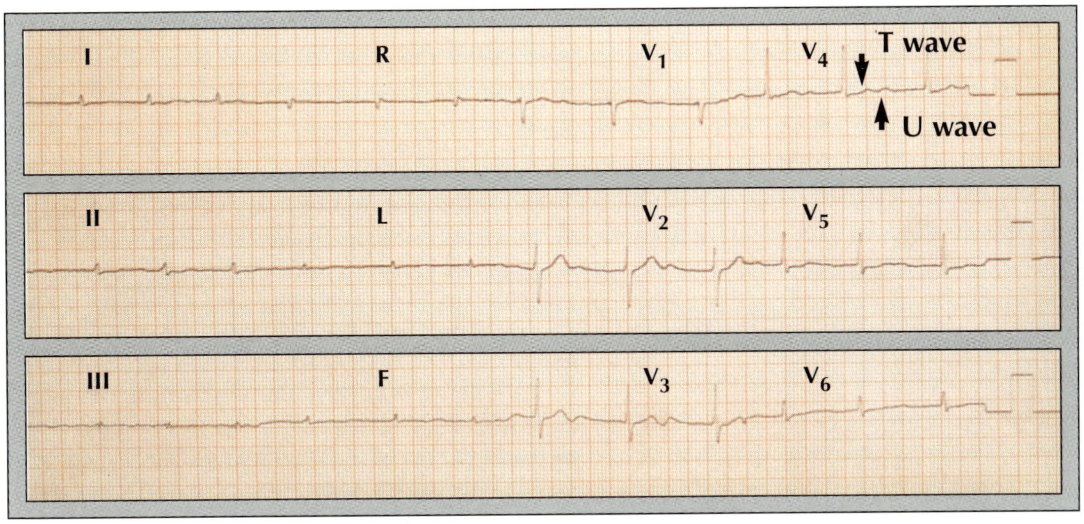

FIGURE 3-11. Prominent U waves as a sign of hypokalemia. In contrast to the U waves shown in Fig. 3-10, the prominent U waves in this 12-lead ECG from a 75-year-old man were due to hypokalemia. The patient's serum potassium level was 2.3 mEq/L. The ECG shows atrial fibrillation with a controlled ventricular response. There is low voltage in the limb leads, and there are prominent U waves in association with a sagging ST segment and attenuation of the T-wave amplitude. In this patient, the ST-TU abnormalities resolved after potassium replacement.

U waves are a normal finding and are best seen in leads V_2 to V_4, in which there are T waves with well-defined terminal segments that are discrete from the beginning of the U waves. Their height is typically 5% to 25% of a normal T wave [9]. The cause of the normal U wave is controversial, but recent observations of the canine ventricle suggest that it may be caused by unmasking of the deep subepicardial layer of M cells from the electrotonic influences of the endocardial and epicardial ventricular myocardium [10,11].

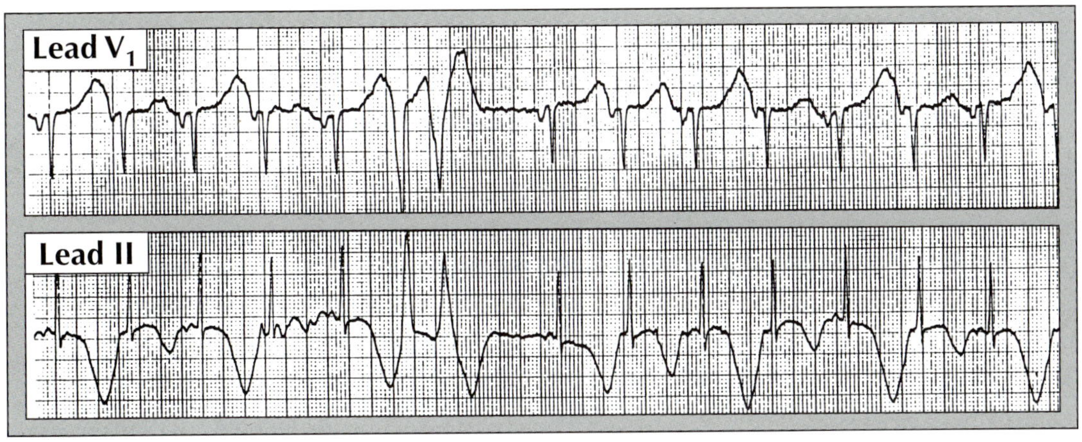

FIGURE 3-12. T-wave alternans as a predictor of ventricular arrhythmias. Subtle electrical alternans on the electrocardiogram primarily involving the ST segment and the T wave (*ie*, the phase of repolarization) may serve as a noninvasive marker of vulnerability to ventricular arrhythmias. Rosenbaum *et al.* [12] prospectively studied 83 patients during electrophysiologic testing, 32 (39%) of whom had inducible sustained ventricular arrhythmias. Most had coronary artery disease, and none had idiopathic long QT syndrome. In patients with inducible ventricular arrhythmias, low-level electrical alternans (a beat-to-beat change in amplitude of <15 μV) was detected over a broad range of physiologic heart rates (from 95 to 150 bpm). Alternans during repolarization was a significant and independent predictor of inducible arrhythmias on electrophysiologic testing (sensitivity, 81%; specificity, 84%; relative risk, 5.2). Of 66 patients followed for up to 20 months, 13 had arrhythmic events. Survival without arrhythmia at 20 months was significantly lower among the patients with T-wave alternans (19%) than among the patients without T-wave alternans (94%) [12].

This figure shows simultaneously recorded rhythm strips of leads V_1 and II from a 61-year-old man being treated with erythromycin for pneumonia. During hospitalization, the patient suffered a thrombotic stroke. The tracings show a sinus rhythm with a ventricular couplet. There is marked T-wave alternans in association with a prolonged QT interval that alternates from 520 to 600 milliseconds, despite fixed RR intervals. The patient subsequently developed torsades de pointes and died.

In contrast to the study by Rosenbaum *et al.* [12], Zareba *et al.* [13] identified T-wave alternans in the electrocardiograms of 30 (1.2%) of 2442 patients with idiopathic long QT syndrome. There was a strong association between prolongation of the corrected QT interval and T-wave alternans. However, logistic regression analysis revealed that T-wave alternans was not a significant predictor of a major cardiac event.(*Courtesy of* Barbara J. Drew, RN PhD, San Francisco, CA.)

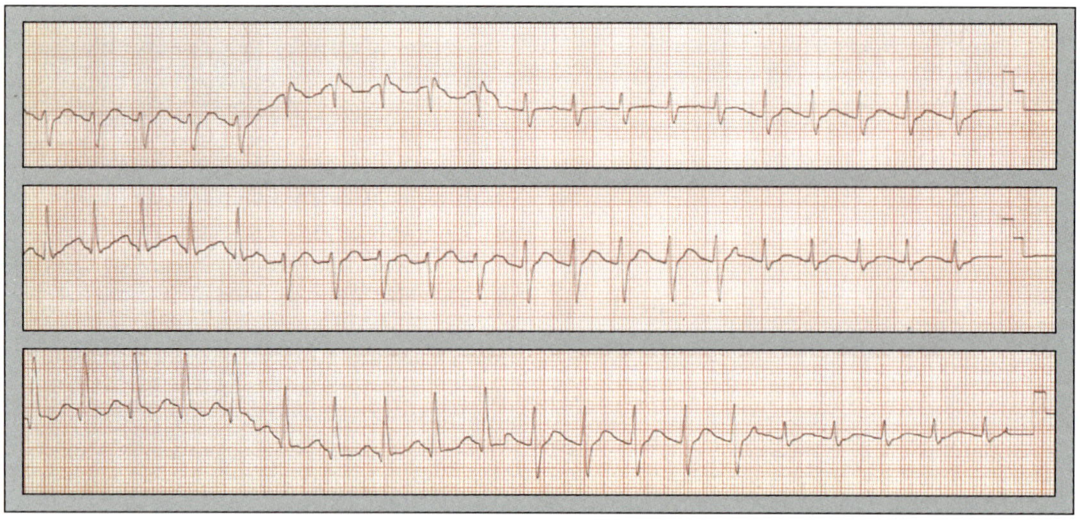

FIGURE 3-13. ECG signs of tricyclic antidepressant overdose as a predictor of ventricular arrhythmias. When applied as a test in the evaluation of 299 patients who presented to the emergency department with drug overdose, three ECG findings allowed for the diagnosis of tricyclic antidepressant overdose with 100% sensitivity, 98% specificity, 66% positive predictive accuracy, 100% negative predictive accuracy, and 97% overall accuracy, even if minimal clinical information was provided [14]. These findings were 1) sinus tachycardia, 2) corrected QT interval of 418 ms or more, 3) the terminal 40 ms of the QRS complex in the frontal plane being between 130° and 270° (corresponding approximately to a terminal S wave in lead I and a terminal R wave in lead aVR). This third finding had both positive and negative predictive values of 1.00. The investigators also reported that a mean frontal plane QRS axis of 90° or more had a positive predictive value of 1.00. A QRS duration 0.10 seconds or more was a predictor of the development of ventricular arrhythmias in 14% of 36 cases in a study by Boehnert and Lovejoy [15], possibly as a result of triggered activity. There was accelerated ventricular rhythm in one case, ventricular bigeminy in one case, and three cases of ventricular tachycardia.

This figure shows the 12-lead ECG of a 25-year-old woman who took an overdose of amitriptyline. There is sinus tachycardia with a 1° atrioventricular block, an intraventricular conduction defect, a corrected QT interval of 550 ms, and the terminal 40 ms of the frontal plane QRS complex at approximately +180°. This patient is at increased risk for development of ventricular arrhythmias.

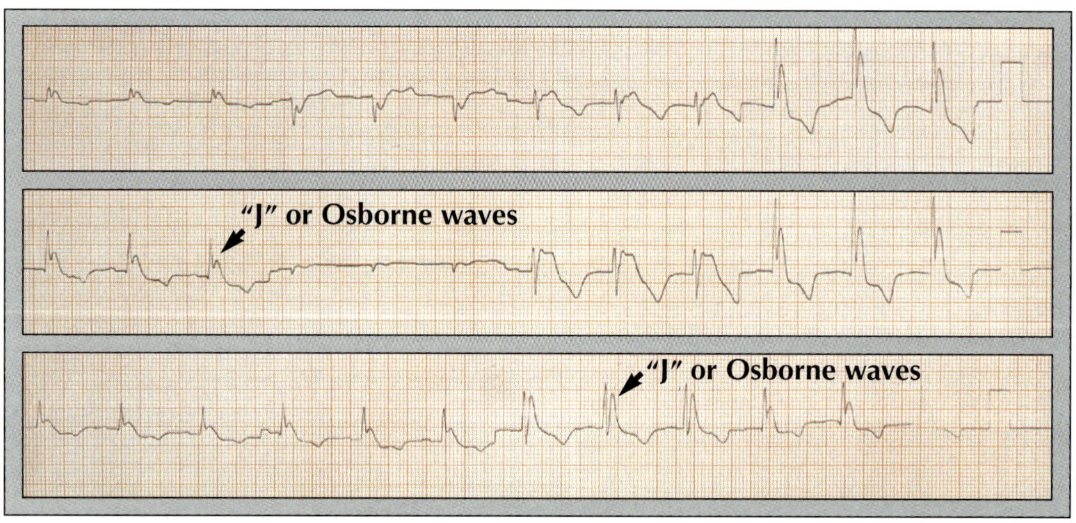

FIGURE 3-14. ECG signs of hypothermia as a predictor of atrial fibrillation (AF) or ventricular fibrillation (VF). Deep hypothermia (temperature <25°C) can be recognized in the ECG by the presence of a characteristic slow wave, called an Osborne or "J" wave, inscribed during the terminal QRS portion, and best seen in the lateral precordial leads, especially V_4. This wave is usually positive in leads with dominant R waves and negative in leads with dominant S waves. There is prolongation of both the PR interval and the QRS duration. The condition causes slowing of the heart rate due to either AF with a slow ventricular response, seen in 50% to 60% of patients, or sinus bradycardia [16].

Moderate hypothermia (*eg*, occurring after exposure to cold) frequently can be suspected in the presence of bradycardia and prolonged QT_c interval. In Schwab's study [17], AF occurred at a mean temperature of 27.2°C (81°F) in patients undergoing rapid induction of hypothermia for surgery.

This figure is a 12-lead ECG from a 20-year-old man who fell unconscious under a sprinkler after he injected heroin intravenously. There is sinus rhythm at a rate of 70 bpm, with prominent Osborne waves. In 10 experiments in dogs, Smith *et al*. [18] showed a 60% decrease in the threshold for VF after the induction of systemic hypothermia. In humans, VF is of imminent concern when the body temperature is less than 30°C. Cardiac arrest can be precipitated by any mechanical stimulation of the heart so that CPR may be contraindicated in a hypotensive but hypothermic patient with an organized cardiac rhythm [19].

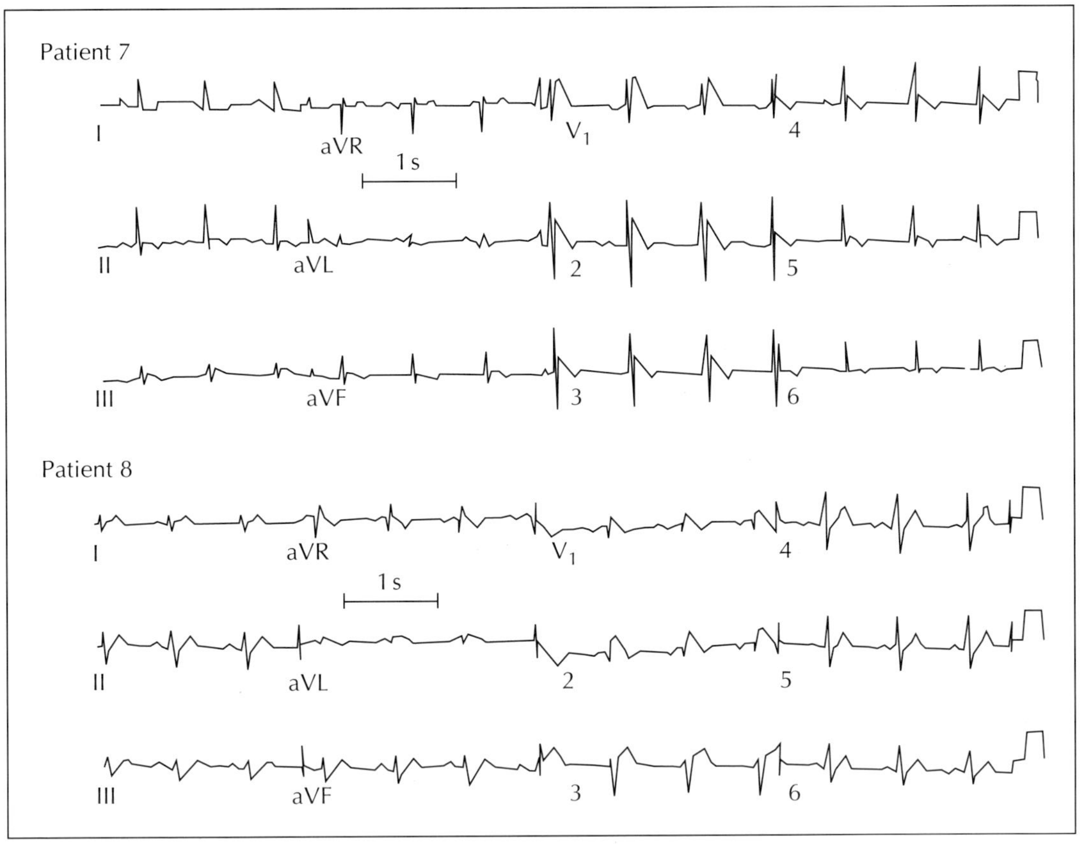

FIGURE 3-15. Right bundle branch block (RBBB) and ST segment elevation in lead V_1 as a predictor of cardiac arrest. Brugada and Brugada [20] recently reported a syndrome characterized by RBBB, persistent ST segment elevation, and sudden cardiac death. Patient ages ranged from 2 to 53 years, and six of the eight were males. All eight patients presented with syncope. ECGs from two of the cases are shown. (*Adapted from* Brugada and Brugada [20]; with permission.)

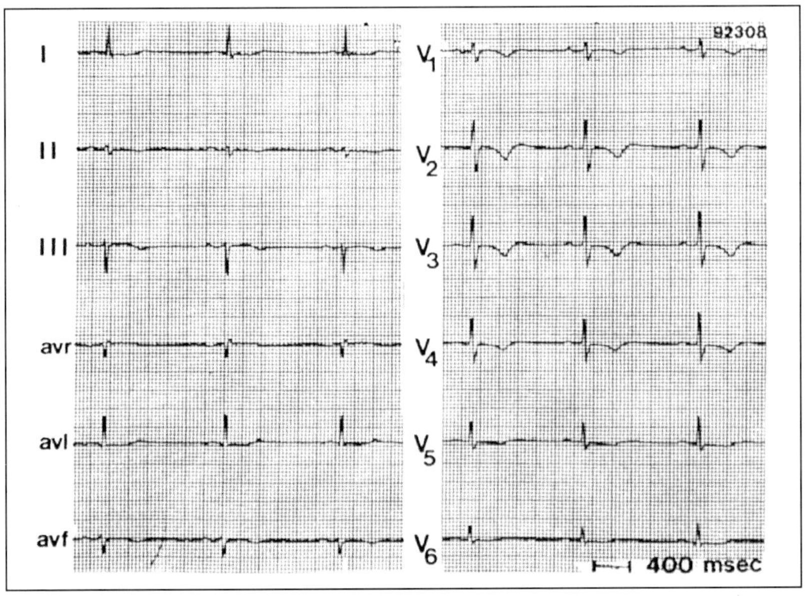

FIGURE 3-16. Precordial T-wave inversion as a predictor of serious ventricular arrhythmias. The most frequent ECG abnormality in symptomatic patients with arrhythmogenic right ventricular dysplasia is the presence of negative T waves in the precordial leads. This 12-lead ECG shows a QRS duration of 110 ms and negative T waves from leads V_1 through V_5 [21,22]. (*Adapted from* Metzger and coworkers [22]; with permission.)

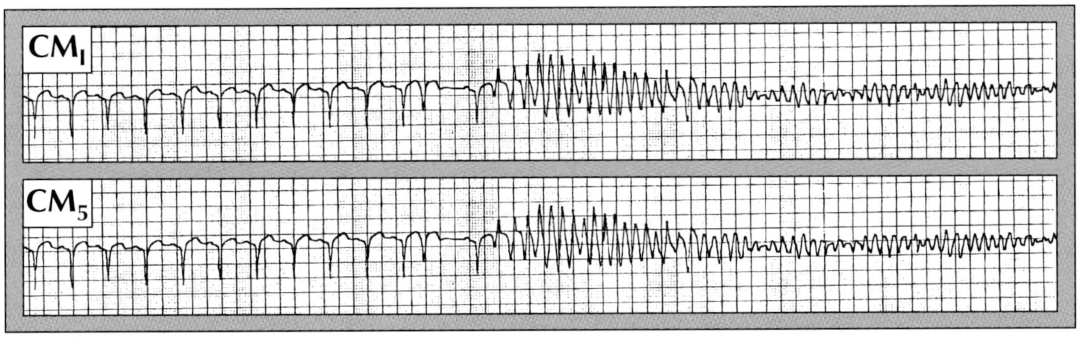

FIGURE 3-17. Acute myocardial ischemia as a predictor of ventricular arrhythmias. Acute myocardial ischemia due to acute coronary occlusion or coronary artery spasm, or to supply-demand mismatch may be arrhythmogenic. Continuous ECG monitoring in a hospitalized patient shows leads CM_1 and CM_5. The baseline rhythm shows sinus tachycardia with 1.5 to 2.0-mm ST segment elevation in lead CM_5. An episode of pause-dependent ventricular fibrillation occurs after a premature ventricular contraction with the "R-on-T" timing.

PREDICTORS OF ATRIOVENTRICULAR BLOCK

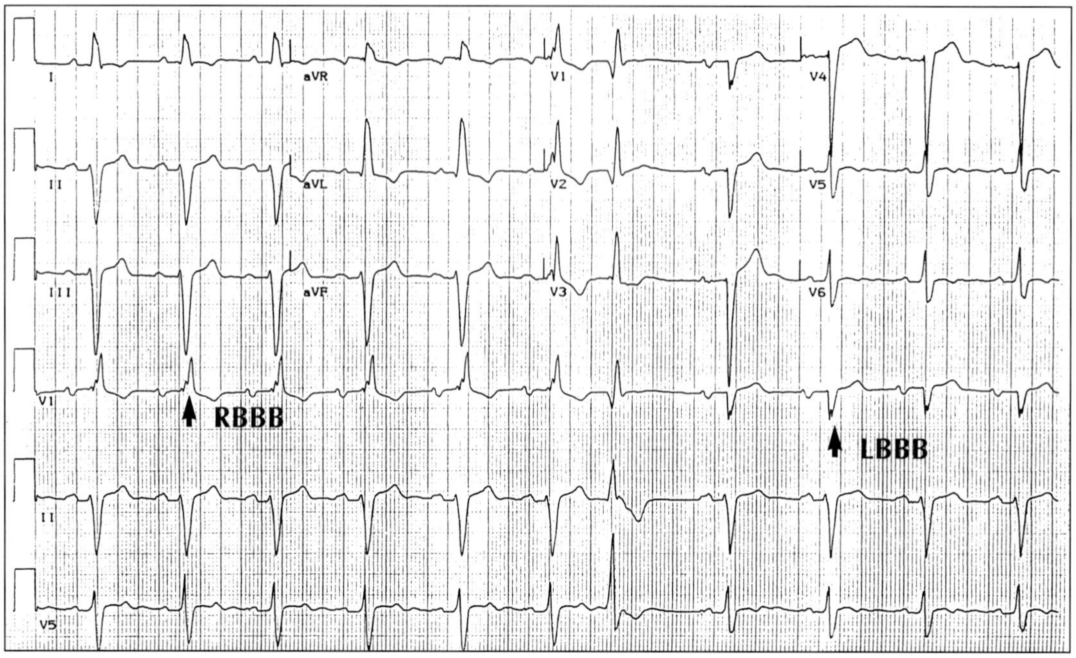

FIGURE 3-18. Alternating bundle branch block. Spontaneous alternating bundle branch block represents the most ominous ECG sign for progression to atrioventricular (AV) block. This phenomenon implies both His-Purkinje instability and pathology involving both bundle branches, the His bundle, or the main trunk of the conducting system. Patients with this pattern have the highest incidence of HV intervals exceeding 100 ms, but it is seldom seen. Although alternating bundle branch block is very insensitive as a predictor, seven (78%) of nine patients who showed this pattern developed high-grade AV block within weeks of this finding. Thus, the presence of alternating bundle branch block mandates insertion of a cardiac pacemaker [4].

This 12-lead ECG from an 82-year-old man shows sinus rhythm with first-degree AV block. There is left atrial abnormality, left ventricular hypertrophy with an old anterior myocardial infarction, and left axis deviation consistent with left anterior fascicular block, as well as alternating periods of right and left bundle branch block, the latter occurring after a premature ventricular complex.

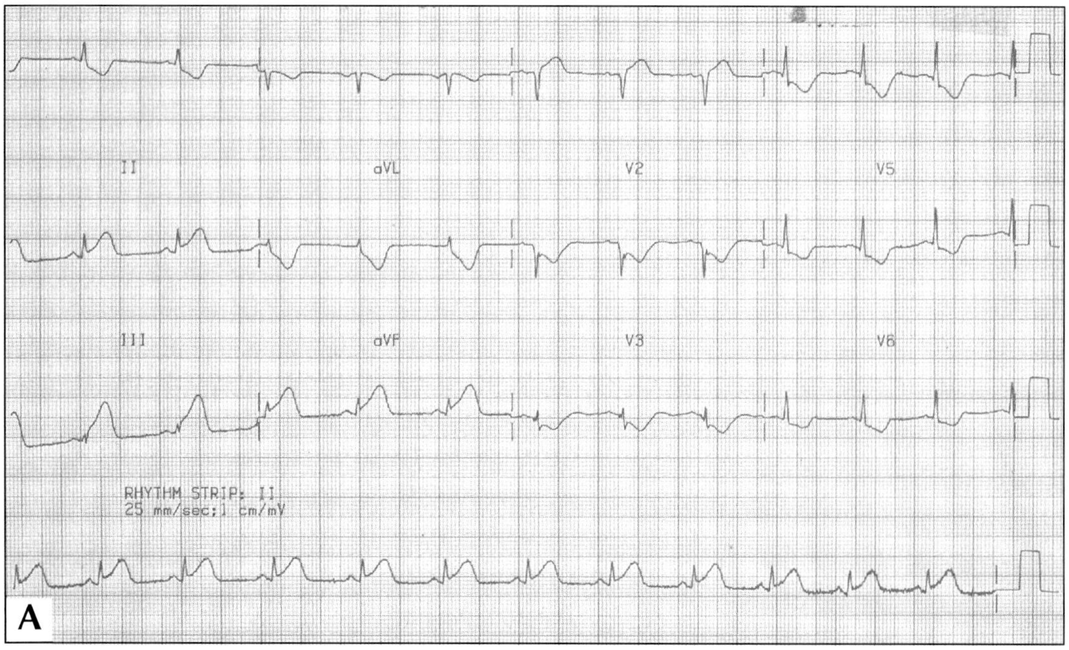

FIGURE 3-19. RV infarction as a predictor of atrioventricular (AV) block. Zehender *et al.* [23] studied 200 consecutive patients admitted to the hospital with acute inferior myocardial infarctions and in 107 patients found ST segment elevation in lead V_{4R}, reflective of right ventricular (RV) involvement. Fifteen patients with RV involvement developed AV block, compared with three who had no RV involvement (P<0.05). **A,** This 12-lead ECG is from a 50-year-old man who presented to the emergency department with crushing substernal chest pain. There is sinus rhythm with acute inferoposterior injury in addition to findings of old anterior myocardial infarction. There is ST-segment elevation in lead V_1. *(continued)*

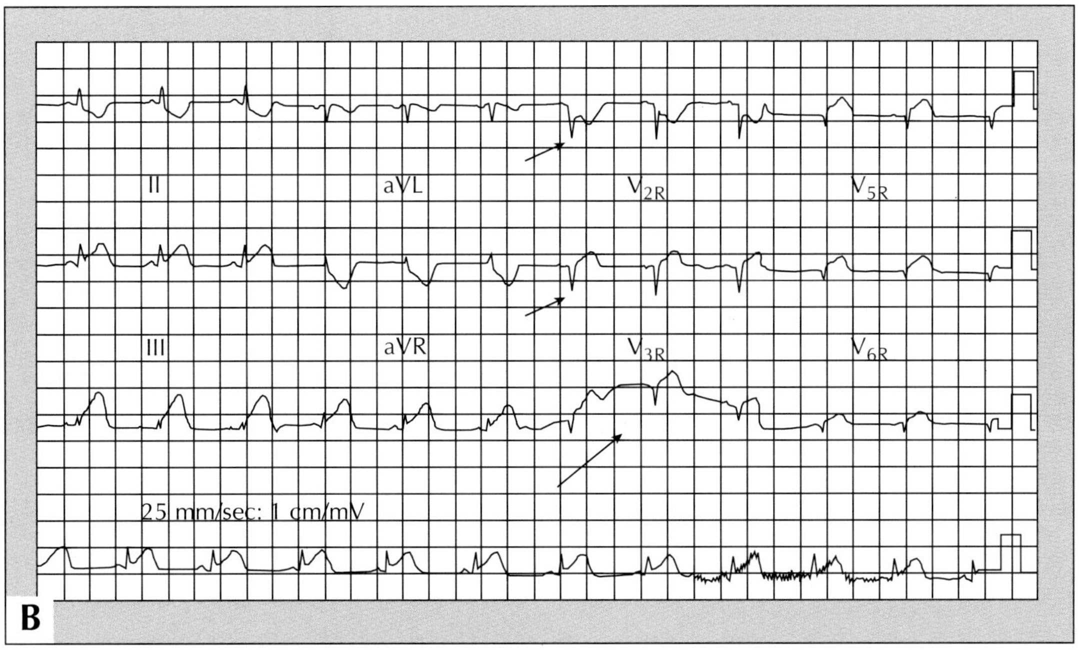

FIGURE 3-19. (*continued*) **B,** A tracing was recorded from the same patient a few moments later, with placement of right-sided chest leads (*arrows*). There is ST-segment elevation in association with QS complexes in leads V_{2R} to V_{6R}, consistent with RV infarction. In the evaluation of patients with acute inferior wall myocardial infarctions, lead V_{4R} should be recorded to detect proximal occlusion of the right coronary artery and right ventricular involvement [24].

PREDICTORS OF MISCELLANEOUS RHYTHM DISTURBANCES

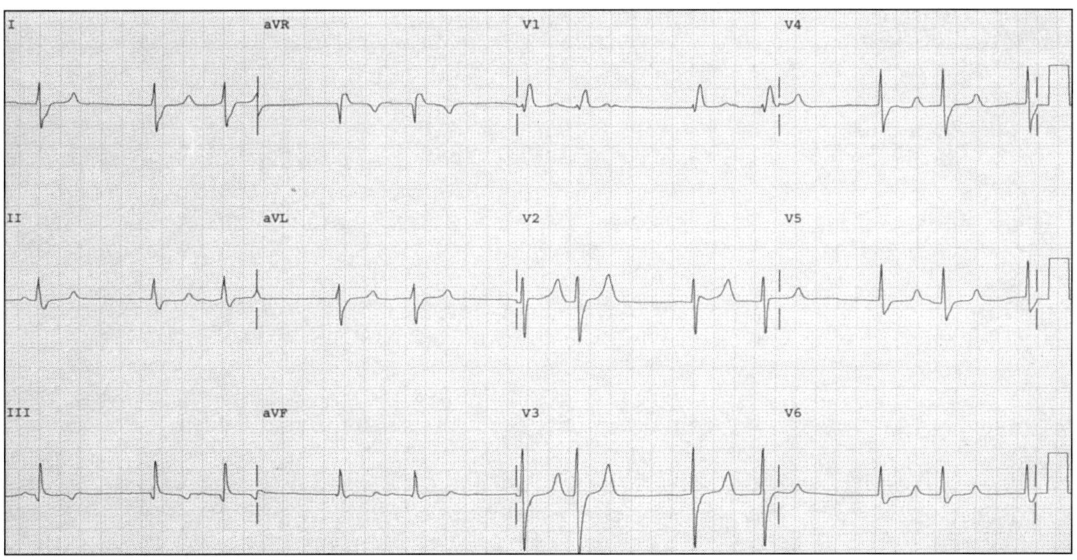

FIGURE 3-20. ECG changes of severe hyperkalemia as a predictor of an agonal sine-wave rhythm. This 12-lead ECG is taken from a 57-year-old woman with a history of renal insufficiency who presented with weakness. Her serum potassium level was 8.0 mEq/L. There is group beating, possibly due to sinoatrial exit block, and a pattern of escape-capture bigeminy. There is complete right bundle branch block which, combined with right axis deviation, suggests left posterior fascicular block. The T waves in the midprecordial leads are peaked and narrow at their base, resulting in an ST segment that is more horizontal than normal.

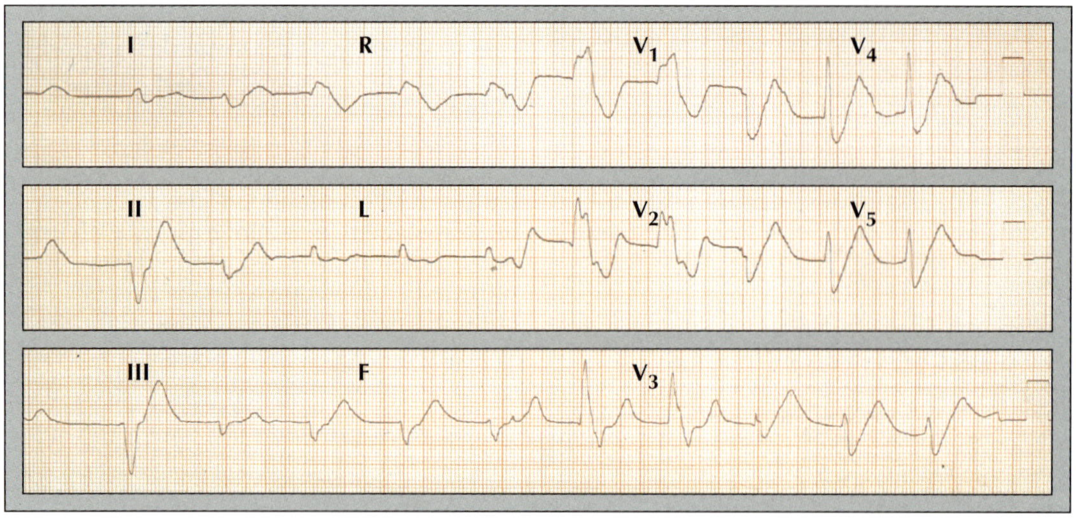

FIGURE 3-21. This 12-lead ECG illustrates severe hyperkalemia with a right bundle branch block–type of intraventricular conduction defect. There are absent P waves and a mean ventricular rate of 65 bpm. Of the two QRS complexes in leads I, II, and III, one shows extreme axis deviation and the other shows left axis deviation, both with a markedly widened and bizarre QRS complex accompanied by slurred S waves in the precordial leads. Leads V_5 and V_6 show an M-shaped pattern consisting of the QRS complex, the ST segment, and the T wave. The T wave in profound hyperkalemia may lose its peaked character and assume a rounded appearance. The QT interval is 600 ms, of which the QRS duration comprises 230 ms. Hyperkalemia interferes with cell-to-cell coupling, leading to ECG patterns of either fascicular block or a markedly widened and bizarre QRS complex.

REFERENCES

1. Kannel WB, Wolf PA: Epidemiology of atrial fibrillation In *Atrial Fibrillation: Mechanisms and Management*. Edited by Falk RH, Podrid PJ. New York: Raven Press; 1992:81–92.
2. Milstein S, Sharma AD, Klein GJ: Electrophysiologic profile of asymptomatic Wolff-Parkinson-White pattern. *Am J Cardiol* 1986, 57:1097–1100.
3. Robles de Medina EO, Bernard R, Coumel P, *et al.* for the WHO/ISFC Task Force: Definition of terms related to cardiac rhythm. *Eur J Cardiol* 1278, 8:127–144.
4. Josephson ME: *Clinical Cardiac Electrophysiology*. Philadelphia: Lea & Febiger; 1993.
5. Klein GJ, Bashore TM, Sellers TD, *et al.*: Ventricular fibrillation in the Wolff-Parkinson-White Syndrome. *N Engl J Med* 1979, 301:1080–1085.
6. Keren A, Tzivoni D, Gavish D, *et al.*: Etiology, warning signs and therapy of torsade de pointes: a study of 10 patients. *Circulation* 1981, 64:1167–1174.
7. Jackman WM, Friday KJ, Anderson JL, *et al.*: The long QT syndromes: a critical review, new clinical observations and a unifying hypothesis. *Prog Cardiovasc Dis* 1988, 31:115–172.
8. Antzelevitch C, Sicouri S, Litovsky SH, *et al.*: Heterogeneity within the ventricular wall: electrophysiology and pharmacology of epicardial, endocardial, and M cells. *Circ Res* 1991, 69:1427–1449.
9. Lepeschkin E: Physiologic basis of the U wave. In *Advances in Electrocardiography*, vol 2. Edited by Schlant RC and Hurst JW. New York: Grune & Stratton, Inc., 1976:353–375.
10. Antzelevitch C, Sicouri S: Clinical relevance of cardiac arrhythmias generated by afterdepolarizations. Role of M cells in the generation of U waves, triggered activity and torsade de pointes. *J Am Coll Cardiol* 1994, 23:259–277.
11. Nesterenko VV, Antzelevitch C: M cells as the basis for the electrocardiographic U wave. *Circulation* 1992, 86(suppl 1):I-302.
12. Rosenbaum DS, Jackson LE, Smith JM, *et al.*: Electrical alternans and vulnerability to ventricular arrhythmias. *N Engl J Med* 1994, 330:235–241.
13. Zareba W, Moss AJ, le Cessie S, *et al.*: T wave alternans in idiopathic long QT syndrome. *J Am Coll Cardiol* 1994, 23:1541–1546.
14. Niemann JT, Bessen HA, Rothstein RJ, *et al.*: Electrocardiographic criteria for tricyclic antidepressant cardiotoxicity. *Am J Cardiol* 1986, 57:1154–1159.
15. Boehnert MT, Lovejoy FH Jr: Value of the QRS duration versus the serum drug level in predicting seizures and ventricular arrhythmias after an acute overdose of tricyclic antidepressants. *N Engl J Med* 1985, 313:474–479.
16. Harumi K, Chen CY: Miscellaneous electrocardiographic topics. In *Comprehensive Electrocardiology: Theory and Practice in Health and Disease*, vol 1. Edited by MacFarlane PW, Veitch Lawrie TD. New York: Pergamon Press; 1989:671–728.
17. Schwab: R, Lewis D, Killurgh J: Electrocardiographic changes occurring in rapidly induced deep hypothermia. *Am J Med Sci* 1964, 248: 290–303.
18. Smith JM, Clancy EA, Valeri CR, *et al.*: Electrical alternans and cardiac electrical instability. *Circulation* 1988, 77:110–121.
19. Weaver WD, Dolack L: Ventricular fibrillation and torsades de pointes. In *Current Practice of Emergency Medicine*, ed 2. Edited by Callaham MI. Philadelphia: B.C. Decker; 1991:483.
20. Brugada P, Brugada J: Right bundle branch block, persistent ST-segment elevation and sudden cardiac death: a distinct clinical and electrocardiographic syndrome. *J Am Coll Cardiol* 1992, 20:1391–1396.
21. Marcus FI, Fontaine GH, Guiradon G, *et al.*: Right ventricular dysplasia: a report of 24 adult cases. *Circulation* 1982, 65:384–387.
22. Metzger JT, de Chillou C, Cheriex E, *et al.*: Value of the 12-lead electrocardiogram in arrhythmogenic right ventricular dysplasia, and absence of correlation with echocardiographic findings. *Am J Cardiol* 1993, 72:964–967.
23. Zehender: M, Kasper W, Kauder E, *et al.*: Right ventricular infarction as an independent predictor of prognosis after acute inferior myocardial infarction. *N Engl J Med* 1993, 328:981-988.
24. Wellens HJ: Right ventricular infarction [editorial]. *N Engl J Med* 1993, 328:1036–1038.

SINUS NODE DISORDERS

4

CHAPTER

Laurence M. Epstein

Although the sinus node is the site of impulse formation, it was the last component of the specialized conducting system to be described in the cardiology literature. In 1907, Keith and Flack [1] noted a compact mass of cells at the junction of the superior vena cava and right atrium. They speculated that "in them the dominating rhythm of the heart is believed to arise." Lewis, by carefully mapping electrical activity in canine hearts [2], then demonstrated that this region was, in fact, the origin of electrical activity. Although subsequent studies have greatly increased our understanding of impulse formation and conduction, areas of controversy remain.

Disorders of sinus node function cover a wide spectrum: patients can present with bradyarrhythmias, tachyarrhythmias, or both. Bradyarrhythmias may be caused by either a failure of impulse formation or impulse conduction, whereas tachyarrhythmias may be due to reentry, enhanced automaticity, or triggered arrhythmias. In 1954, Short [3] described the syndrome of alternating tachycardia and bradycardia, which has since come to be called the "tachy-brady syndrome." The term "sick sinus syndrome" was coined in 1968 by Ferrer [4] and refers to the spectrum of disorders, including symptomatic bradyarrhythmias as well as the tachy-brady syndrome. It is estimated that one in 600 cardiac patients has the sick sinus syndrome and that it is the leading cause of permanent cardiac pacemaker insertion [5].

The cause of sinus node dysfunction is most often termed *idiopathic*, and in the majority of patients the cause is probably degenerative change in the sinus node and atrium. In addition, surgical trauma, coronary artery disease, inflammation, tumor, amyloidosis, and collagen vascular diseases can lead to sinus node dysfunction. Although evidence of sinus node dysfunction can be found on routine electrocardiograms (ECGs), patients most often present with symptoms of inadequate cerebral perfusion or exercise intolerance. Because episodes are often intermittent, it is important to correlate ECG abnormalities with symptoms. Therefore, although a variety of noninvasive and invasive techniques are available to evaluate these patients, ambulatory ECG monitoring, either continuously or with an event recorder, remains the mainstay of evaluation. Therapy most often includes permanent cardiac pacing to prevent bradycardic episodes, and occasionally antiarrhythmic medications and/or ablative procedures to control the tachyarrhythmias. This chapter reviews normal and abnormal sinus node anatomy and physiology as well as the evaluation of patients with symptomatic sinus node dysfunction.

Normal Anatomy and Physiology

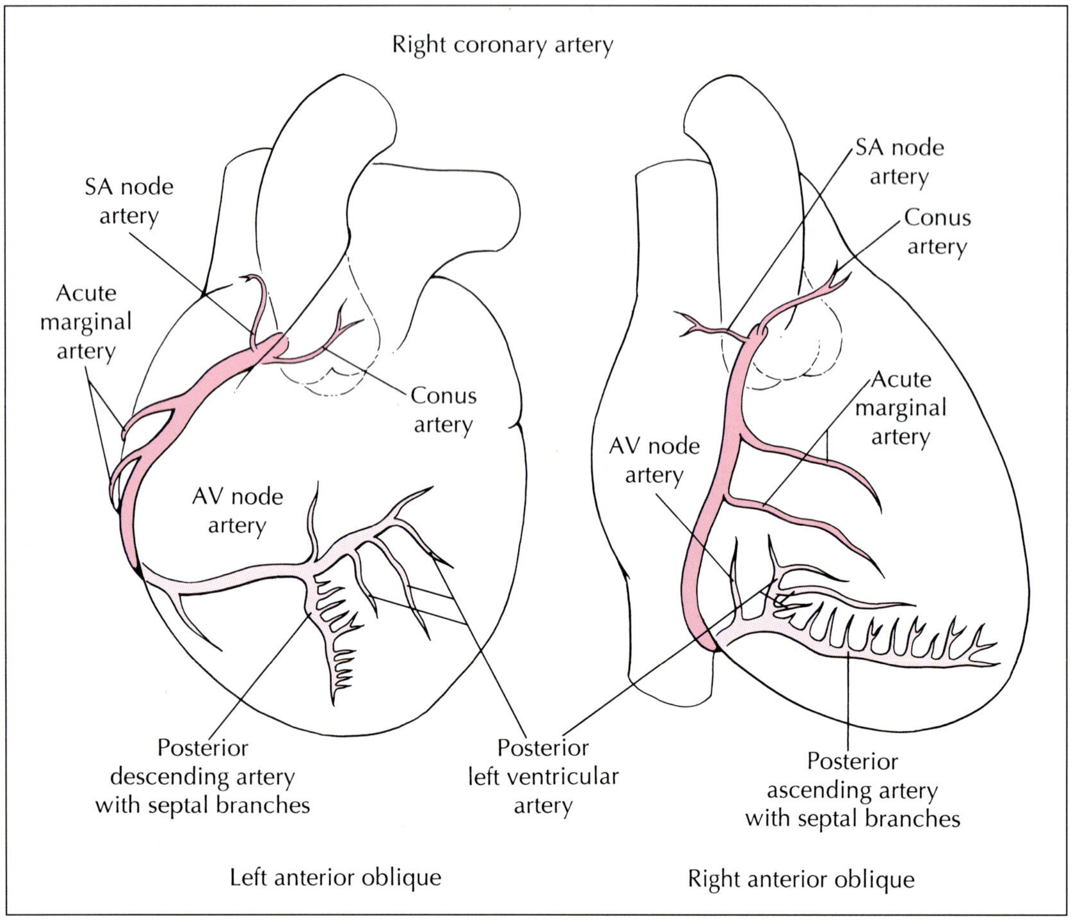

Figure 4-1. The sinoatrial (SA) node and the SA node artery. The SA node is located within the wall of the right atrium at its junction with the superior vena cava. The sinus node receives its blood supply from the sinus node artery, and sinus node cells form clusters around one or more branches of this vessel. In 55% of patients the sinus node artery arises from the proximal 2 to 3 cm of the right coronary artery (RCA; following the takeoff of the conus branch). In 45% of patients it arises from the proximal 1 cm of the left circumflex coronary artery [6]. This figure is a representation of the left anterior oblique and right anterior oblique projections of the anatomy of the RCA. In this example, the SA node artery arises from the proximal RCA.

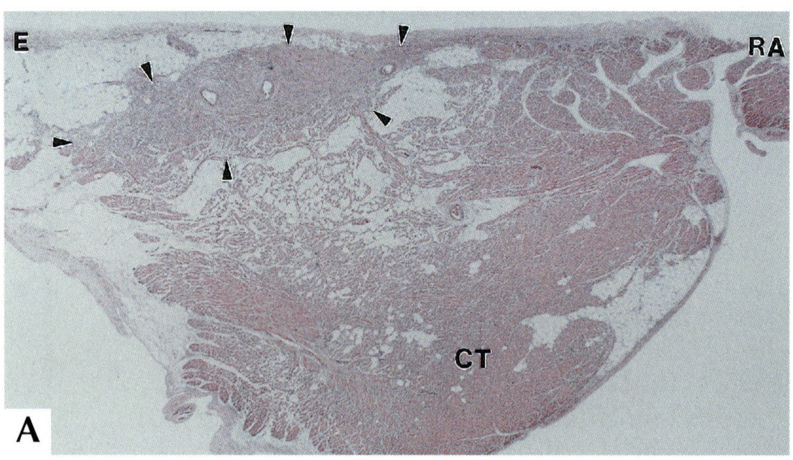

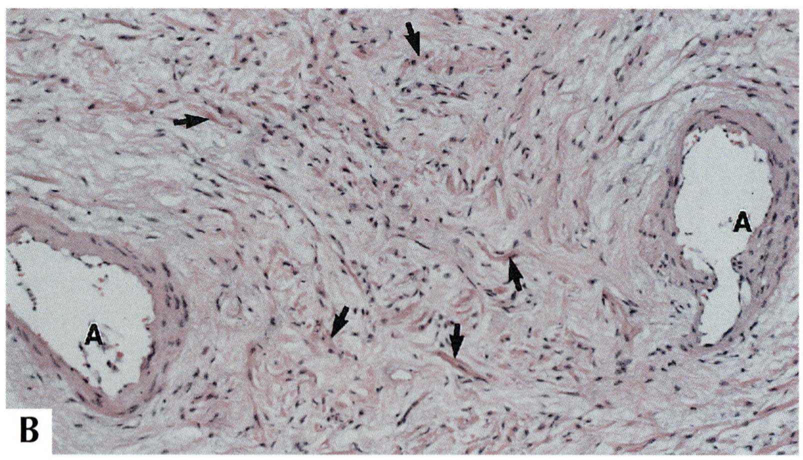

Figure 4-2. Sinus node histology. Photomicrographs of a section through the right atrial wall in the region of the sinus node. **A,** Low-power view in which the sinus node (*arrowheads*), lies adjacent to the epicardial surface (E) and the crista terminalis (CT). **B,** High-power view in which two sinus node arteries (A) are surrounded by rests of sinus node cells (*arrows*) embedded in an extensive matrix of connective tissue. RA—right atrial working muscle.

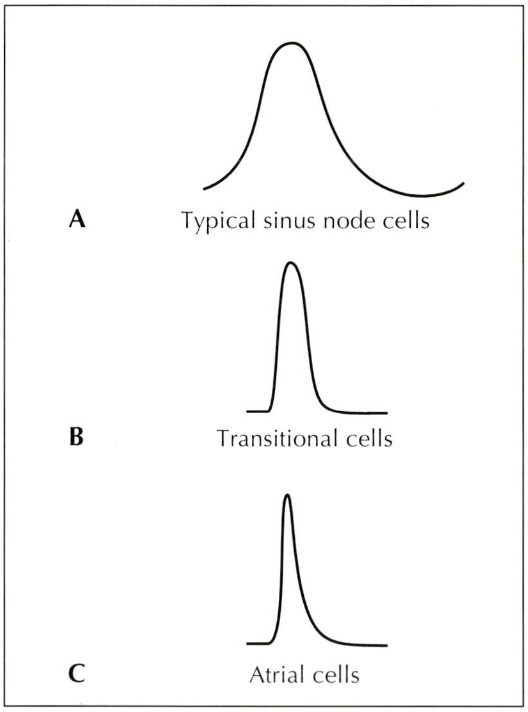

FIGURE 4-3. Action potential for cell types of the sinus node region [7–9]. **A,** Typical sinus node cells consist of small rests of cells surrounded by connective tissue. The cells appear pale (hence called "P" cells) or empty due to poor development of contractile elements. Myofilaments are scarcely present (approximately 20% of volume) and there are no organized myofibrils. **B,** Transitional cells surround the typical sinus node cells. They are a very heterogeneous group of cells. As the distance from the typical nodal cells increases, so does the number of myofibrils. **C,** Atrial cells contain more than 50% organized myofibrils by volume. There are granules (atrial granules) in the perinuclear region that are not present in nodal or transitional cells.

IONIC CURRENTS IN THE SINUS NODE REGION

CURRENT	ION	ROLE
$^{i}Ca_{,f}$	Ca^{2+}	Responsible for the upstroke of the action potential of sinus node cells
Ca/Na exchange ($^{i}NaCa$, ^{i}ti)	$1Ca^{2+}/3Na^{+}$	Partly governs the duration of the repolarization phase by offsetting the outward current
Extremely slow inward current	Ca^{2+}	?
^{i}f	Na^{+}/K^{+}	Partially responsible for diastolic depolarization in cells with a maximum diastolic potential less than 60 mV (transitional cells)
Background current	$?Ca^{2+}/Na^{+}$	Partially responsible for diastolic depolarization (pacemaker current)
^{i}Na	Na^{+}	Largely inactive at diastolic potentials of sinus node cells; increasingly active in the perinodal region (responsible for the more rapid upstroke of the action potential of transitional cells)
^{i}k	K^{+}	Main current responsible for repolarization; slowing of this current may contribute to diastolic depolarization
$^{i}k1$	K^{+}	Virtually absent in sinus node cells; part of the reason sinus node cells are more resistant to hyperkalemia
^{i}f	Na^{+}	Thought to be pacemaker current, decreasing $Ik_i + I_f$, which are thought to generate sinus node discharge, especially at hyperpolarized levels

FIGURE 4-4. Ionic currents in the sinus node region. This table represents the proposed ionic currents (i) involved in the generation and propagation of impulses in the sinus node region [10]. At present, there is only a partial understanding of these currents.

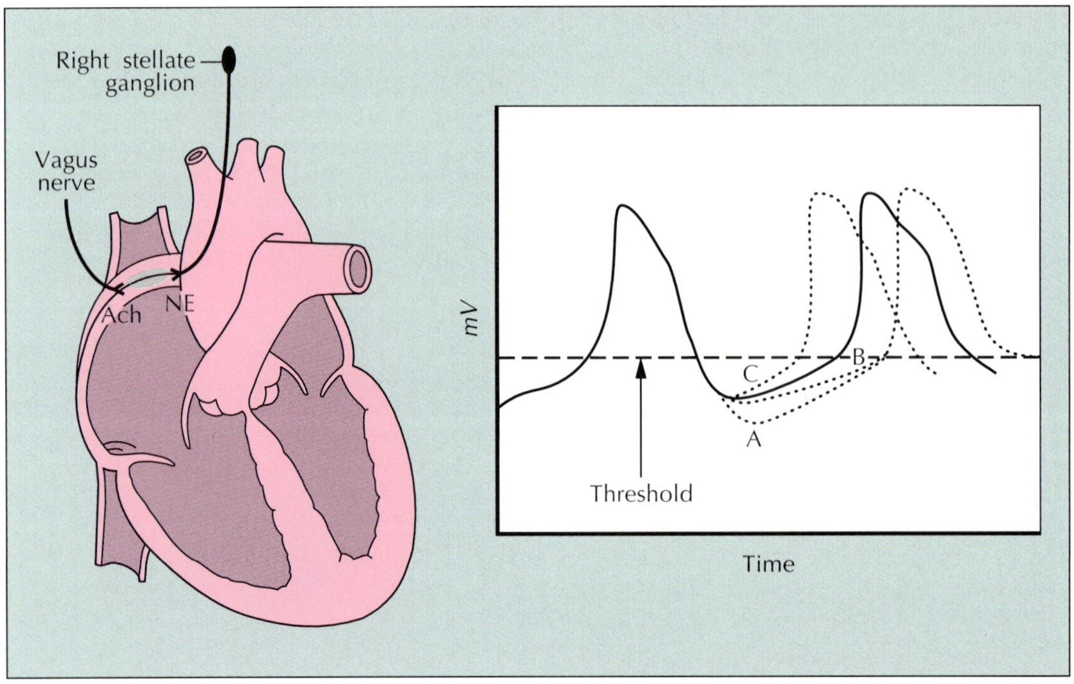

FIGURE 4-5. Autonomic nervous system inputs to the sinus node. Parasympathetic stimulation via the vagus nerve results in the release of acetylcholine (Ach). This produces a *negative* chronotropic response due to a decrease in the maximum diastolic potential (hyperpolarization) (A) and a decrease in the slope of phase and depolarization (B). Sympathetic stimulation via the right stellate ganglion results in norepinephrine (NE) release from the postsynaptic nerve terminals within the sinus node. This produces a *positive* chronotropic response mainly by an increase in the rate of phase 4 depolarization (C).

Modulation of the sinus rate is therefore due to the interactions of the two limbs of the autonomic nervous system (parasympathetic and sympathetic). During sleep and in response to some stimuli (nausea, and in some people, the sight of blood or pain, for example), parasympathetic stimulation predominates, and the heart rate slows. During exercise and in response to fright or to some kinds of pain, sympathetic stimulation predominates, and the heart races.(*Adapted from* Talano and coworkers. [11]; with permission.)

TYPES OF SINUS NODE DYSFUNCTION

SPECTRUM OF SINUS NODE DYSFUNCTION

Abnormalities of impulse formation
- Sinus bradycardia
- Sinus arrest

Abnormalities of impulse conduction
- Sinoatrial exit block

Tachy-brady syndrome
Sinus node reentry
Inappropriate sinus tachycardia
Carotid sinus hypersensitivity

FIGURE 4-6. The spectrum of sinus node dysfunction. Sinus node dysfunction may be due to abnormalities of impulse formation or impulse conduction. An inappropriately slow rate of impulse formation or no sinus impulse formation can cause sinus bradycardia (sinus rate = 60 bpm) or sinus arrest (no sinus P-waves). Each of the entities listed is discussed in detail in this chapter.

CONDITIONS ASSOCIATED WITH SINUS NODE DYSFUNCTION

INTRINSIC	EXTRINSIC
Aging	Hypothermia
Hypertension	Electrolyte abnormalities
Coronary artery disease	Hypothyroidism
Rheumatic heart disease	Abnormalities of autonomic nervous system (carotid hypersensitivity)
Cardiomyopathies	Hyperbilirubinemia
Pericarditis	Drugs
Congenital heart abnormalities	Cardiac glycosides
Collagen vascular disease	β-Adrenergic receptor blockers
Amyloidosis	Calcium-channel blockers
Trauma	Methyldopa
Surgical	Reserpine
Closure of ASD (sinus venosus type)	Lithium carbonate
Mustard procedure	Cimetidine
Placement of caval cannula	Amitriptyline
Tumor	Phenothiazines
Irradiation	

FIGURE 4-7. Conditions associated with sinus node dysfunction. Sinus node dysfunction may be due to a pathologic process that directly involves the sinus node (intrinsic) or other processes and drugs that have secondary effects on the sinus node (extrinsic). ASD—atrial septal defect.

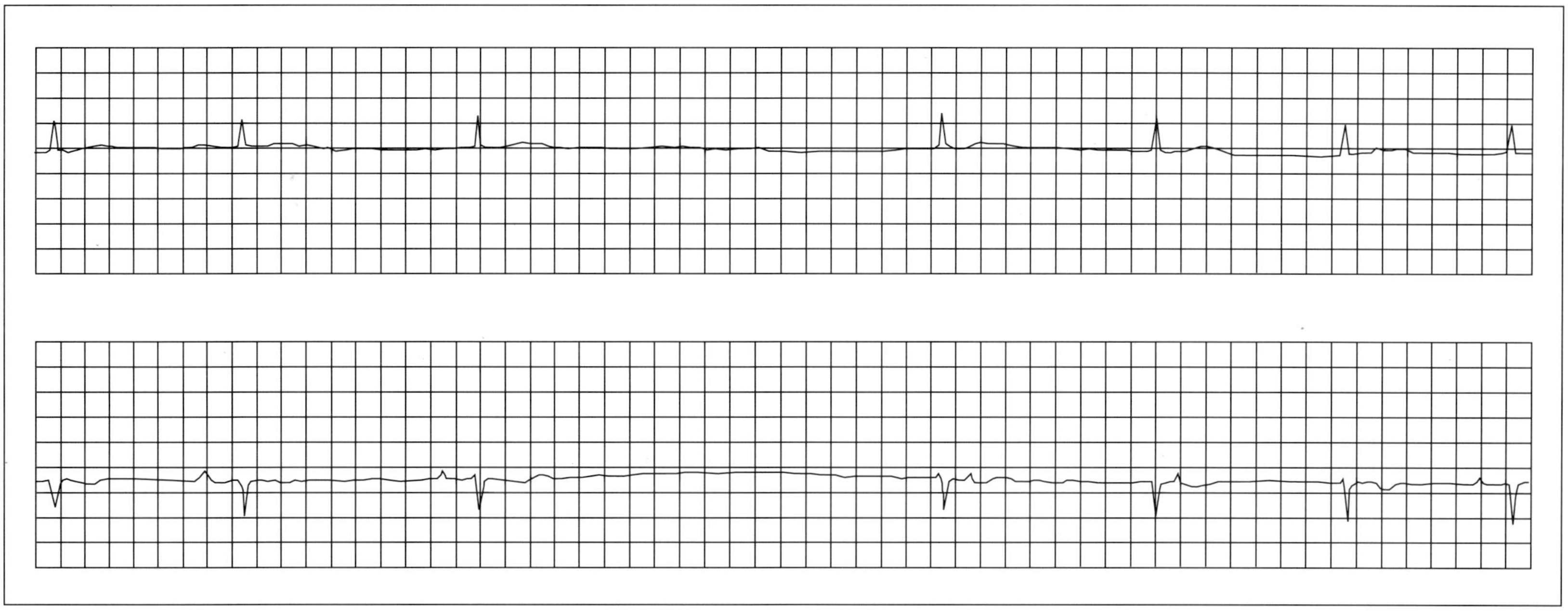

FIGURE 4-8. Failure of impulse generation. Sinus node dysfunction can be manifested as a failure of impulse generation. This can result in sinus bradycardia (defined as sinus rhythm <60 bpm) or sinus arrest. However, this rate is considered normal during sleep or in a trained person at rest. Sinus bradycardia is clinically significant only if it results in failure to meet the patient's metabolic demands. This may result in physical signs such as hypotension or congestive heart failure or symptoms of fatigue, shortness of breath, exercise intolerance, angina, lightheadedness, or even syncope.

Simultaneous leads V_5 (*top*) and V_1 (*bottom*) of a Holter recording from an 85-year-old woman with a history of syncope. Both sinus bradycardia (38 bpm) and sinus arrest (4.2-second pause) with a junctional escape rhythm are represented. (*Adapted from* Evans [12]; with permission.)

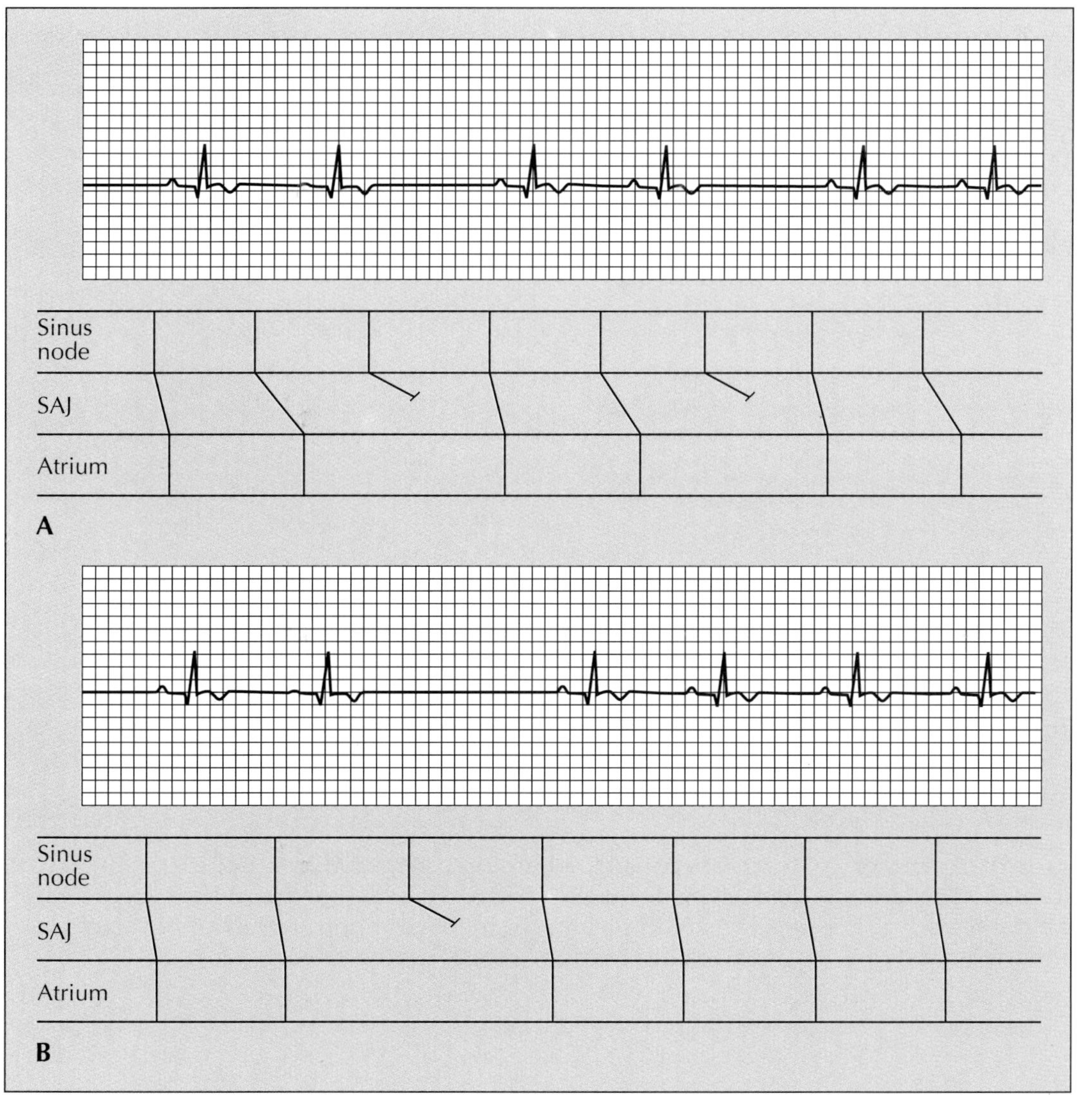

FIGURE 4-9. Abnormalities of impulse conduction. Sinus pauses can be due to sinoatrial exit block of the impulse generated from the primary pacemaker cells in the node itself or at the sinoatrial junction.

Block may be manifested in one of two forms. **A,** A typical Wenckebach pattern, with progressive slowing of conduction (in the sinoatrial junction [SAJ]), resulting in progressive shortening of the P-wave–P-wave interval, ending in a sinus pause (blocked impulse). The pause is less than twice the shortest atrial cycle length. **B,** Sudden block, with no prior evidence of conduction slowing, may be observed. In this setting the pause is equal to twice the atrial cycle length (Mobitz II SA block). In *A,* Wenckebach block in the SAJ can be seen. There is progressive slowing (represented by a deceased slope) of conduction in the SAJ prior to block (beats 3 and 6). In *B,* there is no change in conduction through the SAJ. Block (beat 3) occurs suddenly. (*continued*)

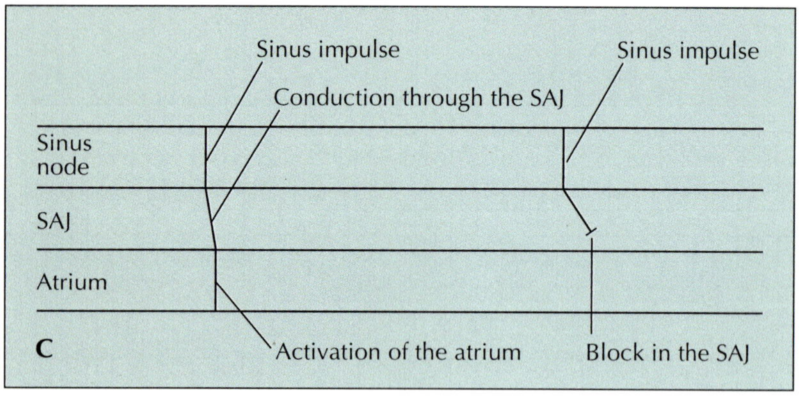

FIGURE 4-9. (*continued*) **C**, A ladder diagram with explanation. Throughout this chapter, ladder diagrams are used to demonstrate electrophysiologic phenomena. Each horizontal area represents a region within the heart. Impulse origin and conduction are represented by the vertical (or slanting) lines. Conduction block is represented by a vertical line with a perpendicular line at the end of it.

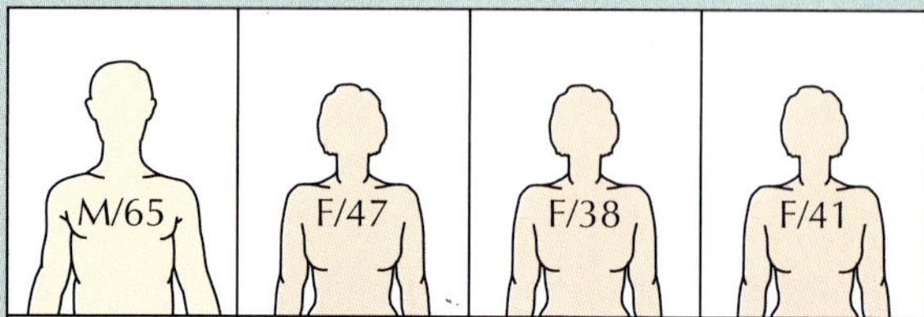

Sex/Age, *y*	M/65	F/47	F/38	F/41
Associated heart disease	Aortic valve sclerosis	Mitral valve disease	Mitral valve disease	None
Heart rate, *bpm* Sinus rhythm	28–48	35–75	22–43	35–45
Atrial tachycardia *Atrial*	220–250	180–130	260	270
Ventricular	60–120	90–180	50–65	110

FIGURE 4-10. The tachy-brady syndrome. In 1954, Short [3] described a syndrome characterized by periods of profound bradycardia alternating with episodes of tachycardia, which today is known as the *tachy-brady* syndrome. In addition, in these four patients, Short described a major concern in patients with this disorder: pauses associated with tachycardia termination that can cause syncope and cerebrovascular accidents due to emboli related to paroxysmal atrial fibrillation. Because permanent cardiac pacing to treat bradycardia was not available, but ventricular rate could be controlled with digitalis, Short believed that a means of inducing and maintaining atrial fibrillation in humans would be an invaluable way of preventing the life-threatening consequences of sinus pauses. (*Adapted from* Short [3]; with permission.)

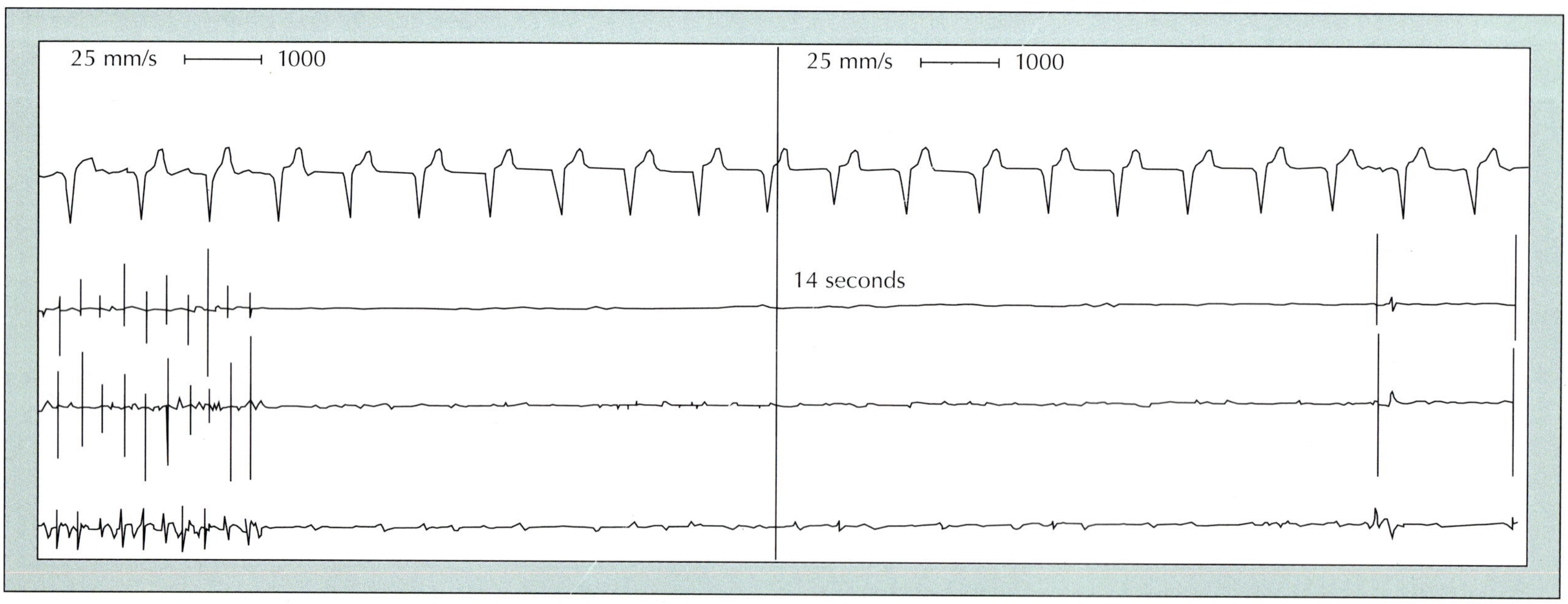

FIGURE 4-11. *Tachy-brady syndrome* is the common term for the syndrome of alternating bradycardia and tachycardia. This figure shows surface lead V_1 and V_3 intracardiac right atrial recordings in a patient with atrial fibrillation/flutter and sinus node dysfunction. This patient had multiple syncopal episodes and ultimately underwent complete atrioventricular junction ablation and VVI pacemaker implantation. In this example, termination of tachycardia resulted in a 14-second atrial pause.

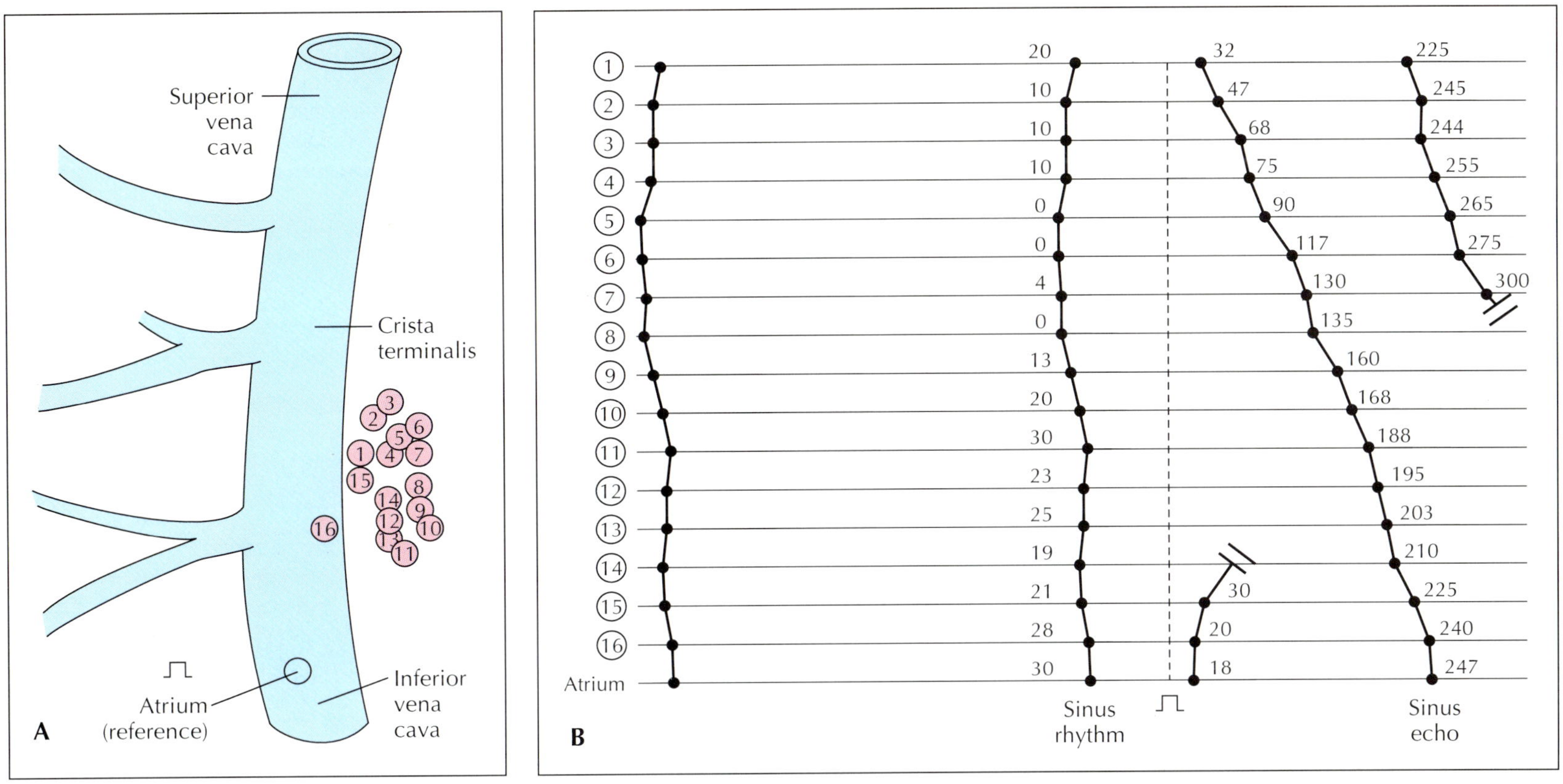

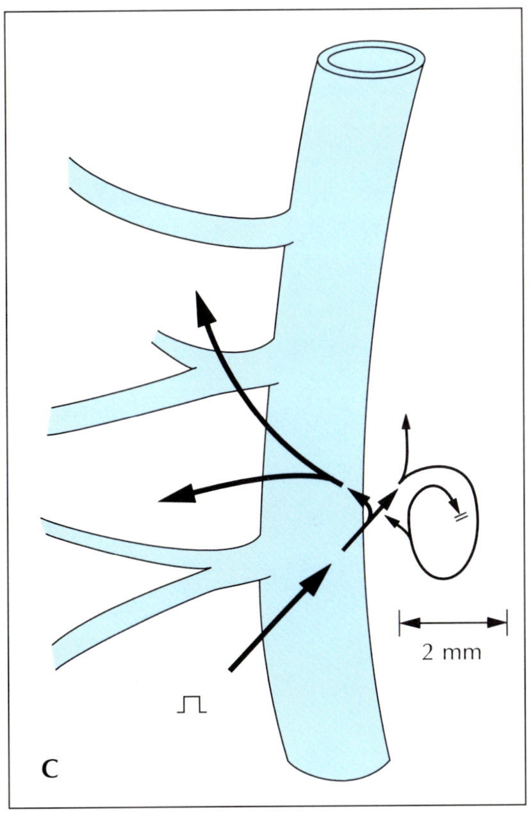

FIGURE 4-12. Sinus node reentry. Although reentry within the sinus node had been postulated for some time, it was not demonstrated until 1979. This illustration is from an experiment in isolated rabbit right atrial tissue. **A,** The locations of 16 intracellular recordings from sinus node cells and one atrial reference (atrium) electrode are shown. **B,** Activation from the 16 sinus node sites and one atrial site. Numbers represent activation times (ms). On the left, a sinus impulse that conducts to the atrium. The second beat results in repeat activation in the sinus region (reentry) and a repetitive response (echo). **C,** A schematic representation of the activation pattern demonstrated in *B*. (*Adapted from* Allessie and Bonke [13]; with permission.)

STEPS IN DIAGNOSING SINUS NODE REENTRY

- The P wave morphology must be identical or almost identical to the P wave morphology during sinus rhythm
- A right-sided accessory atrioventricular connection must be excluded
- The tachycardia must be initiated, reproducibly, by an appropriately timed atrial premature beat
- The return cycle following the premature beat must be short such that A_1–A_3 is significantly shorter than A_1–A_1

FIGURE 4-13. Common criteria for the diagnosis "sinus node reentry." Clinically, sinus node reentry presents as a paroxysmal supraventricular tachycardia with abrupt initiation and termination. Although these criteria are suggestive of sinus node reentry, they represent only indirect evidence. Unfortunately, current technologic limitations prevent the direct recording of sinus node reentry in humans [14].

DIAGNOSING INAPPROPRIATE SINUS TACHYCARDIA

Identifiable causes of sinus tachycardia are excluded

Inappropriate sinus tachycardia is defined as

- P-wave axis and morphology during tachycardia, which resemble baseline ECG
- Lack of initiation or termination of the tachycardia by a critically timed atrial premature stimulus
- Initiation of tachycardia with isoproterenol or aminophylline
- Resetting curve not inconsistent with sinus node reentry (flat or downsloping)

FIGURE 4-14. Inappropriate sinus tachycardia is a diagnosis of exclusion. Therefore, identifiable causes of sinus tachycardia must be excluded. This disorder appears to have a neurocardiac component. As opposed to catecholamine excess, a component of the underlying mechanism appears to be an enhanced responsiveness to sympathetic or catecholamine stimulation by pacemaker cells. ECG—electrocardiogram.

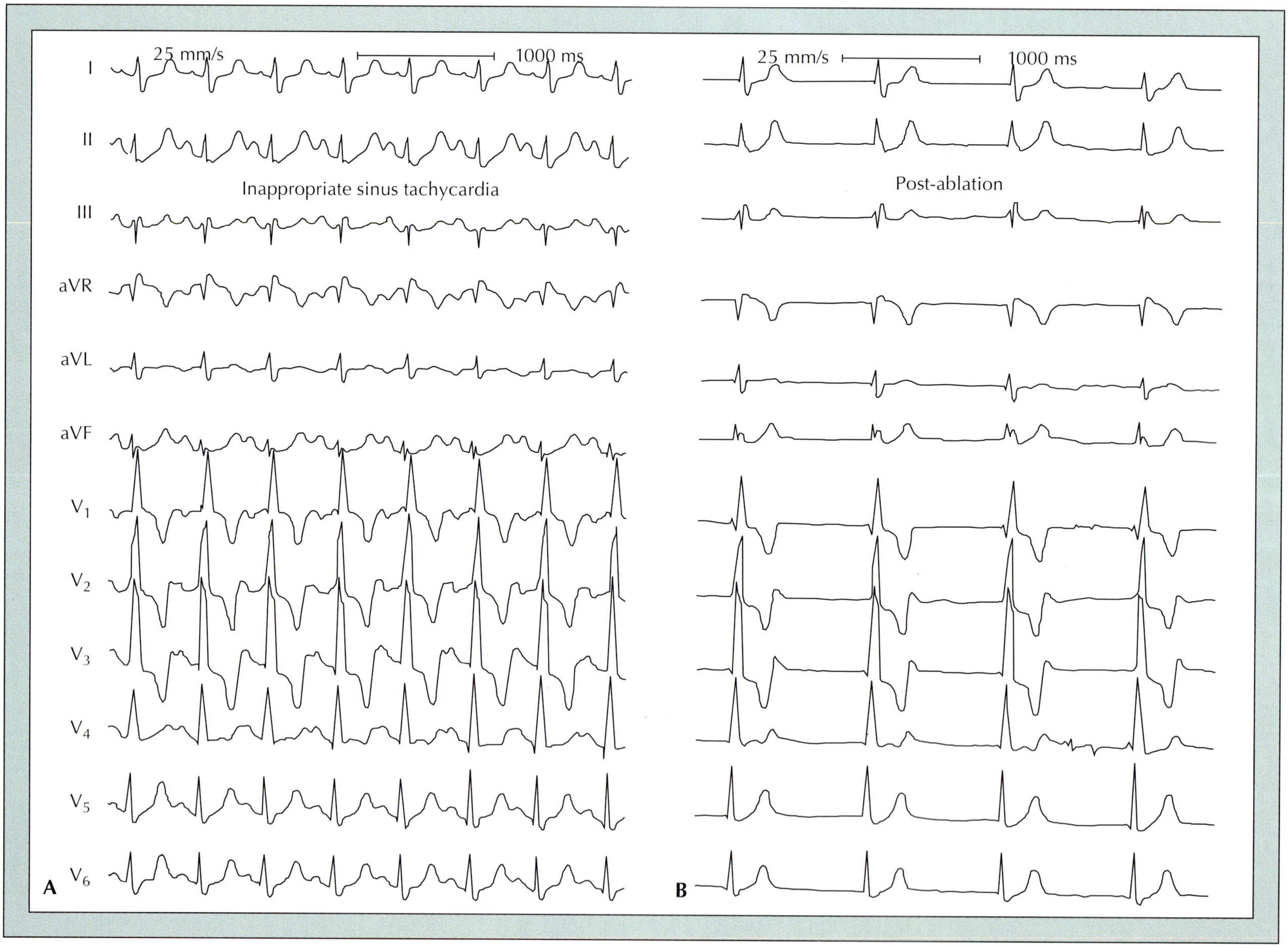

FIGURE 4-15. Inappropriate sinus tachycardia often can be difficult to treat, and in many cases even combination drug therapy fails to control this arrhythmia adequately. Transcatheter sinus node ablation and/or modification using radiofrequency energy appears to be a treatment option in patients with this refractory arrhythmia. **A,** A 12-lead electrocardiogram from a patient with drug-resistant inappropriate sinus tachycardia. **B,** Following sinus node ablation the patient initially had a junctional rhythm, but within a week a stable atrial rhythm that appropriately responded to exercise was evident.

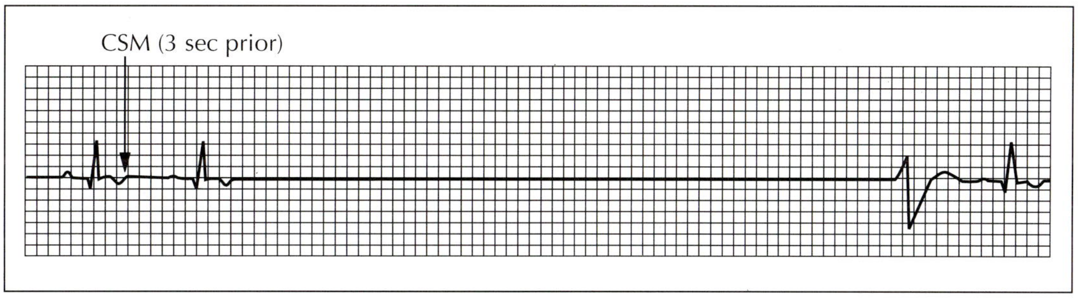

FIGURE 4-16. Carotid sinus hypersensitivity. Increased pressure in or on the carotid body results in a reflex increase in vagal tone. This results in sinus slowing and pauses up to as much as 3 seconds. In some patients an excessive reflex response may result in decreased cerebral blood flow due to 1) a cardiac vagotonic component, resulting in sinus bradycardia, sinus arrest, atrioventricular block, and even asystole; 2) a vasodepressor component, resulting in venous pooling and diminished venous return; or 3) both. In this electrocardiogram from a 65-year-old patient with repeated syncopal episodes, left carotid sinus massage (CSM) results in a prolonged episode of asystole associated with lightheadedness. The pause is followed by a ventricular escape beat.

EVALUATION OF SINUS NODE DYSFUNCTION

TECHNIQUES FOR EVALUATING SINUS NODE DYSFUNCTION

NONINVASIVE

- 12-Lead ECG
- Ambulatory ECG
  - Continuous (24–48 h)
  - Event recorder
- Carotid sinus massage
- Exercise stress testing
- Pharmacologic interventions
  - Atropine
  - Propranolol
  - Isoproterenol

INVASIVE

- Sinus node recovery time
- Sinoatrial conduction time
  - Indirect (Strauss, Narula methods)
  - Direct (sinus node ECG recording)

FIGURE 4-17. Methods for evaluating sinus node dysfunction. The evaluation of sinus node dysfunction may include both noninvasive and invasive techniques, which are discussed in detail in the following figures. ECG—electrocardiogram.

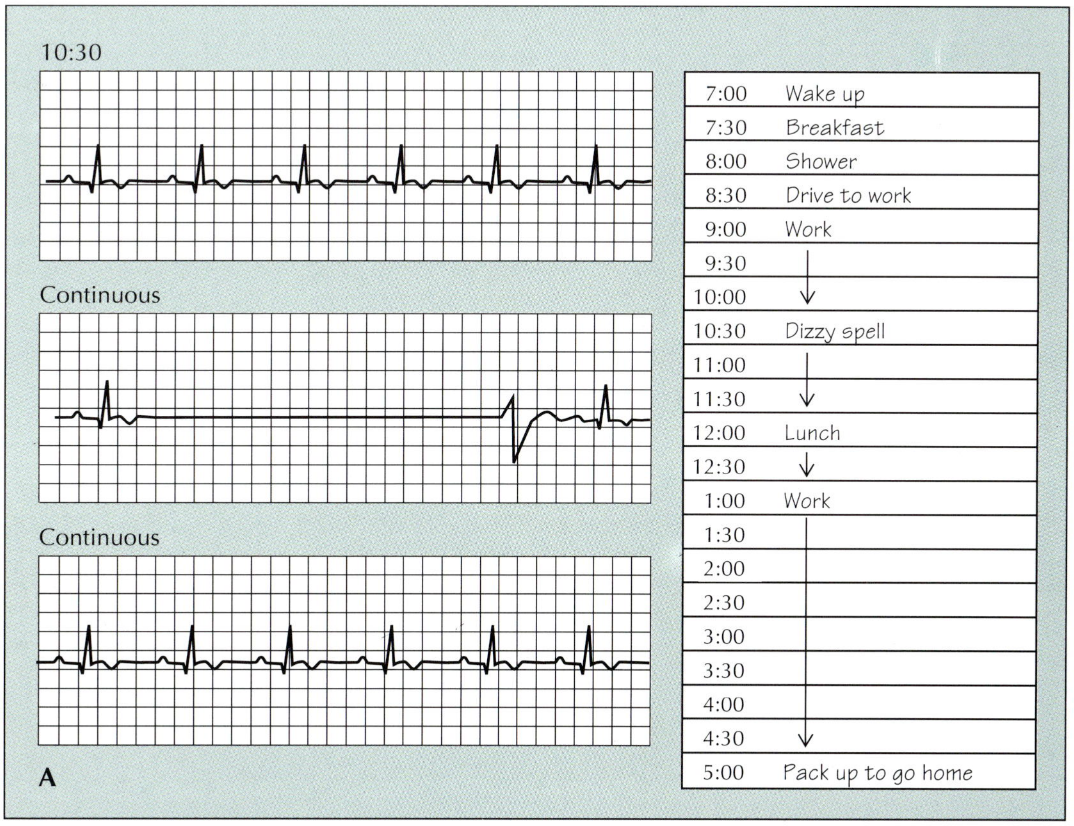

FIGURE 4-18. Ambulatory electrocardiographic (ECG) monitoring, whether continuous (*ie*, Holter) or event-related (event recorder), is the most helpful technique for diagnosing symptomatic sinus node dysfunction. These examples of a continuous portion of the Holter recording and accompanying diaries from two patients show that symptoms may or may not correlate with the arrhythmia. **A**, Ambulatory ECG monitoring can be used to document that symptoms are related to arrhythmic episodes, in which case appropriate therapy can be instituted. (*continued*)

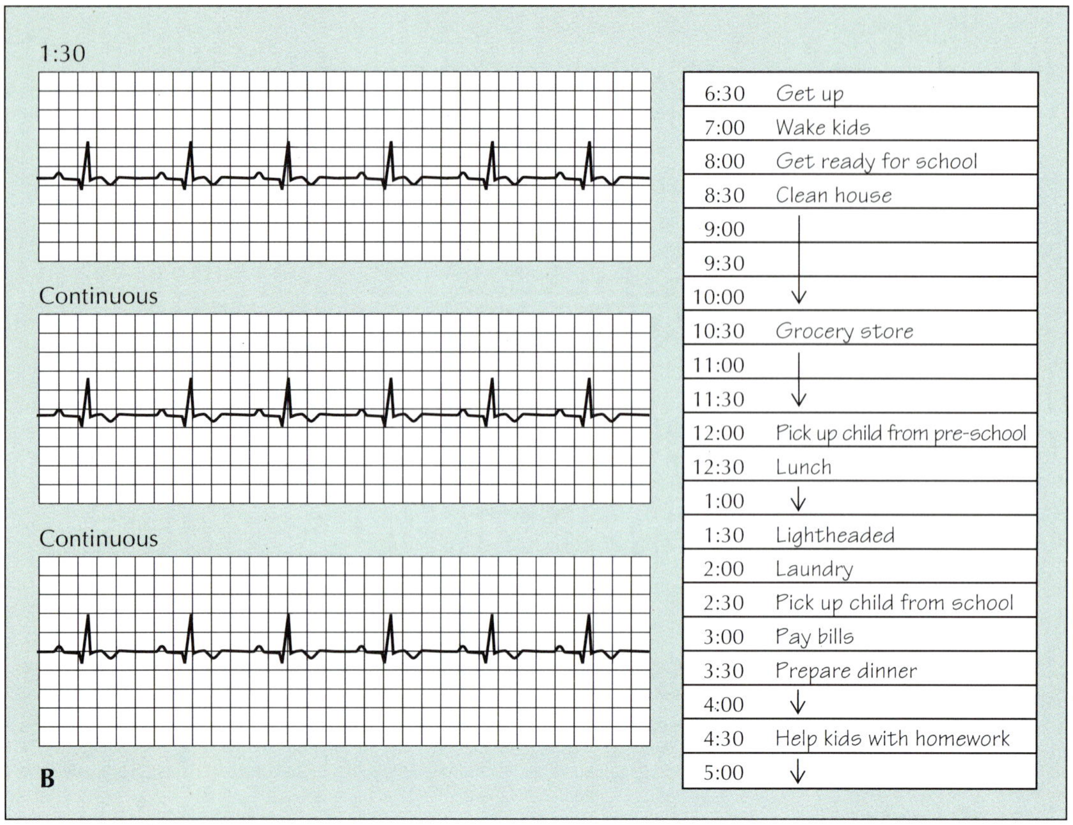

Figure 4-18. (*continued*) **B**, Symptoms may be unrelated to arrhythmia, in which case an alternative diagnosis can be sought.

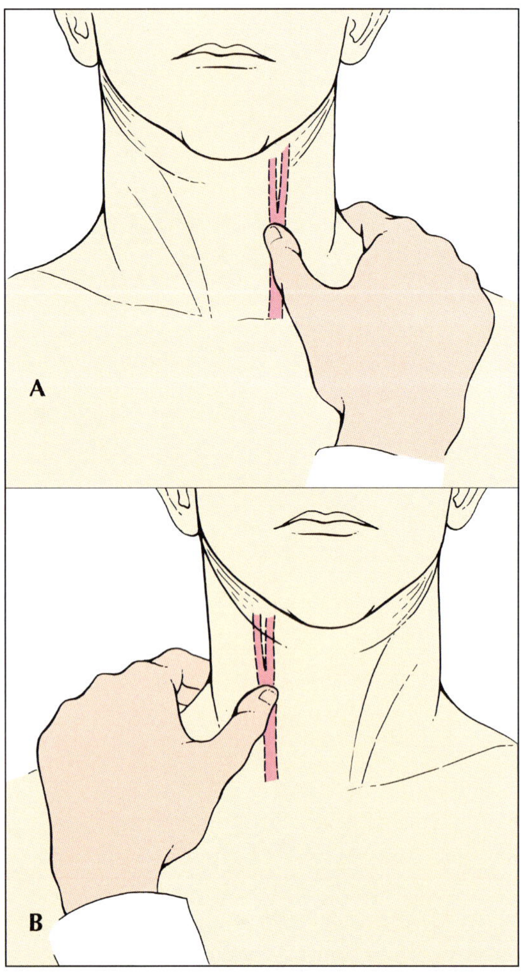

Figure 4-19. The carotid sinus is found in both carotid arteries and is involved in the regulation of blood pressure. Normally, increases in blood pressure stimulate the carotid sinuses, resulting in an increase in parasympathetic tone and a decrease in sympathetic tone. This can lead to heart rate slowing and vasodilatation. Carotid sinus hypersensitivity is a disorder in which external stimulation of the carotid sinus (by a tight collar, for example) results in an exaggerated response, including sinus bradycardia, sinus pauses or asystole, or vasodilation.

In response to carotid sinus massage, patients with greater than a 3-second pause in heart rate that replicates their clinical symptoms are said to have carotid sinus hypersensitivity. An example of left (**A**) and right (**B**) carotid sinus massage is shown. It is important to test both sides individually because only one may show an abnormal response. (*Adapted from* Perloff [15]; with permission.)

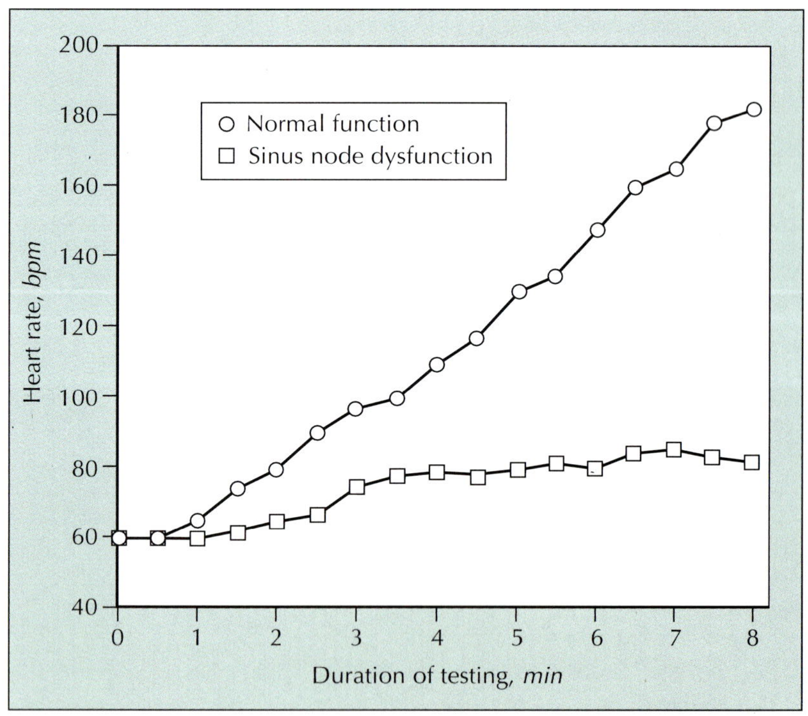

Figure 4-20. Exercise stress testing has proven relatively insensitive in diagnosing sinus node disorder in symptomatic patients. However, exercise stress testing can be used to evaluate chronotropic competence. Patients with chronotropic incompetence often present with dyspnea on exertion or limited exercise tolerance. This figure shows the chronotropic responses in a patient with normal sinus node function and a patient with sinus node dysfunction manifested as chronotropic incompetence.

PHARMACOLOGIC INTERVENTIONS FOR ASSESSMENT OF SINUS NODE DISORDERS

DRUG	STUDY	DOSAGE	RESPONSE: NORMAL	RESPONSE: ABNORMAL	COMMENTS
Atropine	Dauchot and Gravenstein [16]	1.0 mg	>17% decrease in cycle length	<25% increase in sinus rate	Relatively easy, safe; helpful only if positive
	Eckberg *et al.* [17]	0.04 mg/kg	>15% increase in HR		
	Lekieffre *et al.* [18]	0.03 mg/kg	HR >90 bpm		
	Medvedowsky and Barnay [19]	0.04 mg/kg	HR >85 bpm		
Isoproterenol	Mandel *et al.* [20]	3 mg/min	>25% increase in HR	<25% increase in sinus rate	Helpful if positive; may be dangerous in patients with ventricular arrhythmias or CAD
	Strauss *et al.* [21]	Variable	Based on dose required for 20% increase in HR		
Propranolol	Eckberg *et al.* [17]	0.2 mg/kg	≥12% decrease in HR	>20% decrease in sinus rate	May be dangerous in patients with marked bradycardia or decreased LV function
	Vasquez *et al.* [22]	0.1 mg/kg	≥12% decrease in HR		
Atropine + propranolol	Jose and Collison [23]	0.04 mg/kg + 0.2 mg/kg	IHR=118.1-(0.57 × age); SD depends on age	>10% decrease in age-predicted rate	Wide variability
	Tonkin and Heddle [24]	0.03 mg/kg + 0.15 mg/kg	IHR=118.1-(0.57 × age); SD depends on age		

FIGURE 4-21. Pharmacologic interventions for the assessment of sinus node disorders. A variety of pharmacologic interventions can be used to assess sinus node competence. Included in this table are agents that either enhance or block autonomic activity in the heart. Although abnormal responses may suggest sinus node dysfunction, these interventions are neither sensitive nor specific. CAD—coronary artery disease; HR—heart rate; IHR—intrinsic heart rate; LV—left ventricular; SD—standard deviation [25,26,26a].

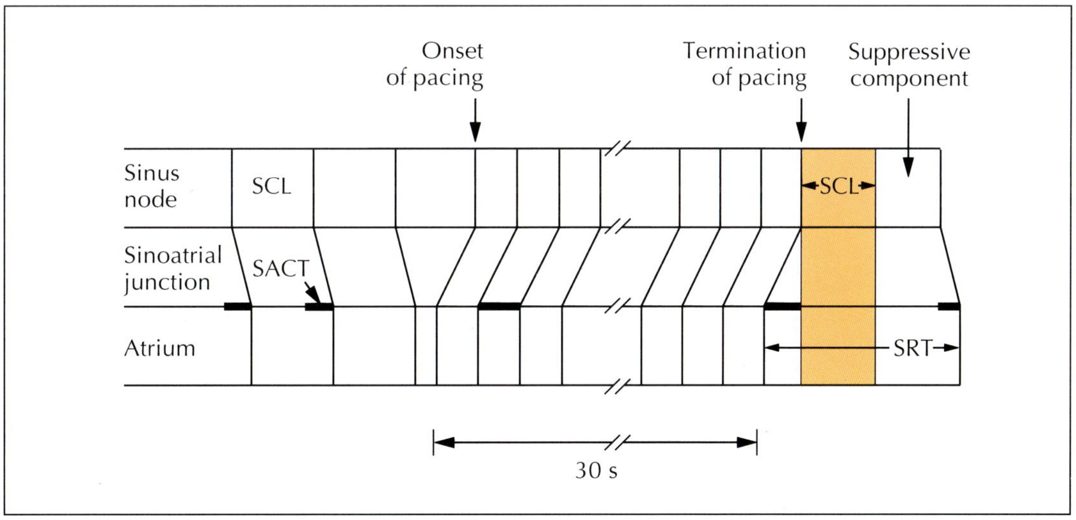

FIGURE 4-22. Sinus node recovery time (SRT). By pacing the atrium at rates progressively faster than the sinus rate (atrial decremental pacing), the SRT can be determined. Rapid stimulation of the sinus node may suppress intrinsic automaticity, resulting in a delay in the post-pacing response. This ladder diagram depicts events during decremental atrial pacing to assess sinus recovery time. At the termination of pacing, the SRT, as determined from recordings in the atria, actually consists of three elements: retrograde atriosinus conduction, the intranodal cycle length (which is an interval equal to the basic sinus cycle length [SCL] plus an interval resulting from overdrive suppression), and antegrade sinoatrial conduction. The length of sinoatrial conduction time (SACT) is emphasized periodically with a thickening of the rung between the sinoatrial junction and the atrium. (*Adapted from* Reiffel [27]; with permission.)

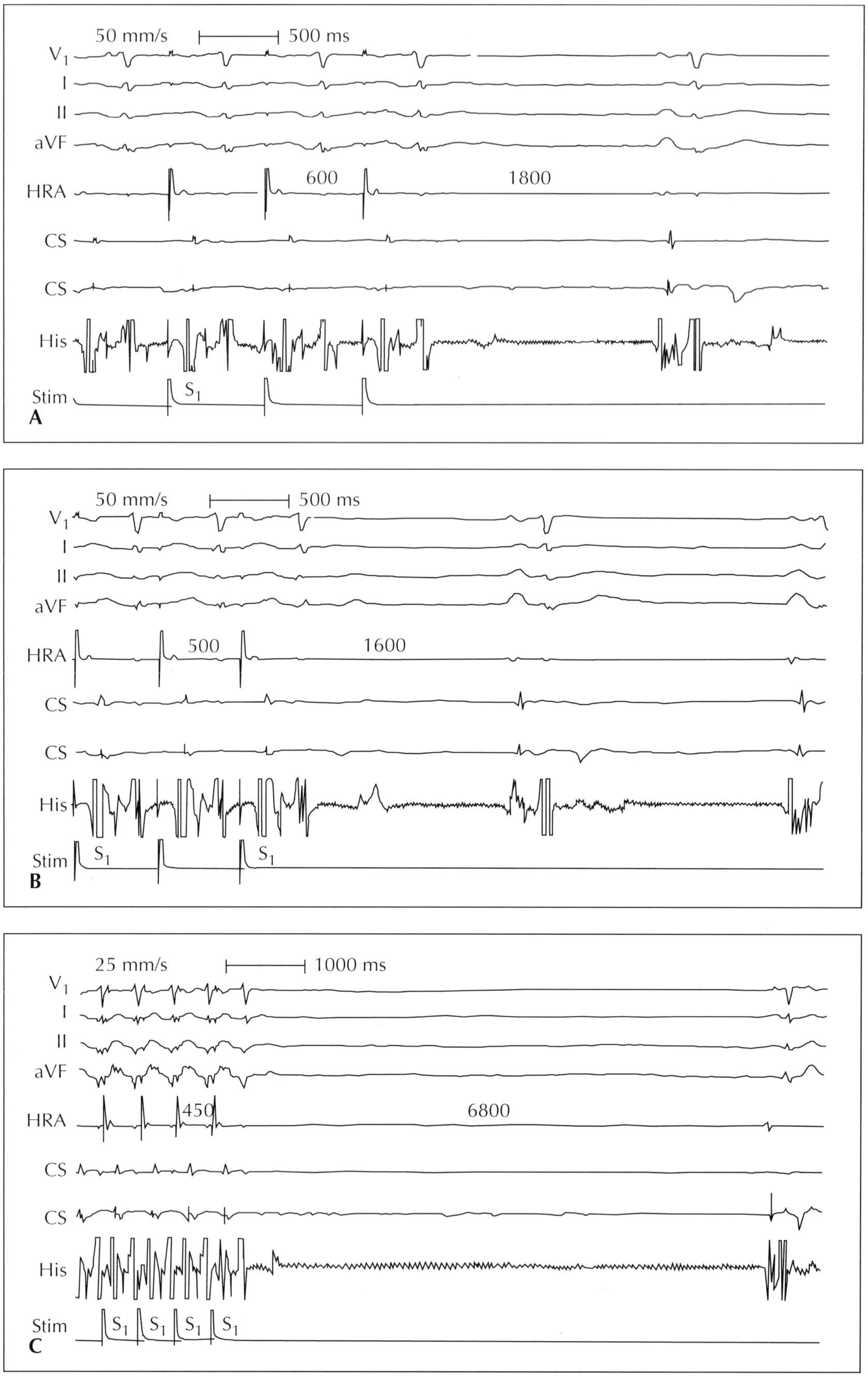

FIGURE 4-23. Sinus node recovery time (SRT). As the rate of atrial pacing increases, the SRT will be prolonged due to increasing overdrive suppression and potentially an increased sinoatrial conduction time. At the paced atrial rate whereby sinus node entrance block occurs, the SRT will shorten. Secondary pauses (pauses following the first return sinus beat) also may occur following atrial overdrive pacing and are an indication of sinus node dysfunction. **A** through **D,** These examples show the SRT associated with four paced rates. The maximum SRT occurs with atrial pacing at a cycle length of 450 ms (C). (*continued*)

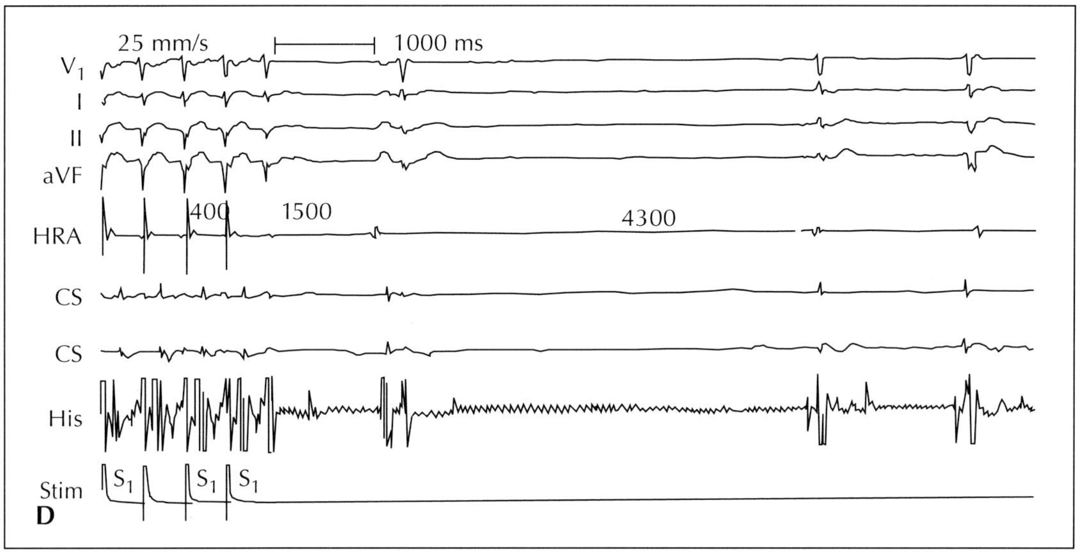

FIGURE 4-23. (*continued*) In addition, an example of a secondary pause can be seen following atrial pacing at a cycle length of 400 ms (*D*). Surface leads V_1, I, II, and aVF and intracardiac recordings from the high right atrium (HRA) and coronary sinus (CS) are shown.

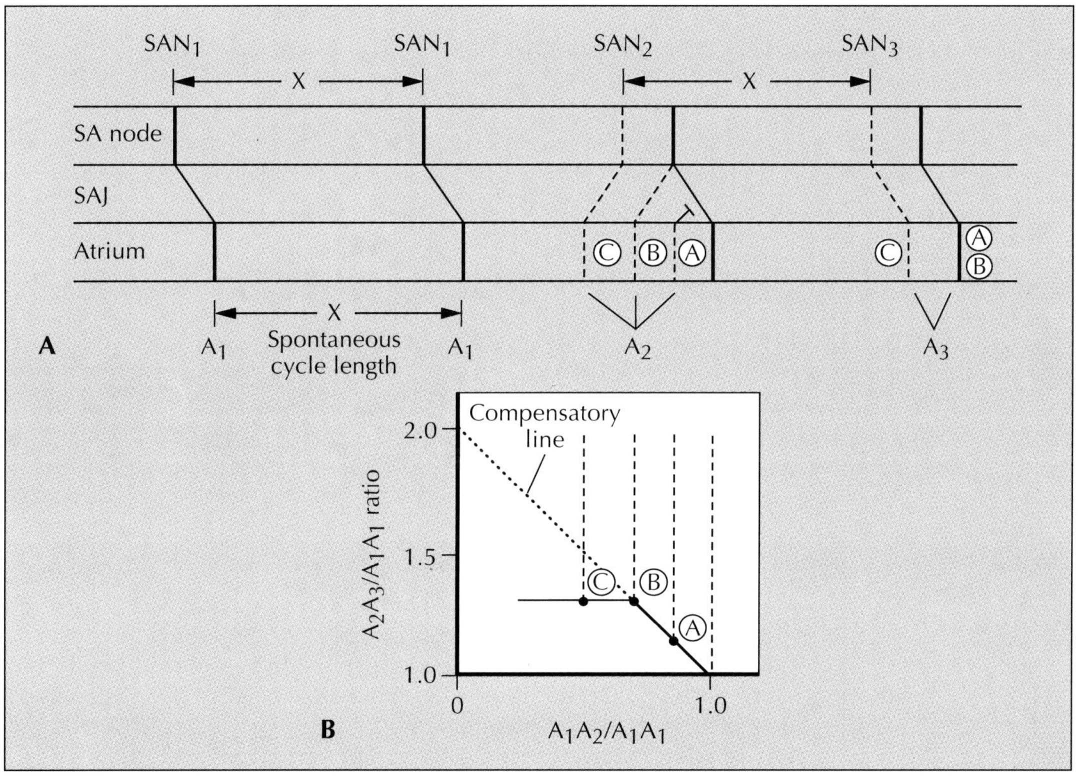

FIGURE 4-24. Sinoatrial conduction time (SACT): atrial extrastimulus method [28]. **A,** Derivation of antegrade sinoatrial conduction time (SACT A + R). A_1A_1 is spontaneous cycle length; A_2 is atrial premature depolarization (APD), and A_2A_3 is the atrial return cycle. This technique is based on the assumption that $SAN_1SAN_1 = A_1A_1 = SAN_2SAN_3$. Therefore, the difference between A_2A_3 and A_1A_1 is the antegrade and retrograde SACT (between atrium and SAN and SAN and atrium). **B,** This graph shows A_2A_3/A_1A_1 plotted against A_1A_2/A_1A_1. A late APD (point A) is followed by a compensatory response, where $A_1A_3 = 2A_11A_1$, which falls on the compensatory line. An early APD (point C) is followed by a less-than-compensatory response, which falls on the plateau below the compensatory line. Point B marks the transition between compensatory and less-than-compensatory responses. SAJ —sinoatrial junction; SAN—sinoatrial node. (*Adapted from* Strauss and coworkers [28]; with permission.)

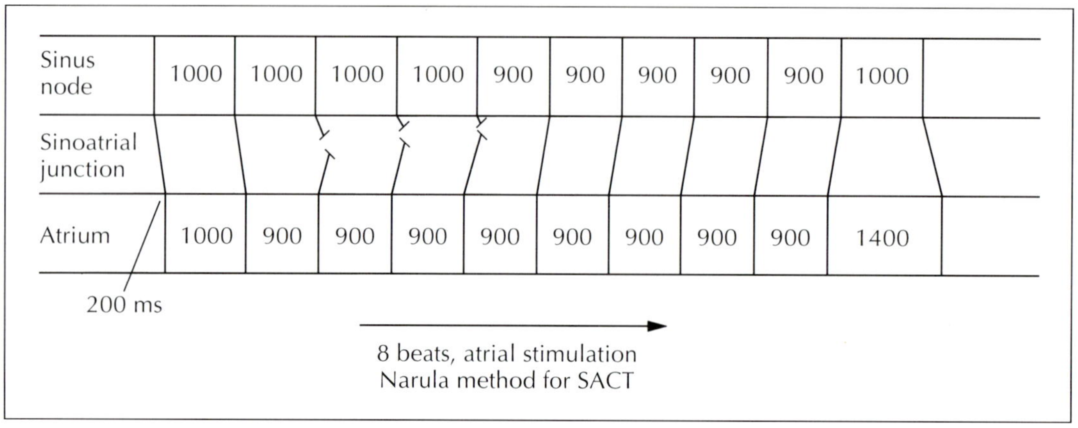

FIGURE 4-25. Sinoatrial conduction time (SACT): constant atrial pacing method. In 1978, Narula *et al.* [29] addressed the problem of the interference of sinus arrhythmia with SACT estimation by suggesting a new approach to the calculation of SACT: slow atrial pacing. They reasoned that short trains (eight beats) of slow atrial pacing (at rates only 10 bpm above the shortest sinus cycle length) would overcome sinus arrhythmia, stabilize the sinus cycle length, and probably not significantly suppress sinus node automaticity. This ladder diagram depicts events during the Narula method for assessing SACT. Atrial pacing is being performed at a cycle length of 900 ms, and unidirectional SACT is assumed to be 200 ms (which is prolonged). (*Adapted from* Reiffel [27]; with permission.)

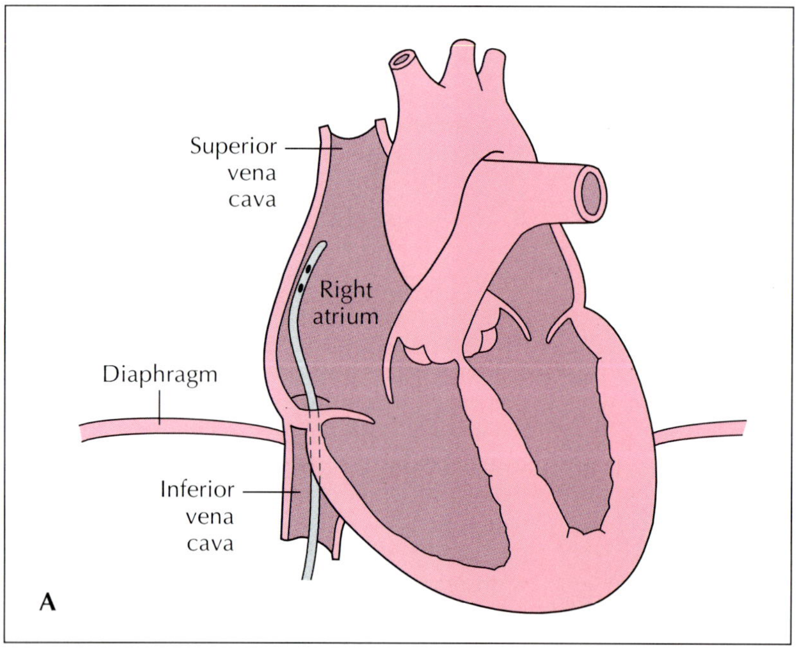

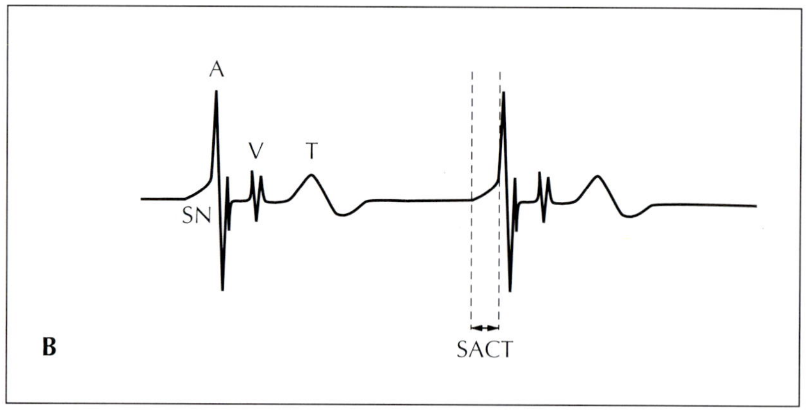

FIGURE 4-26. The sinus node electrocardiogram (SNE) can be directly recorded in humans, so an accurate measure of sinoatrial conduction time (SACT) therefore can be made [30]. **A,** Catheter location for recording the SNE. The SNE can be recorded during a diagnostic electrophysiologic study. Shown here is the position of an electrode catheter, which is introduced via a femoral vein to record an SNE. The catheter is advanced to the superior vena cava (at which point electrical signals will disappear). The catheter is then slowly withdrawn along the crista terminalis until the SNE is seen. **B,** A schematic representation of an SNE used to measure the SACT directly. On the SNE, atrial (A) and ventricular (V) depolarization, as well as the T wave (T) and sinus node (SN) potential are identified. In the second beat the SACT is defined. (*Adapted from* Reiffel and coworkers [30]; with permission.)

SENSITIVITY AND SPECIFICITY OF INVASIVE TESTS FOR SINUS NODE DYSFUNCTION

	SENSITIVITY, *n/TOTAL (%)*		SPECIFICITY, *n/TOTAL (%)*	
STUDY	CSRT/SRT	SACT	CSRT/SRT	SACT
Reiffel *et al.* [31]	12/23 (56)	7/13 (54)	22/25 (88)	22/25 (88)
Gupta *et al.* [32]	3/17 (18)	NA	15/15 (100)	NA
Pop and Fleischmann [33]	46/67 (69)	NA	108/110 (98)	NA
Seipel *et al.* [34]	NA	36/57 (63)	NA	78/136 (57)
Bethge *et al.* [35]	9/35 (26)	NA	14/16 (87)	NA
Szatmary *et al.* [36]	2/4 (50)	3/4 (75)	5/5 (100)	5/5 (100)
Benditt *et al.* [37]	11/39 (28)	NA	20/44 (45)	NA
Total	84/185 (45)	46/74 (62)	204/215 (95)	105/166 (63)

FIGURE 4-27. Sensitivity and specificity of invasive tests for sinus node dysfunction. Although evaluation of corrected or uncorrected sinus node recovery time (CSRT and SRT) and sinoatrial conduction time (SACT) yields a reasonable specificity, the sensitivity is poor. Therefore, these tests are useful only in patients in whom sinus node dysfunction is highly suspected based on clinical grounds but electrocardiographic documentation is not available. Invasive electrophysiologic study also may be helpful in diagnosing other causes of symptoms in patients suspected of having sinus node dysfunction, such as atrioventricular block, supraventricular arrhythmias, and ventricular arrhythmias. Criteria for an abnormal test are CSRT greater than 525 ms, SRT greater than 1600 ms, and SACT greater than 206 ms. NA—not available. (*Adapted from* Benditt and coworkers [25] and Talano and coworkers [26]; with permission.)

THERAPEUTIC OPTIONS FOR SINUS NODE DISORDERS

DIAGNOSIS	THERAPY
Symptomatic sinus node dysfunction (bradycardia, chronotropic incompetence, sinus arrest, sinoatrial exit block)	AAIR pacing when no evidence of AV conduction disease DDDR pacing with evidence of AV conduction disease
Tachy-brady syndrome	Type I or III antiarrhythmics to treat atrial arrhythmias β-Blockers, calcium-channel blockers, and/or digoxin to control ventricular response VVI or DDD pacing for bradycardic episodes (drug used to treat atrial arrhythmia may worsen bradyarrhythmias and precipitate the need for cardiac pacing) AV junction ablation with DDDR or VVIR pacing in patients whose ventricular response is difficult to control
Sinus node reentry	β-Blockers, calcium-channel blockers Type I and III antiarrhythmics Catheter ablation (sinus node modification)
Inappropriate sinus tachycardia	β-Blockers, calcium-channel blockers Catheter ablation (sinus node ablation/modification)
Carotid sinus hypersensitivity	Pindolol, Norpace Cardiac pacing Avoidance of tight collars

FIGURE 4-28. Therapeutic options for sinus node disorders. Pacing nodes are standard. AAIR—rate-responsive atrial pacing; AV—atrioventricular; DDD—dual chamber pacing; DDDR—rate-responsive dual chamber pacing; VVI—ventricular pacing; VVIR—rate-responsive ventricular pacing.

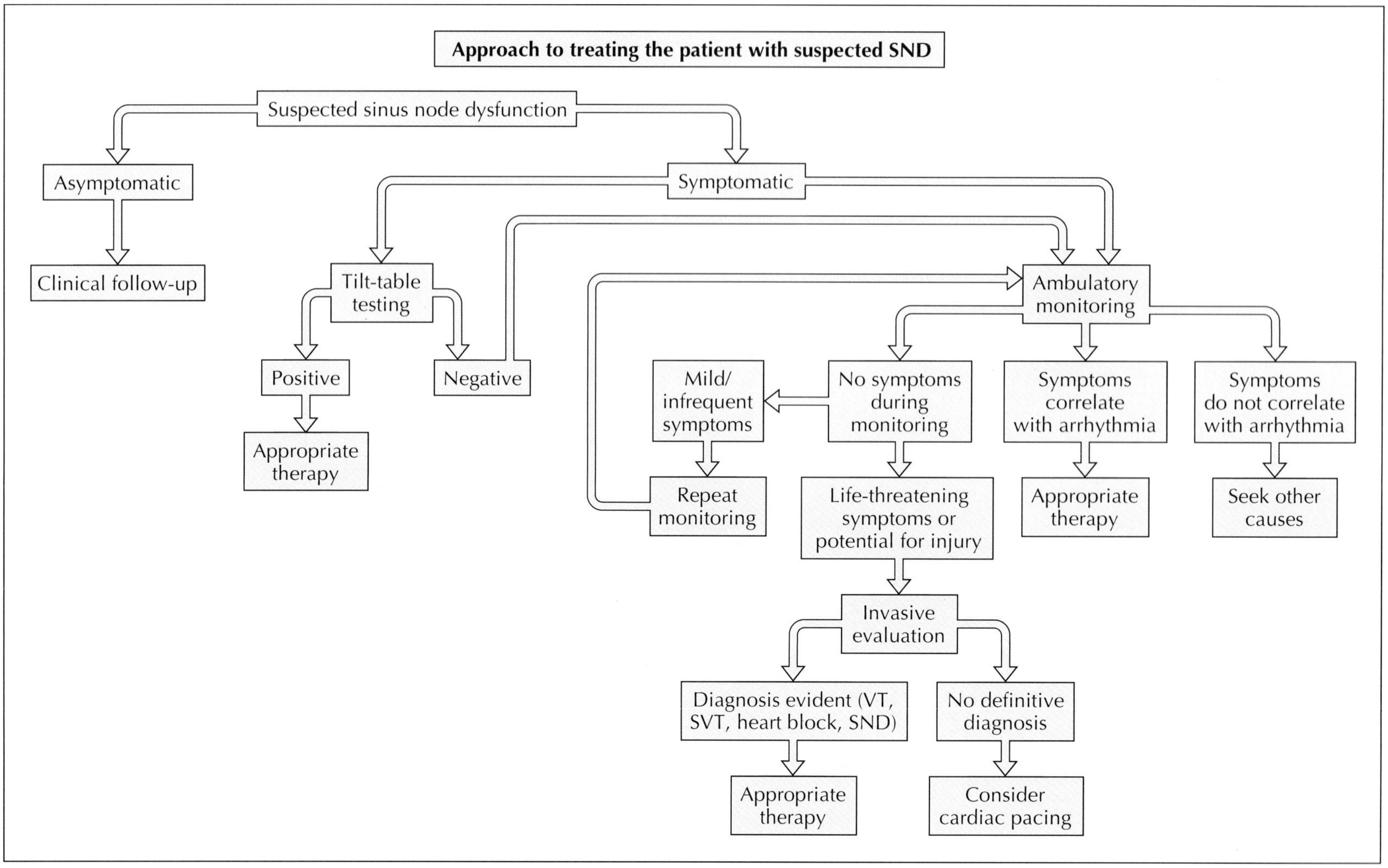

FIGURE 4-29. The approach to diagnosing and treating sinus node dysfunction (SND). In patients with suspected SND, the correlation with symptoms is crucial. The presence of bradycardia alone is not an indication for treatment. In symptomatic patients, a careful history may reveal diagnostic clues. In patients with syncope or syncope associated with standing, a tilt-table test may be in order. In patients with frequent symptoms, 24-hour monitoring is often diagnostic. When symptoms are less frequent, an event-type recorder may be more useful. If symptoms do not correlate with cardiac arrhythmias, other causes (*ie*, neurologic) should be sought. If no symptoms occur during monitoring but the patient has recurrent syncope or has been injured during episodes, a more invasive evaluation is indicated. SVT—supraventricular tachycardia; VT—ventricular tachycardia. (*Adapted from* Gomes [38]; with permission.)

REFERENCES

1. Keith A, Flack M: The form and nature of the muscular connections between the primary divisions of the vertebrate heart. *J Anat Physiol* 1907, 41:172–189.
2. Lewis T: The pacemaker of the mammalian heart, as ascertained by electrocardiographic curves. *J Physiol* 1910–1911, 41:9–10.
3. Short DS: The syndrome of alternating bradycardia and tachycardia. *Br Heart J* 1954, 16:208–214.
4. Ferrer MI: The sick sinus syndrome in atrial disease. *JAMA* 1968, 206:645–646.
5. Kulbertus HE, de Leval-Rutten F, Demoulin JC: Sino-atrial disease: a report on 13 cases. *J Electrocardiol* 1973, 6:303–312.
6. Grossman WG, ed: *Cardiac Catheterization and Angiography*. Philadelphia: Lea & Febiger; 1991.
7. Anderson RH, Yen HS, Becker AE, *et al*.: The development of the sinoatrial node. In *The Sinus Node: Structure, Function and Clinical Relevance*. Edited by Bonke FIM. The Hague: Martinus Nijhoff; 1978:166–182.
8. Janse MJ, Tranum-Jensen J, Kleber AG, *et al*.: Techniques and problems correlating cellular electrophysiology and morphology in cardiac nodal tissues. In *The Sinus Node: Structure, Function and Clinical Relevance*. Edited by Bonke FIM. The Hague: Martinus Nijhoff; 1978:183–194.
9. Masson-Pevet M, Bleeker WK, Mackaay AJC, *et al*.: Ultrastructural and functional aspects of the rabbit sinoatrial node. In *The Sinus Node: Structure, Function and Clinical Relevance*. Edited by Bonke FIM. The Hague: Martinus Nijhoff; 1978:195–211.
10. Bouman LN, Jongsma HJ: Structure and function of the sino-atrial node: a review. *Eur Heart J* 1986, 7:94–104.
11. Talano, JV. Euler D, Randall WC, *et al*.: Sinus node dysfunction: an overview with emphasis on autonomic and pharmacologic considerations. *Am J Med* 1978, 64:773—781.
12. Evans T: *Electrocardiographic Test Set: Basic Electrocardiography and Cardiac Arrhythmias*, ed 2. Copyright © 1993 by Thomas Evans.

13. Allessie MA, Bonke FIM: Direct demonstration of sinus node reentry in the rabbit heart. *Circ Res* 1979, 44:557–568.

14. Bonke FIM, Kirchof CJH, Allessie MA: Sinus node reentry. In *Cardiac Electrophysiology: From Cell to Bedside*. Edited by Zipes DP, Jalife J. Philadelphia: W.B. Saunders Co; 1990.

15. Perloff JK: Physical examination of the heart. *Circulation*, ed 2. Philadelphia: W.B. Saunders Co; 1990.

16. Duchot P, Gravenstein JS: Effects of atropine on the electrocardiogram in different age groups. *Clin Pharmacol Ther* 1971, 12:274–280.

17. Eckberg DL, Drabinsky M, Braunwald E: Defective cardiac parasympathetic control in patients with heart disease. *N Engl J Med* 1971, 285:877–883.

18. Lekieffre J, Libersa C, Caron J, *et al.*: Electrocardiographic aspects of sinus node dysfunction: use of the Holter electrocardiographic recording. In *Cardiac Arrhythmias: From Diagnosis to Therapy*. Edited by Levy S, Scheinman MM. Mount Kisco, NY: Futura; 1984:73–86.

19. Medvedowsky J-L, Barnay C: Electrophysiologic study of sinus node function: role of the autonomic nervous system: indications for pacing. In *Cardiac Arrhythmias: From Diagnosis to Therapy*. Edited by Levy S, Scheinman MM. Mount Kisco, NY: Futura; 1984:87–105.

20. Mandel WJ, Laks MM, Obayashi K: Sinus node function: evaluation in patients with and without sinus node disease. *Arch Intern Med* 1975, 135:388–394.

21. Strauss HC, Bigger JT Jr, Saroff AL, *et al.*: Electrophysiologic evaluation of sinus node function in patients with sinus node dysfunction. *Circulation* 1976, 53:763–767.

22. Vasquez M, Chuquimia R, Shantha N, *et al.*: Clinical electrophysiological effects of propranolol on normal sinus node function. *Br Heart J* 1979, 41:709–715.

23. Jose AD, Collison D: The normal range and the determinants of the intrinsic heart rate in man. *Cardiovasc Res* 1970, 4:160–166.

24. Tonkin AM, Heddle WF: Electrophysiological testing of sinus node function. *PACE Pacing Clin Electrophysiol* 1984, 7:735–748.

25. Benditt DG, Milstein S, Goldstein M, *et al.*: Sinus node dysfunction: pathophysiology, clinical features, evaluation and treatment. In *Cardiac Electrophysiology: From Cell to Bedside*. Edited by Zipes DP, Jalife J. Philadelphia, W.B. Saunders Co; 1990:708–734.

26. Talano JV, Euler D, Randall WC, *et al.*: Sinus node function: an overview with emphasis on autonomic and pharmacologic consideration. *Am J Med* 1978, 64:773–781.

26a. Desai JM, Scheinman MM, Strauss HC, *et al.*: Electrophysiologic effects of combined autonomic blockade in patients with sinus node disease. *Circulation* 1981, 63(4):953–960.

27. Reiffel JA: Electrophysiologic evaluation of sinus node function. *Clin Cardiol* 1986, 4:401–416.

28. Strauss HC, Scheinman MM, LaBarre A, *et al.*: Programmed atrial stimulation and rapid atrial pacing in patients with sinus pauses and sinoatrial exit block. In *The Sinus Node*. Edited by Bonke FIM. The Hague: Martinus Nijhoff; 1978:56–64.

29. Narula OS, Somet P, Javler R: Significance of the sinus node recovery time. *Circulation* 1972, 45:140–158

30. Reiffel JA, Gang E, Gliklich J, *et al.*: The human sinus node electrogram: a transvenous catheter technique and a comparison of directly measured and indirectly estimated sinoatrial conduction time in adults. *Circulation* 1980, 62:3124–3134.

31. Reiffel JA, Ferrick K, Zimmerman J, *et al.*: Electrophysiologic studies of the sinus node and atria. In *Cardiovascular Clinics*. Edited by Brest AN. Philadelphia: F.A. Davis; 1985:37–59.

32. Gupta PK, Lichstein E, Chadda KD, *et al.*: Appraisal of sinus nodal recovery time in patients with sick sinus syndrome. *Am J Cardiol* 1974, 34:265–270.

33. Pop T, Fleischmann D: Measurement of sinus node recovery time after atrial pacing. In *The Sinus Node: Structure, Function and Clinical Relevance*. Edited by Bonke FIM. The Hague: Martinus Nijhoff; 1978:23–35.

34. Seipal L, Breithardt G, Leunder C: Programmed atrial stimulation used for the calculation of sinoatrial conduction time (SACT) in man. In *The Sinus Node: Structure, Function and Clinical Relevance*. Edited by Bonke FIM. The Hague: Martinus Nijhoff; 1978:36–45.

35. Bethge C, Gebhardt-Seehausen U, Mullges W: The human sinus nodal electrogram: techniques and clinical results of intra-atrial recordings in patients with and without sick sinus syndrome. *Am Heart J* 1986, 112:1074–1082.

36. Szatmary L, Medvedowsky J-L, Barnay C, *et al.*: Electrophysiological classification of normal and pathological sinus node function. *Acta Med Acad Sci Hung* 1982, 39:47–61.

37. Benditt DG, Strauss HC, Scheinman MM, *et al.*: Analysis of secondary pauses following termination of rapid atrial pacing in man. *Circulation* 1976, 54:436–441.

38. Gomes JA: The sick sinus syndrome and evaluation of the patient with sinus node disorders. In *Cardiology*. Edited by Parmley W, Chatterjee K. Philadelphia: J.B. Lippincott Co; 1988:1–16.

Supraventricular Tachycardia

5

CHAPTER

Harlan R. Grogin

Advances in catheter ablative techniques have emphasized the importance of discerning the mechanism of supraventricular rhythms. It is no longer adequate to identify a narrow complex tachycardia as a "paroxysmal supraventricular tachycardia." Classifying the tachycardia by its mechanisms and origin allows the clinician to choose proper antiarrhythmic drug therapy or decide whether catheter ablation is appropriate. In this chapter, we will review the different types of supraventricular tachycardia and correlate them with their 12-lead electrocardiographic appearances and electrophysiologic mechanisms.

Atrioventricular nodal reentry, atrioventricular reciprocating tachycardia using an accessory atrioventricular connection, atrial flutter, and certain atrial tachycardias are due to reentry. In reentrant rhythms, there is a common circuit that has the following characteristics: (1) at least two pathways with different conduction properties, (2) unidirectional block in one of the pathways, and (3) return of retrograde conduction in the blocked pathway after it is no longer refractory. Arrythmias, using a reentrant mechanism, are reliably induced in the laboratory. Rhythms due to abnormal automaticity are less reliably induced in the electrophysiology laboratory. Atrial tachycardias due to abnormal automaticity may be difficult to induce or characterize in the laboratory either with programmed extrastimulation or with the infusion of isoproterenol. Arrhythmias due to triggered activity resulting from early or delayed after-depolarizations are more reliably induced with pacing than arrhythmias due to abnormal automaticity, but their significance in supraventricular arrhythmias remains unclear.

The role of electrophysiologic studies in supraventricular rhythms is to (1) identify the tachycardia and mechanism, (2) assess the efficacy of drugs, if appropriate, and (3) assess the role of catheter ablation. While a 12-lead electrocardiogram may be ambiguous as to the origin of the tachycardia, electrophysiologic studies give an exact diagnosis. The initiation and termination of the tachycardia, the effect of critically timed premature atrial or ventricular complexes on the tachycardia, the effect of bundle branch block on the tachycardia cycle length, and the response to adenosine all contribute to the characterization of the mechanism.

The role of Mahaim conduction in supraventricular tachycardia was elucidated in 1937 when Mahaim [1] described tracts connecting the atrioventricular (AV) node and ventricular myocardium as well as discrete connections from the fascicles to the ventricles. Mahaim conduction is characterized by gradual increases in the AV interval at the same time as the development of a left bundle branch block and a shortening of the His-ventricular (HV) interval in response to atrial overdrive pacing. In addition, the right bundle branch potential is seen to precede the His deflection during preexcited complexes.

Preexcited tachycardia is manifested by antegrade conduction over the pathway to the right bundle branch with retrograde activation of the His bundle, the AV node, and the atrium. Early studies were interpreted as showing a nodoventricular origin of these pathways with insertion into either the right bundle branch or the right ventricle. More recently, excellent evidence on the basis of electrophysiologic studies, surgery, and catheter ablation has definitely established that right atriofascicular fibers crossing the tricuspid annulus serve as the basis for typical Mahaim conduction in most, if not all, of these patients [2–5]. However, there is also evidence, using radiofrequency catheter techniques, for the existence of septal (probable nodoventricular) bypass tracts with Mahaim physiology [6].

ECG Localization

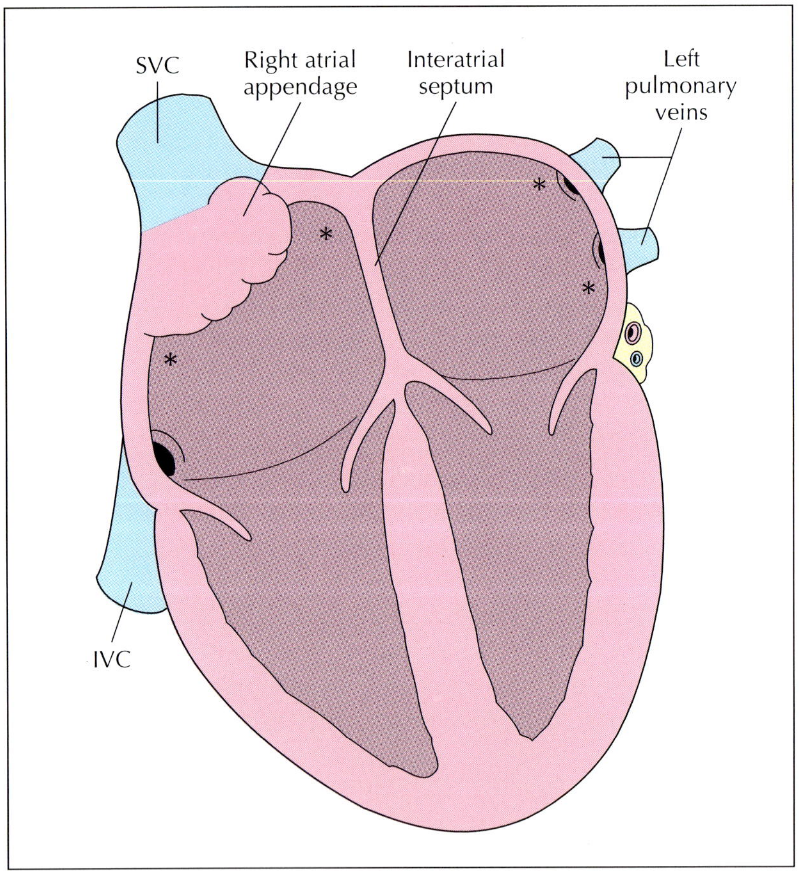

Figure 5-1. Location of atrial tachycardias. Whether from a microreentrant or automatic mechanism, atrial tachycardias may come from a variety of locations in either the right or left atrium (*asterisks*). The most common locations are around the crista terminalis, right atrial appendage, near the pulmonary veins entering into the left atrium, and, in patients with congenital heart disease, along atrial septal defect suture lines or surgical scar lines. SVC—superior vena cava; IVC—inferior vena cava.

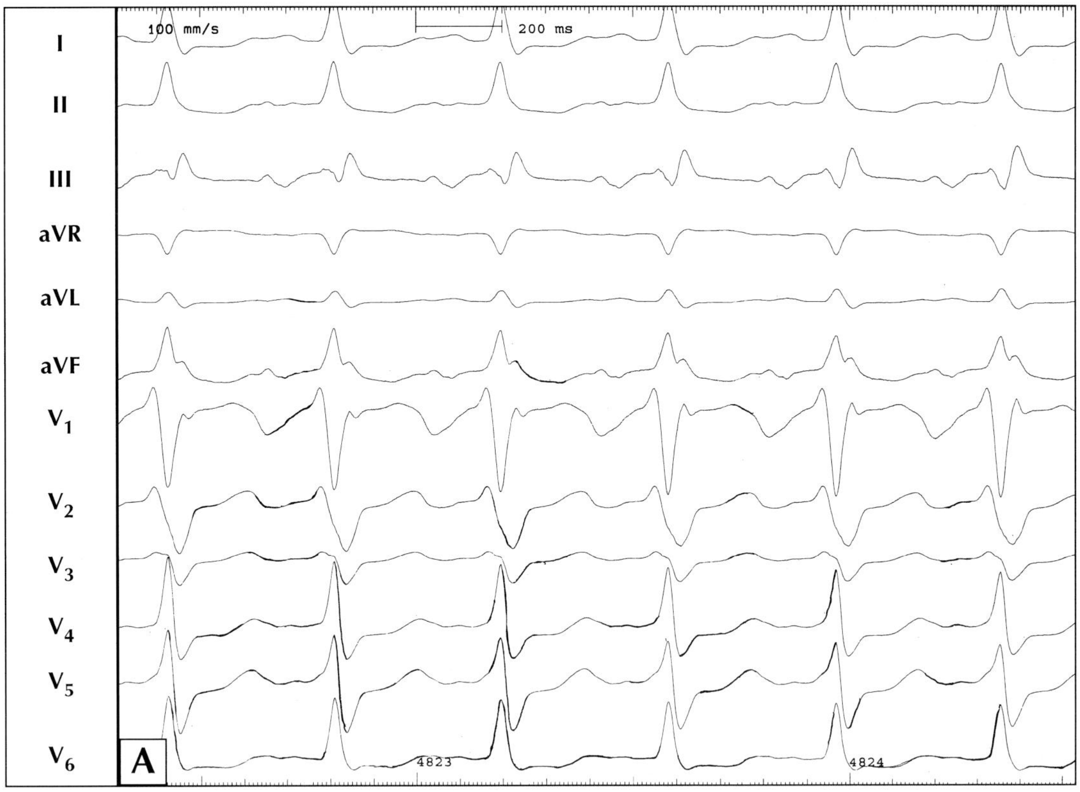

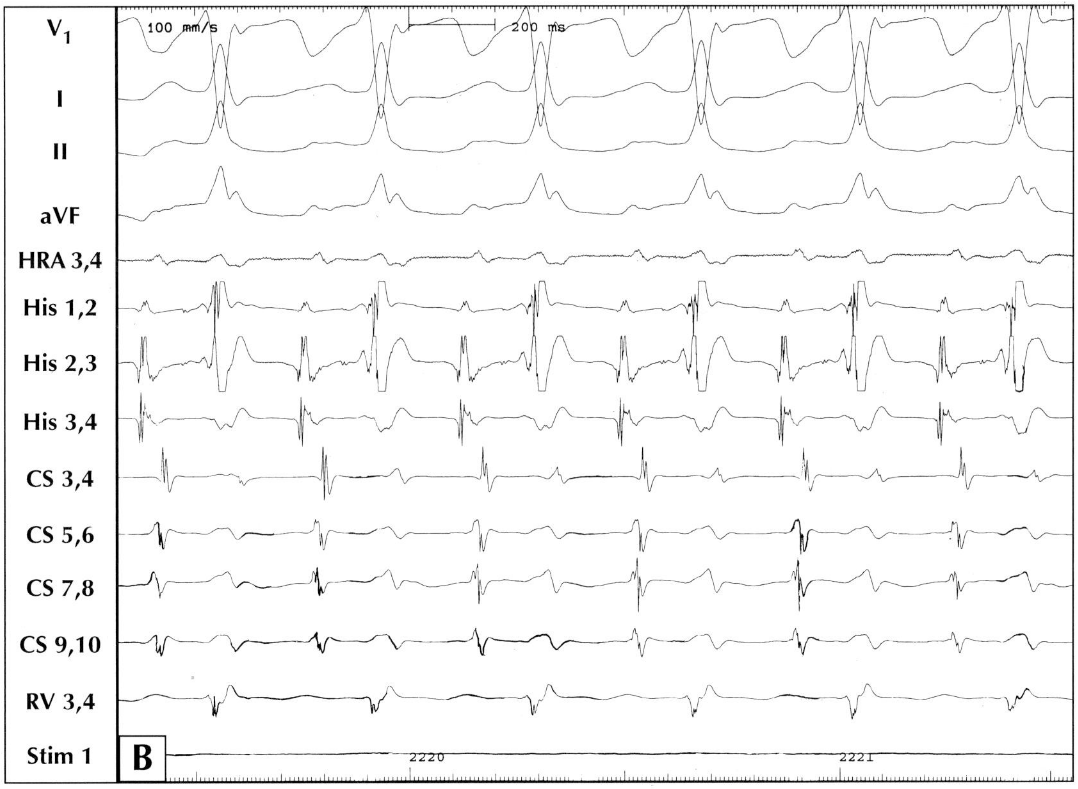

FIGURE 5-2. Atrial tachycardia. **A**, 12-lead electrocardiogram (ECG) of an atrial tachycardia. This ECG shows a narrow complex tachycardia with a rate of 130 beats per minute. Note the upright P waves in leads II, III, aVL, and aVF, and negative P wave in lead V1. The relationship between the P wave and the QRS complex is consistent with a long RP tachycardia. The differential diagnosis of a long RP tachycardia includes atypical atrioventricular (AV) node reentry, a slowly conducting bypass tract, or an atrial tachycardia. From the intracardiac recordings in **B** we clearly see the atrial and ventricular ECG relationship. Atrial intracardiac electrograms from the coronary sinus (CS) catheter, along the left atrioventricular groove, come after the right septal (His bundle) electrograms. Tachycardia initiation required isoproterenol and was induced with programmed stimulation. (Surface leads are V_1, I, II, and aVF. Intracardiac leads include high right atrium (HRA 3,4), His bundle recording (His 1,2–His 3,4), CS recordings (CS 3,4–CS 9,10), and right ventricular apex. (*continued*)

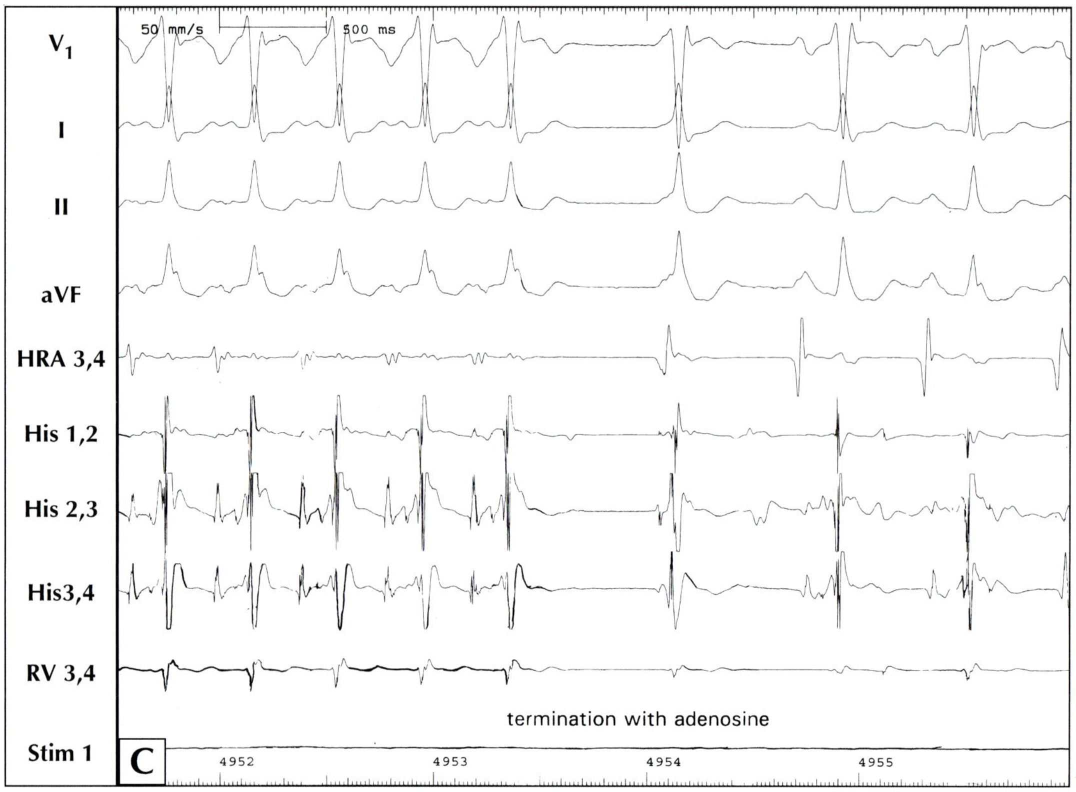

FIGURE 5-2. *(continued)* In **C** the tachycardia was terminated with adenosine. There was no evidence for an accessory pathway or dual AV nodes. These findings are consistent with an adenosine-sensitive atrial tachycardia. Note, the first beat after the tachycardia is terminated in a junctional beat.

MECHANISMS

ATRIAL TACHYCARDIAS BY MECHANISM

	TRIGGERED	AUTOMATICITY	REENTRY
Programmed stimulation: initiation/termination	+	-	+
Reliably induced with EPS	+/-	-	+
Coupling interval of extrastimulus to first tachycardia beat	Direct	-	Inverse
Reset response	Flat, decrease-increase	Increase; flat or decrease	Flat; increase-decrease
CL dependence	+	-	-
Fractionated signals	-	-	+
Warm-up period	+/-	+	-

FIGURE 5-3. Atrial tachycardias by mechanism. Information presented in this table emphasizes the electrophysiologic differences among various tachycardias. Triggered tachycardias are due to early or late membrane after-depolarizations that initiate the tachycardia. Early afterdepolarization–triggered arrhythmias are usually brought on by pauses and may be provoked by a pause protocol. Delayed afterdepolarization–triggered arrhythmias are usually triggered over a precise pacing rate. In both, there is a direct relationship between the paced rate and the tachycardia cycle length or in the relationship between the premature stimulus and the first beat of tachycardia. Triggered rhythms may respond to overdrive pacing but seldom to premature stimulation. The cycle length (CL) of the tachycardia is directly related to the coupling interval of the extrastimulus that initiates the tachycardia and the first beat of the tachycardia. Since the tissue is "normal," only the impulse formation is abnormal, and there are usually no fractionated signals. Another arrhythmia due to abnormal impulse formation is an automatic arrhythmia, which is initiated as a result of the influence of catecholamines or other stimuli on membrane potentials. Compared with triggered and reentrant arrhythmias, automatic arrhythmias are not induced or terminated by programmed stimulation and may have a warm-up period in which the CL is variable. Reentrant arrhythmias are most reliably initiated and terminated by pacing. There is usually a fixed or functional zone of poor conduction around which the electrical impulses travel and which also gives fractionated signals. The first beat of the tachycardia is usually inversely proportional to the extrastimulus used to initiate the tachycardia. Coupling interval—the time in msec from the last paced complex used to induce the tachycardia to the first beat of the tachycardia. Fractionated signals—electric signals indicating nonhomogeneous conduction. Reset response—the altering influence of a single premature complex during a regular tachycardia. The premature complex may cause the next beat of the tachycardia to be earlier, later, or not changed. EPS—electrophysiologic stimulus; - —not reliable; + —reliable.

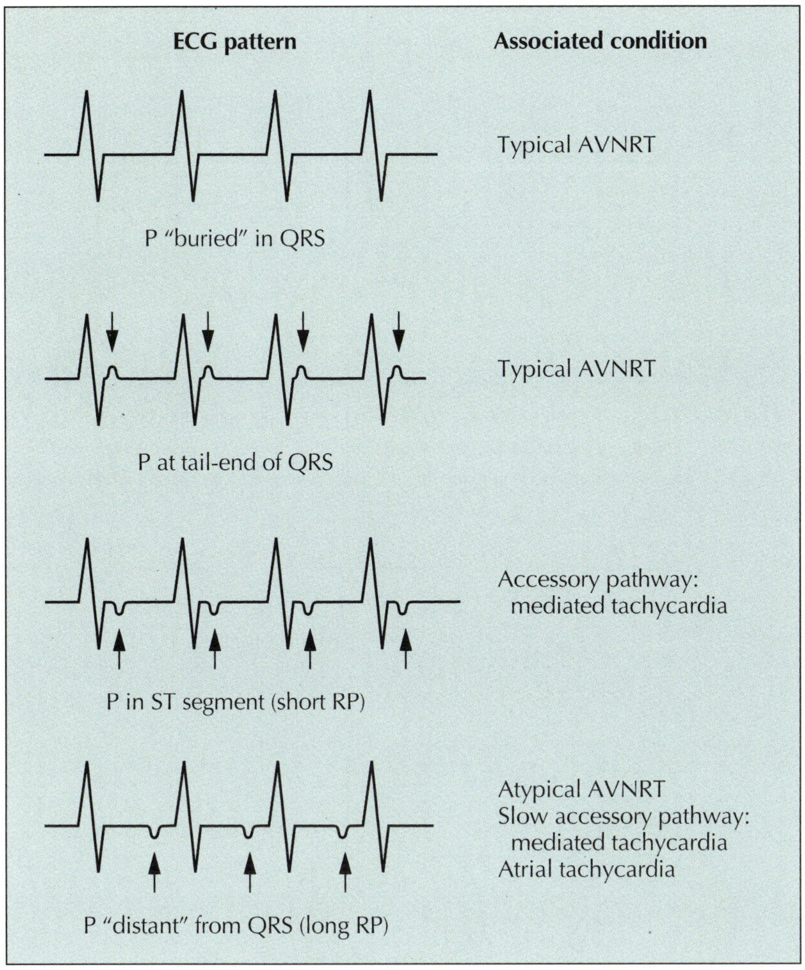

FIGURE 5-4. Electrocardiographic patterns of narrow complex tachycardias. The most important clue to the mechanism of a narrow complex tachycardia is the relationship of the P wave to the QRS complex. No visible P wave often means that the P wave is buried in the QRS complex. This is usually due to typical atrioventricular (AV) nodal reentry. With typical AV nodal reentry, the P wave may also be located just at the start or end of the QRS complex, giving a qRs or Rsr′ pattern. When the P wave is located close to the previous QRS complex, it is identified as a short-RP tachycardia. This is often seen with accessory pathway–mediated tachycardia and is due to retrograde atrial activation over the accessory pathway. The P wave may also be far from the previous QRS complex and classified as a long-RP tachycardia. If the P wave is inverted, it may be the result of atypical AV node reentry, or it may be using a slowly conducting accessory pathway in the retrograde direction. AVNRT—atrioventricular nodal reentry tachycardia; ECG—electrocardiogram.

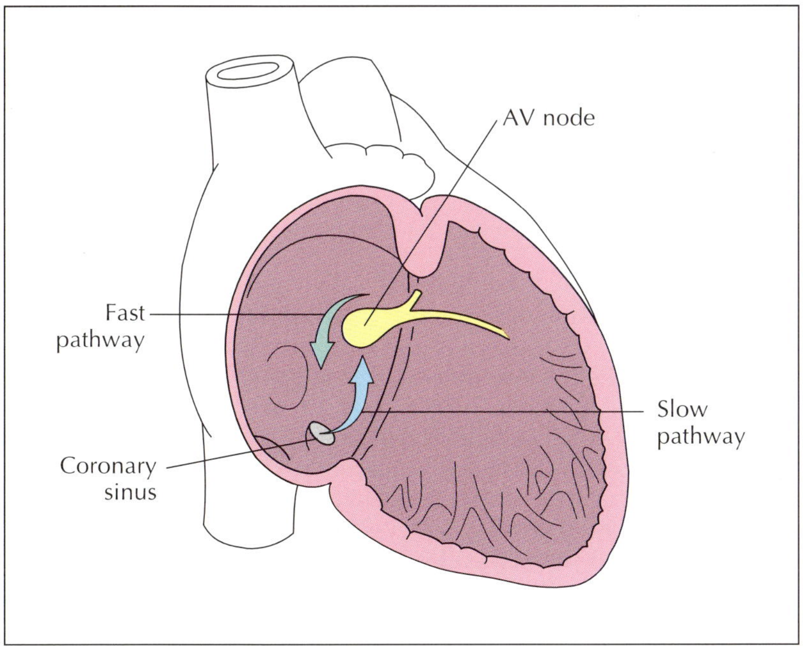

FIGURE 5-5. Diagram of atrioventricular (AV) nodal reentry. Although AV node anatomy and function are incompletely understood, patients with dual AV nodal physiology may be considered to have functional slow and fast AV nodal pathways. Slow pathway fibers begin in or around the coronary sinus (CS) os posteriorly and travel superiorly and anteriorly to converge on the compact AV node, which is in the superior interventricular septum. Fast pathway fibers travel superior and anterior to the compact AV node.

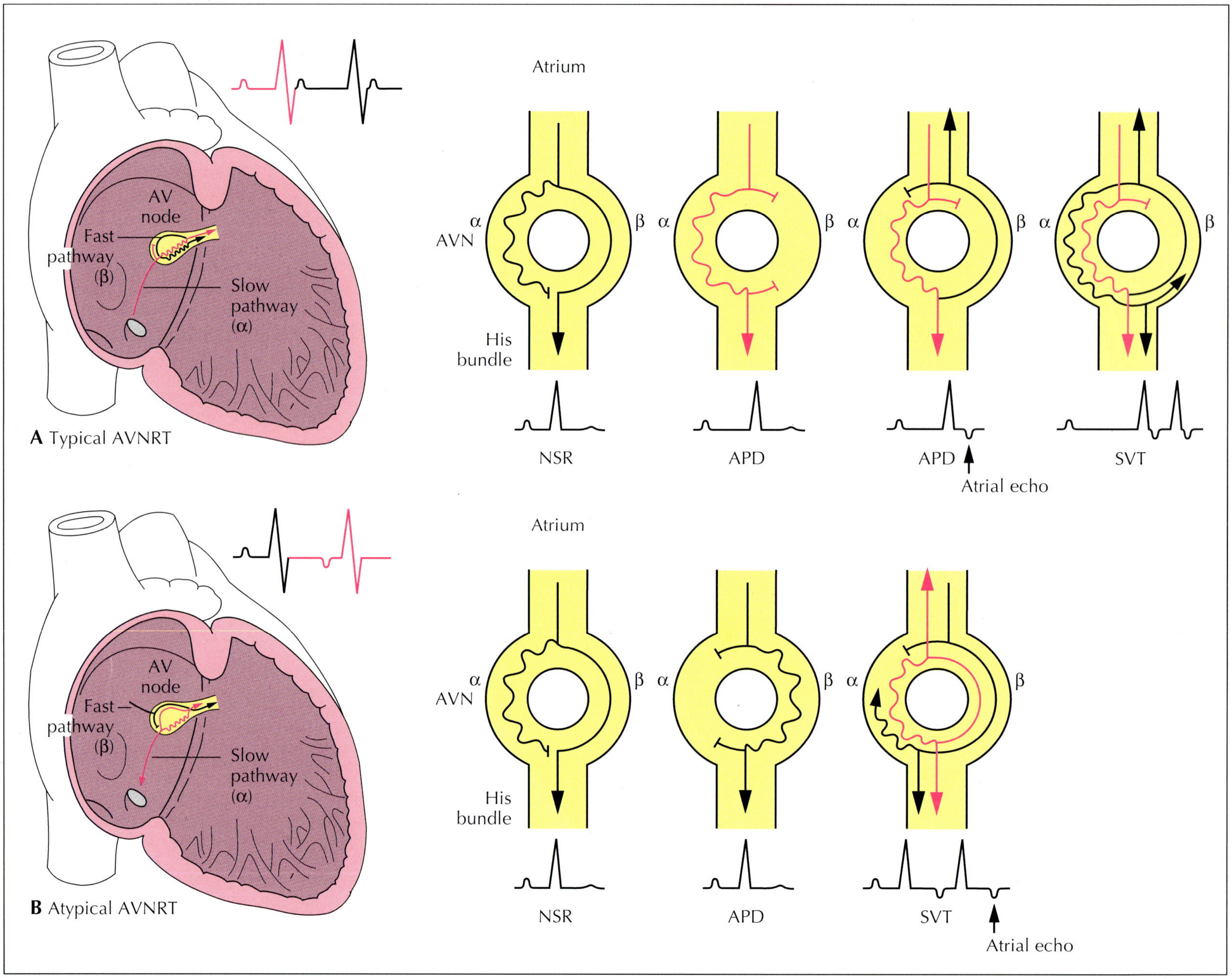

FIGURE 5-6. Schema for typical and atypical atrioventricular node reentrant tachycardia (AVNRT). Typical atrioventricular (AV) node reentry is shown in **A**. An impulse from the atrium enters the AV node and travels down both the slow and fast pathway. It quickly travels down the fast pathway resulting in activation of the ventricles with a short PR interval and results in the blocking of the impulse from the slow pathway when it reaches the terminal portion of the AV node since the tissue is still refractory. An atrial premature depolarization (APD) results in the conduction of the impulse down the slow pathway and thus longer PR interval. It blocks in the fast pathway since that tissue has a longer refractory period. If the tissue of the fast pathway regains conduction, the impulse after traveling down the slow pathway can return retrogradely back to the atrium via the fast pathway resulting in an atrial echo beat. A key component of the circuit is that the retrograde impulse finds the fast pathway no longer refractory. For this to occur, there must be a suitable delay in antegrade conduction over the slow pathway. The QRS complex is narrow because the ventricle is being activated via the normal HPS. Retrograde activation over the fast pathway happens quickly, and on the surface electrocardiogram, the retrograde P wave is usually "buried" or at the tail end of the QRS complex. This can give the appearance of a "pseudo" right bundle branch pattern in lead V_1. This is a short-RP tachycardia. **B** demonstrates that when the circuit is reversed, as during atypical AV node reentry, antegrade conduction occurs over the fast pathway and retrograde conduction over the slow pathway. In atypical AV node reentry, an APD is conducted over the fast pathway. The PR interval remains short. If there is retrograde activation over the slow pathway to the atrium, then SVT may be initiated. The QRS complex remains narrow because activation of the ventricle is still via the normal HPS. Retrograde atrial activation over the slow pathway takes longer compared with conduction over the fast pathway, resulting in a long-RP interval. This is a long-RP tachycardia. α—slow pathway; β—fast pathway. NSR–sinus rhythm; SVT–supraventricular tachycardia.

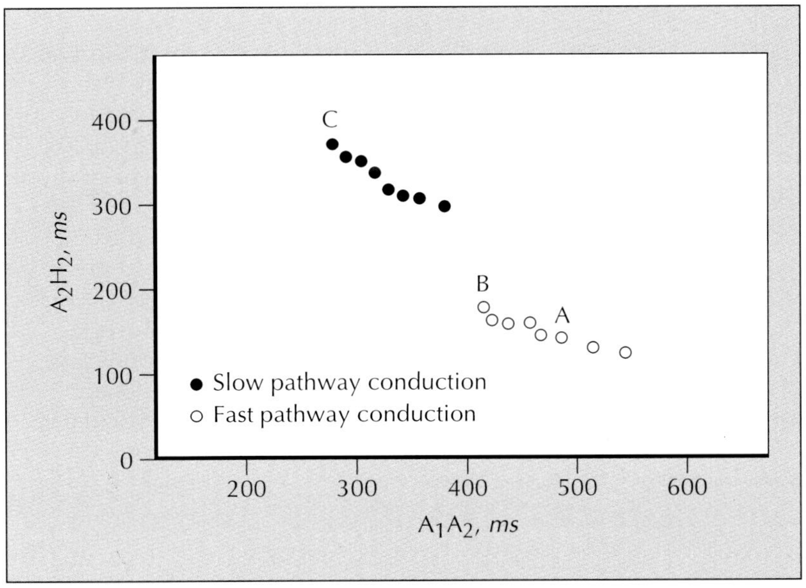

FIGURE 5-7. Dual atrioventricular (AV) conduction curves. Premature atrial extrastimuli (A_2) are inserted during a fixed drive cycle length to determine the effective refractory period (ERP) of the fast and slow pathways in a patient with dual AV nodal pathways. As the premature A_2 interval is made shorter, the A_1A_2 interval decreases. The A_2H_2 increases as a result of a decremental AV nodal conduction. At point *A*, conduction is over the fast pathway and the A_2H_2 conduction times are short but increase with increasing prematurity of the extrastimulus. At point *B*, conduction fails in the fast pathway, thus reaching the fast pathway ERP. However, slow pathway conduction continues because its refractory period is shorter. Thus, there is a discontinuity in the curve as conduction switches from the fast to the slow pathway. Eventually, at point *C*, the ERP of the slow pathway is reached, and there is no AV conduction. Patients with normal AV conduction have a smooth curve with no discontinuity. (A_1A_2—the interval in ms between the drive atrial cycle length (A_1) and the premature atrial extrastimulus (A_2); A_2H_2—the interval in ms between the premature atrial extrastimulus (A_2) and its associated His bundle deflection (H_2).

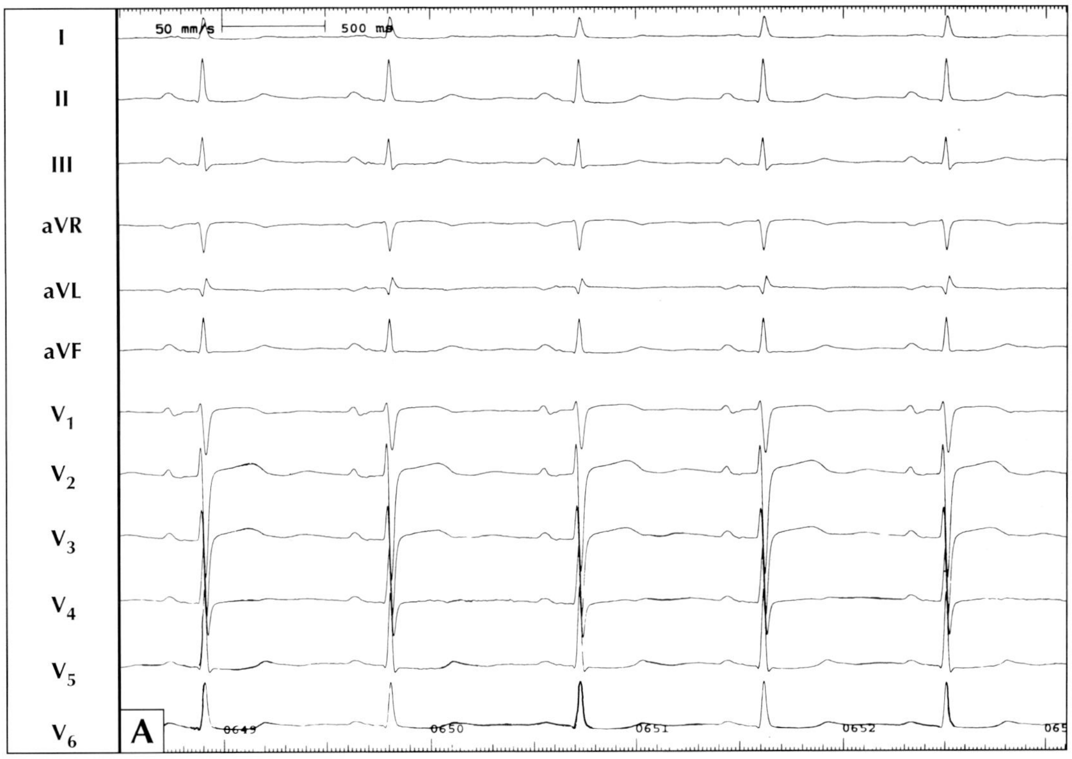

FIGURE 5-8. Typical atrioventricular (AV) node reentry. **A**, The electrocardiogram demonstrates sinus rhythm. Note the configuration of the QRS morphology in lead V1 and lead III. (*continued*)

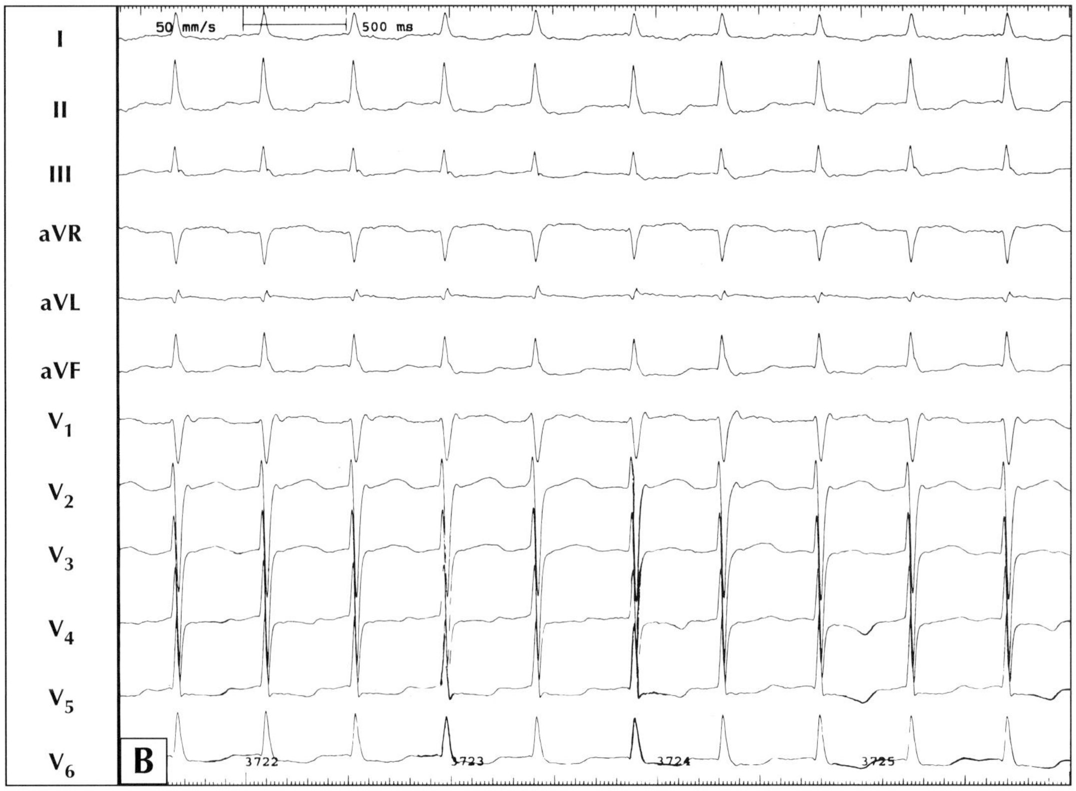

FIGURE 5-8. *(continued)* In **B**, a narrow complex tachycardia is seen at the rate of 150 beats per minute. Compared with sinus rhythm, there is now an r′ or "pseudo" right bundle branch block pattern in lead V_1. This is also seen in lead III. This pattern represents atrial activation over the retrograde fast pathway. In QRS complex 5 there is no r′ in lead V_1. Since retrograde atrial activation is dissociated from ventricular activation in this beat, conduction via an atrioventricular connection is not a possibility, since an atrioventricular connection requires 1:1 atrioventricular conduction.

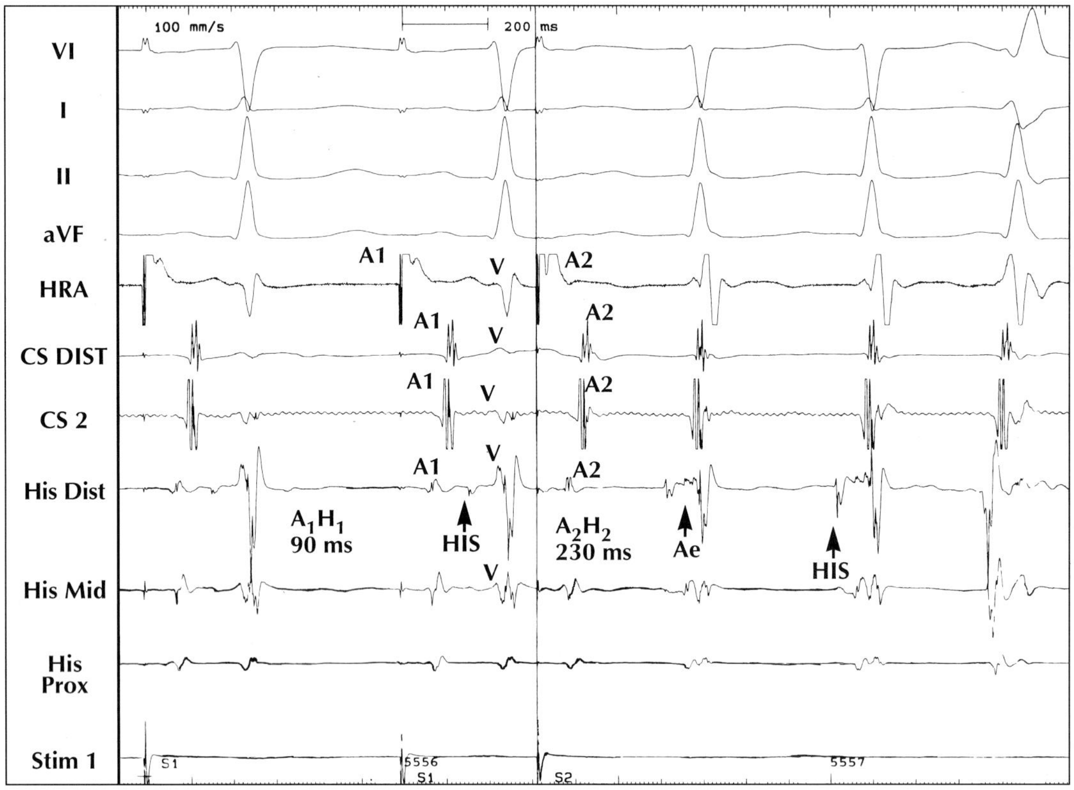

FIGURE 5-9. Initiation of atrioventricular nodal reentry with an atrial extrastimulus. Atrial pacing is performed at a cycle length of 600 ms, and an atrial premature beat (A_2) is given at 290 ms. Note that on the surface leads the atrioventricular (AV) time during the drive is 210 ms and that of the A_2 beat is 400 ms. This is caused by the jump from the fast to the slow pathway. Conduction proceeds over the slow pathway antegradely and retrogradely over the fast pathway, causing an atrial echo beat (Ae). Earliest retrograde activation is at the location of the His catheter (*arrow*) and occurs prior to atrial activation near the coronary sinus (CS) catheter. This occurs because the fast pathway breakthrough is anterior and superior in the AV septum. The CS os is posterior and inferior to the His catheter, and activation occurs later (surface leads V_1, I, II, and aVF, and intracardiac electrocardiograms HRA, CS, and His.) A_1—atrial drive cycle length; A_2—atrial premature extrastimulus; A_1H_1—AH interval associated with the drive cycle length; A_2H_2—AH interval associated with the premature extrastimulus; His—His bundle deflection; V—ventricular electrogram.

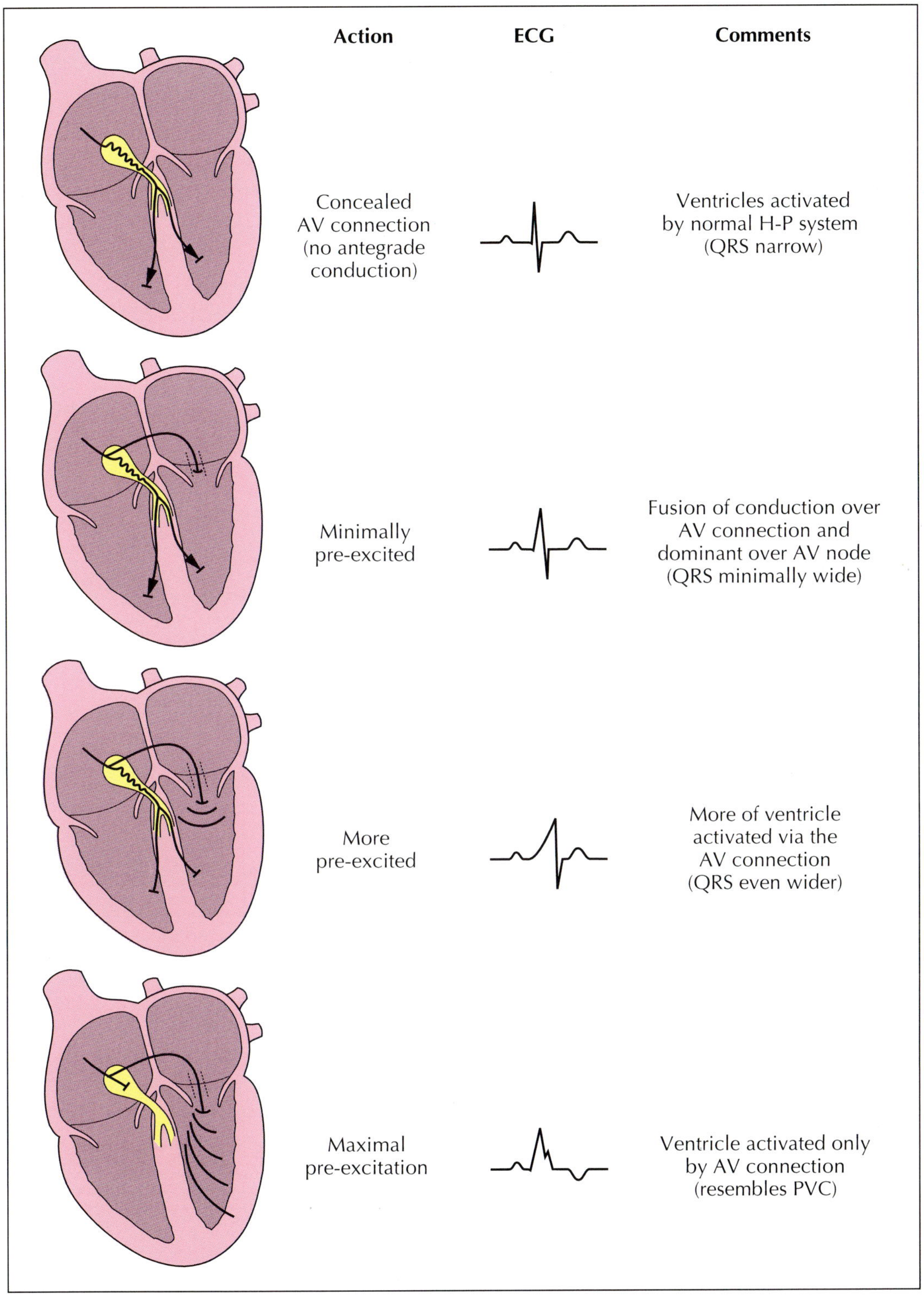

FIGURE 5-10. Conduction over an accessory pathway. The morphology of a QRS complex in patients with an accessory pathway (AP) is an excellent example of fusion. Conduction over an AP is influenced by drugs, sympathetic states, and its location along the atrioventricular annulus. If there is no antegrade conduction, the AP may still conduct in the retrograde direction but is considered concealed, because it is not apparent on the ECG. When conduction over the AP is minimal and atrioventricular (AV) node conduction predominates, the QRS becomes a fusion of conduction over the AV node–His-Purkinje system and the AP. When conduction to the ventricle over the AP predominates compared with AV nodal conduction, the QRS represents a fusion of conduction over the AV node–HPS and the AP, but the larger the portion of the ventricle activated by the AP, the wider the QRS complex appears. If ventricular activation is only over the AP, as with maximally preexcited tachycardias, it is difficult to distinguish the complex from ventricular tachycardia. H-P—His Purkinje; LA—left atrium; LV—left ventricle; PVC—premature ventricular complex; RA—right atrium; RV—right ventricle.

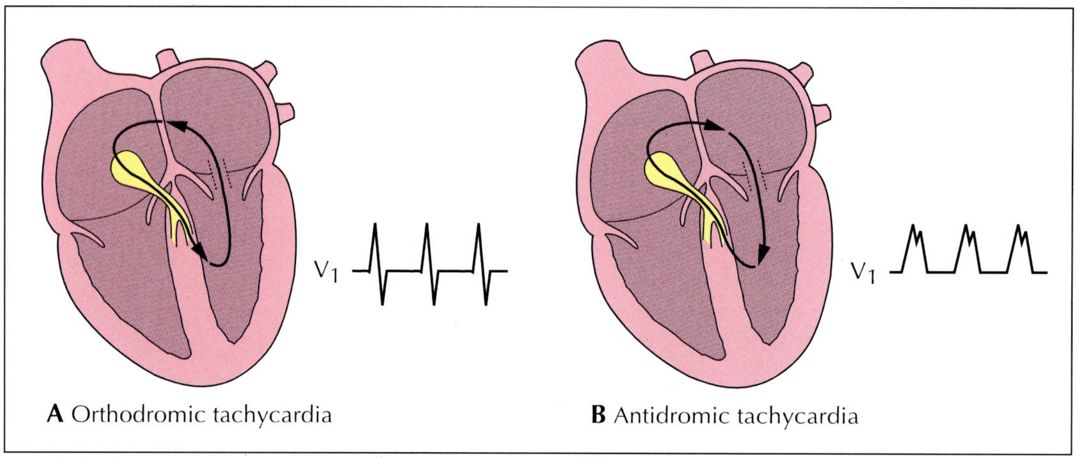

FIGURE 5-11. Tachycardia circuits utilizing an accessory pathway. When antegrade conduction is over the atrioventricular (AV node–His-Purkinje system (HPS) and retrograde conduction is over the AP, the QRS complex is narrow and is called an orthodromic AV reentry tachycardia (**A**). The retrograde P wave is further away from the QRS complex compared with typical AV node reentry, because the time (and distance) it takes to travel over the HPS and the AP is longer than the retrograde fast pathway conduction in AV node reentry. Most orthodromic tachycardias are short-RP tachycardias. When conduction is antegrade over the AP with retrograde conduction over the AV node, *ie*, an antidromic tachycardia, the QRS morphology is wide because of ventricular activation spread through muscle to muscle connections. The appearance of the QRS complex demonstrates maximal preexcitation (**B**).

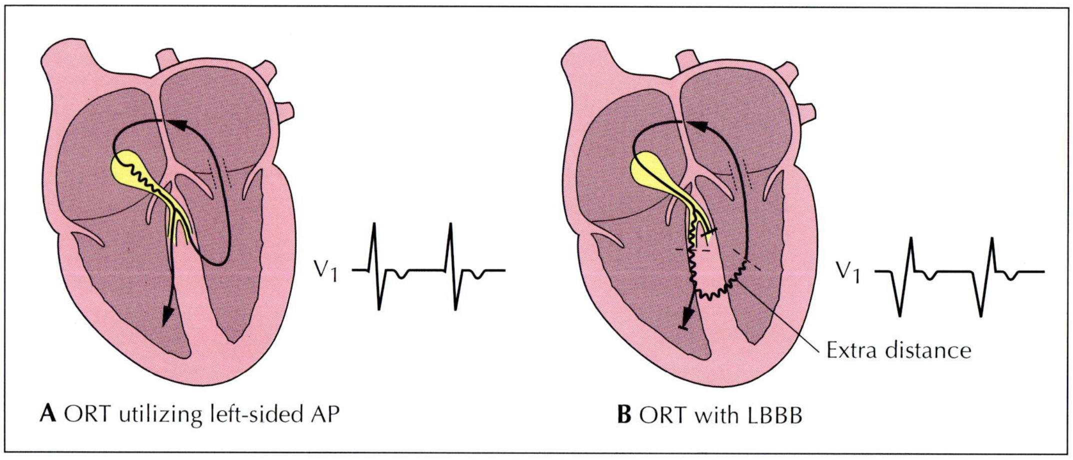

FIGURE 5-12. The effect of bundle branch block on an orthodromic tachycardia. An orthodromic tachycardia (ORT) involves antegrade conduction over the atrioventricular (AV) node and the His-Purkinge system (HPS), giving a narrow complex tachycardia, with retrograde conduction back to the atrium via the accessory pathway (AP). If a patient with an ORT circuit utilizing a left-sided AP (**A**) develops a left bundle branch block (LBBB) (**B**), the antegrade impulse can only travel down the right bundle and then through the septum before it reaches the left-sided AP. This increases the circuit length and hence increases the tachycardia cycle length, the time it takes for the impulse to traverse the circuit. There is also an increase in the VA time, *ie*, the time from ventriclar activation until the atrium is retrogradely activated, because the distance the impulse travels is longer. Similarly, if a patient with tachycardia using a right-sided AP develops a right bundle branch block, the tachycardia will slow down and the VA interval will lengthen. Thus, in a patient with a tachycardia utilizing an anteroseptal AP, a right bundle branch block will slow the tachycardia.

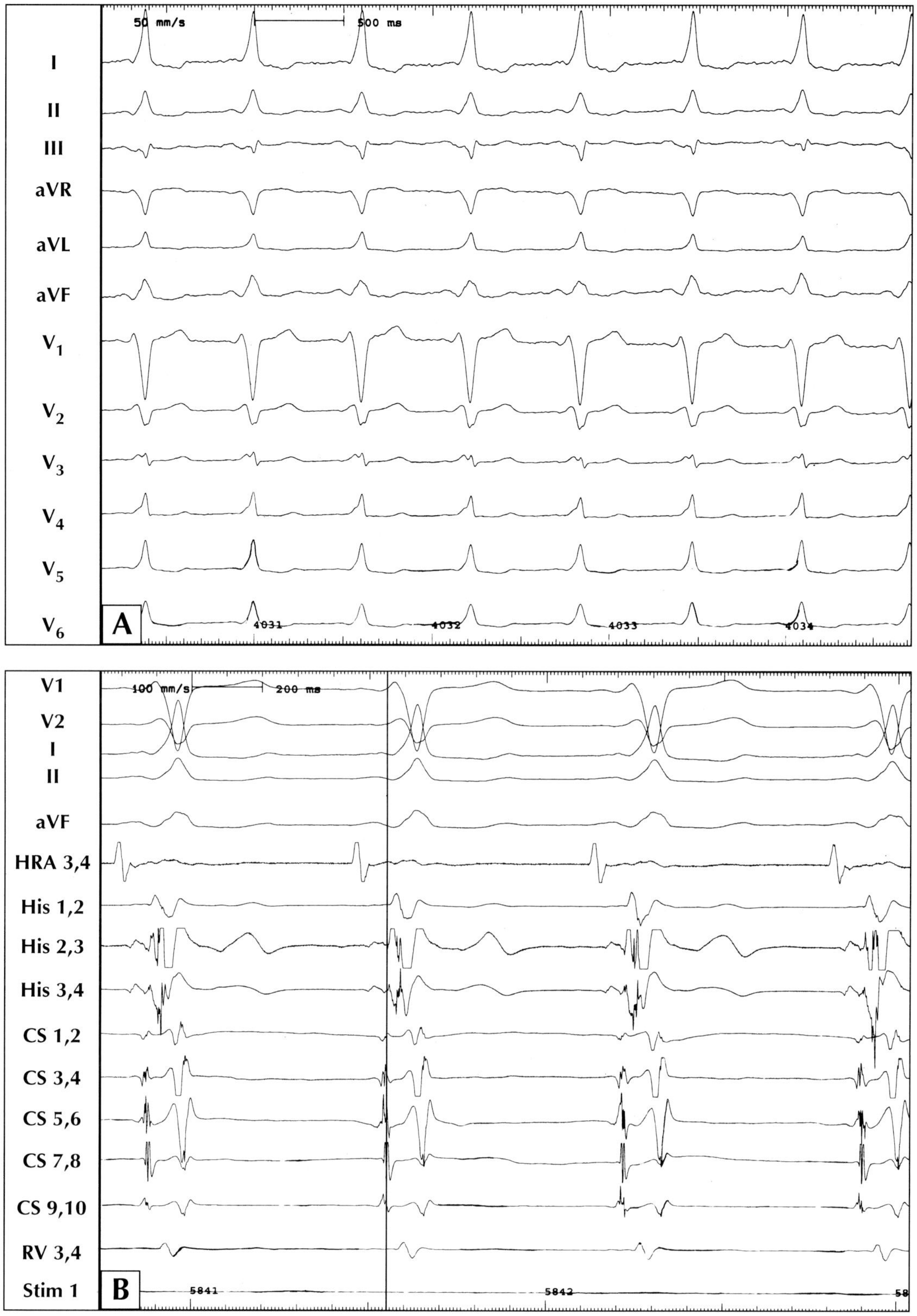

FIGURE 5-13. Intracardiac recordings from a patient with a right-sided accessory pathway. **A**, A 12-lead electrocardiogram (ECG) is shown. Note the positive delta waves in II and aVF, and isoelectric waves in III. **B**, Four surface leads are shown with intracardiac recordings from the high right atrium (HRA), His bundle position, coronary sinus (CS) os, and right ventricle. A line is drawn perpendicular to the onset of the delta wave, which represents the initiation of ventricular activation. Note, the ventricle is activated before activation of the atrioventricular (AV) node. The short HV interval signifies evidence of ventricular preexcitation. The AV interval on the His catheter is short, suggesting it is near the accessory process (AP). This is consistent with a right anteroseptal AP. *(continued)*

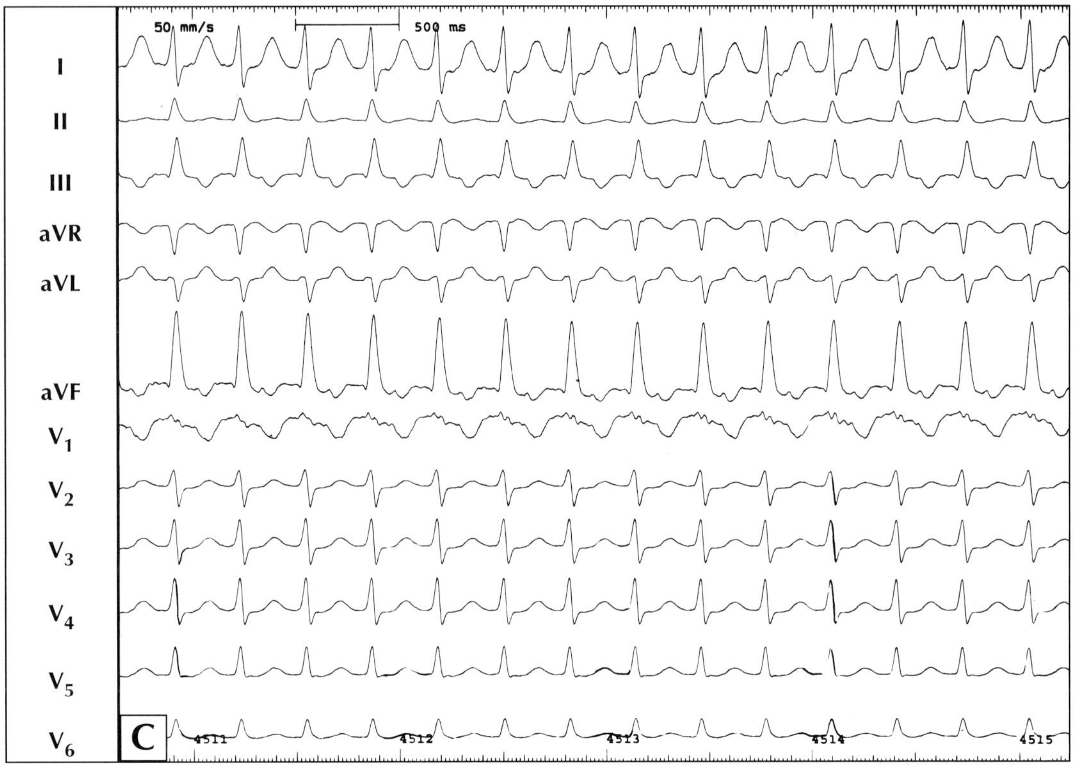

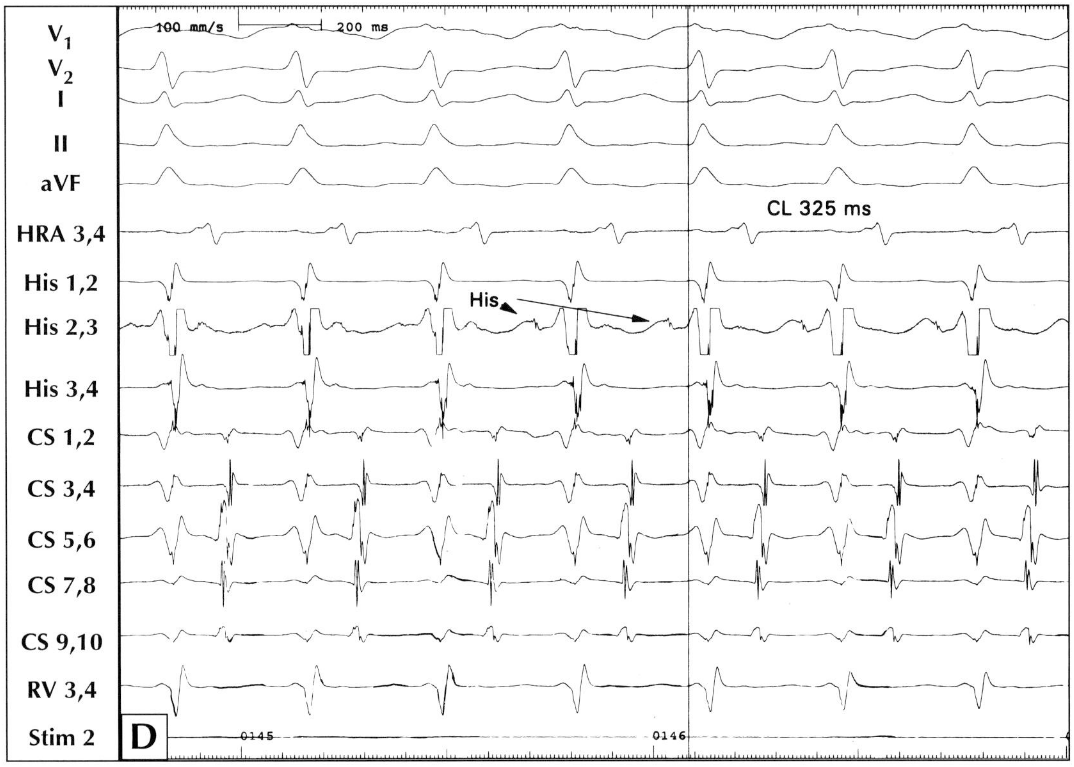

FIGURE 5-13. (*continued*) **C**, A 12-lead ECG of an orthodromic tachycardia with a cycle length of 325 ms is shown. Compared with sinus rhythm, the complexes are narrower because the ventricle is being activated only by the AV node-HPS with no antegrade AP conduction. There is no fusion over the AP. **D**, Intracardiac electrogram during tachycardia. The HV interval is normal. The *arrows* indicate the His bundle electrogram. Retrograde conduction is retrograde over the AP. The earliest right atrial activation is in the His catheter, as with sinus rhythm, well before atrial activation from the left atrium, consistent with a right anteroseptal AP.

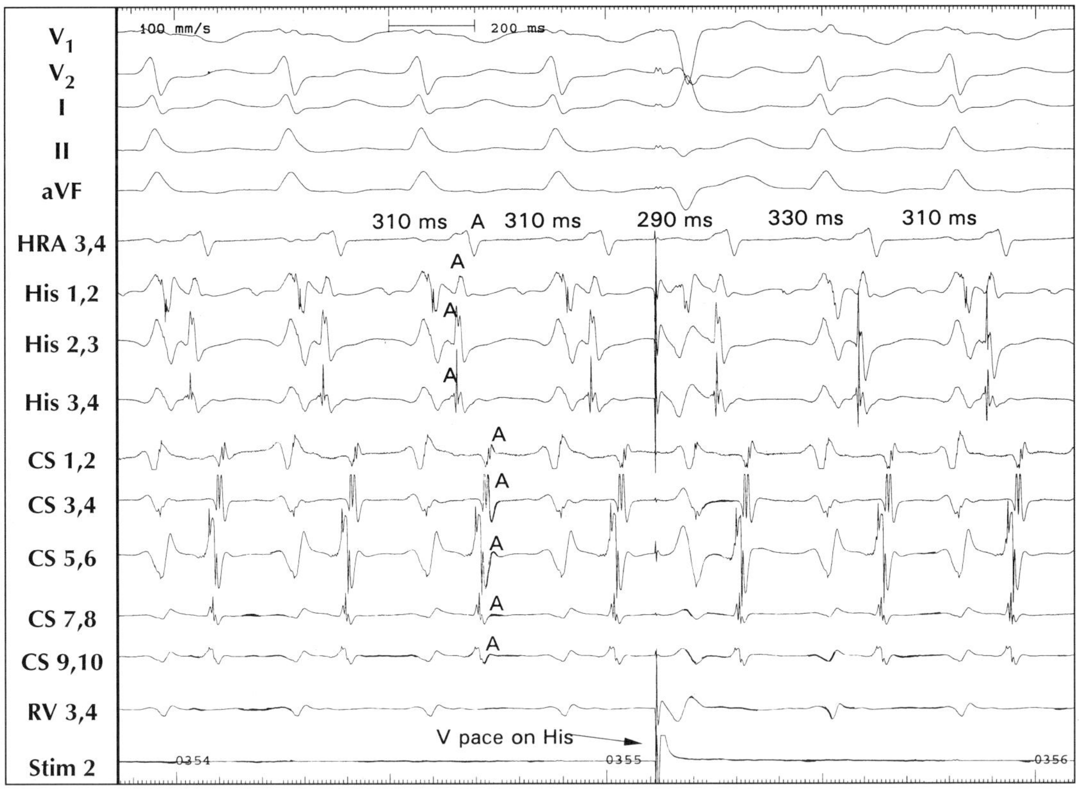

FIGURE 5-14. A premature ventricular depolarization is introduced when the His bundle is refractory. During the narrow complex orthodromic tachycardia shown in Figure 5-13, a premature ventricular complex (PVC) occurred just at the onset of the His bundle electrogram. The PVC cannot travel retrogradely to the atrium via the atrioventricular (AV) node because the His bundle is refractory. However, atrial activation in the high right atrium is advanced. This is because the PVC was able to travel retrogradely to the atrium via the accessory process (AP). Thus, a premature ventricular depolarization during His refractoriness and a narrow complex tachycardia that pulls in the following atrial electrogram proves the presence of an AP. The same retrograde sequence in response to ventricular premature stimulation suggests that the pathway is part of the circuit. A—atrial electrogram.

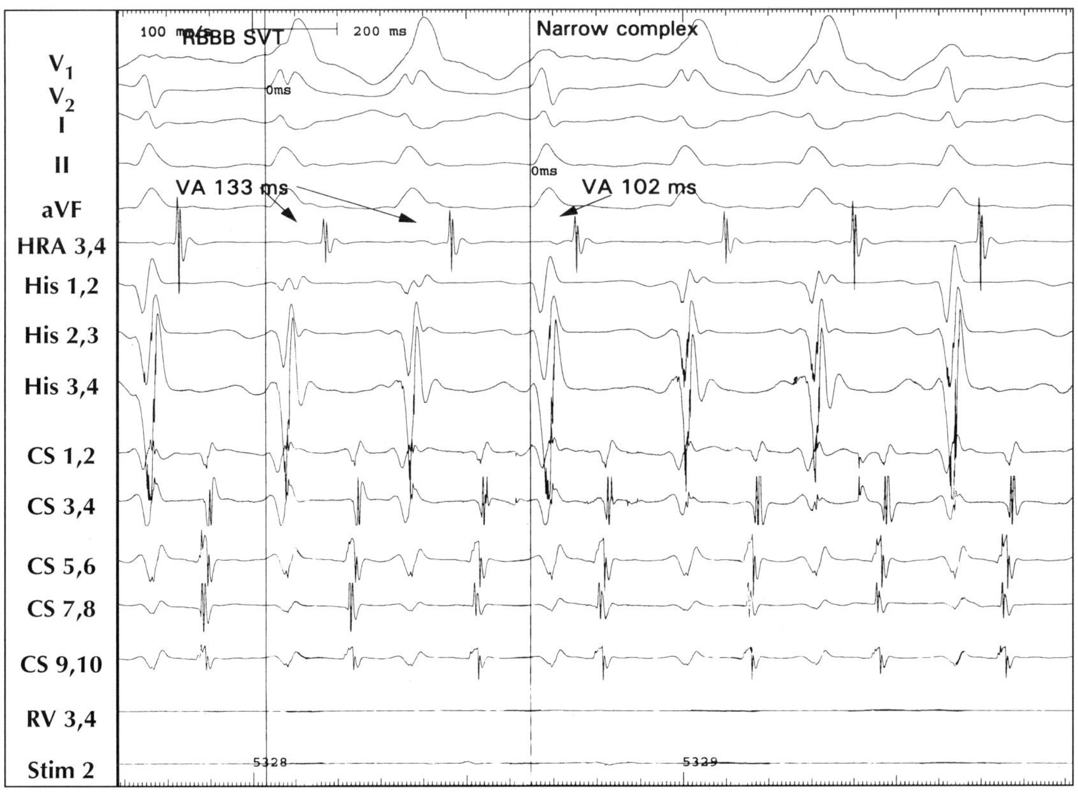

FIGURE 15-15. Right bundle branch block (RBBB) in a patient with a right-sided accessory pathway (AP). Shown are the intracardiac recordings from a patient with an orthodromic atrioventricular (AV) reentrant tachycardia utilizing a right-sided accessory pathway. The right-sided AP is being used in the retrograde direction (*see* Figure 5-12). The second and third complexes have an RBBB morphology, while the fourth complex is narrower. During tachycardia, antegrade conduction is over the atrioventricular (AV) node, and retrograde conduction is over a right anteroseptal AP. The electrogram from ventricular and atrial recordings on the His bundle catheter is almost fused because it is close to the AP. An impulse traveling antegradely down the AV node with right bundle conduction block must travel over the left bundle and across the left septum before reaching the AP. The increased distance thus slows down the tachycardia circuit, specifically, the VA interval is increased. SVT—supraventricular tachycardia.

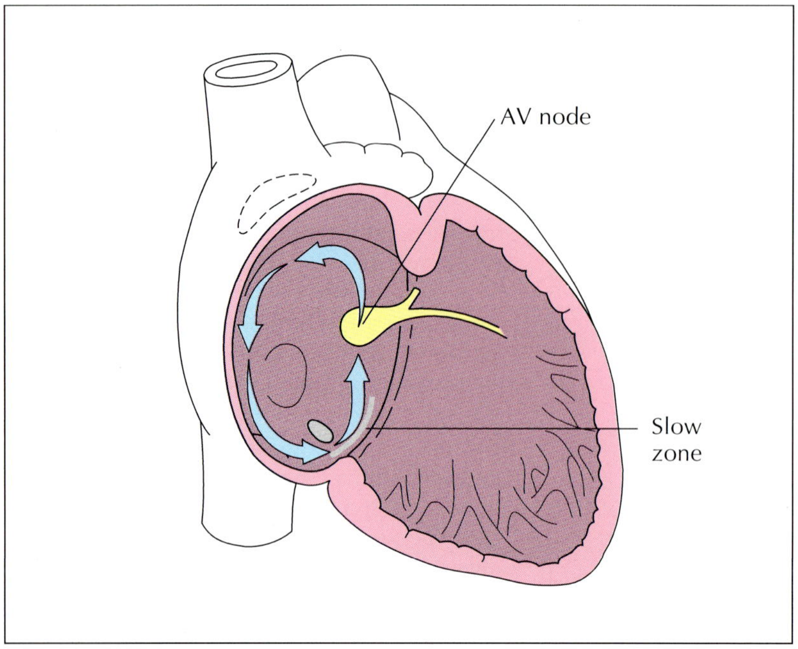

FIGURE 5-16. Atrial flutter circuit. With atrioventricular (AV) nodal reentry, AV reentry utilizing an accessory pathway, and a reentrant atrial tachycardia, there is usually a defined circuit which, if interrupted, can terminate the tachycardia. We now have learned that atrial flutter is a macro reentrant circuit in the right atrium. The circuit involves conduction in a counterclockwise (or clockwise) direction from the low posterior right atrium near the tricuspid valve annulus (TA), the posteroseptal region near the coronary sinus os, the interatrial septum, the high lateral right atrium, and down the crista terminalis to the isthmus between the inferior vena cava and the TA. The region of the posterior right atrium is thought to be the slow zone of conduction in the circuit. Evidence that supports this theory are data showing that atrial flutter can be entrained with atrial pacing. This has led to the development of techniques allowing electrophysiologists to ablate the critical regions of the circuit causing atrial flutter, thus, rendering the circuit inoperable.

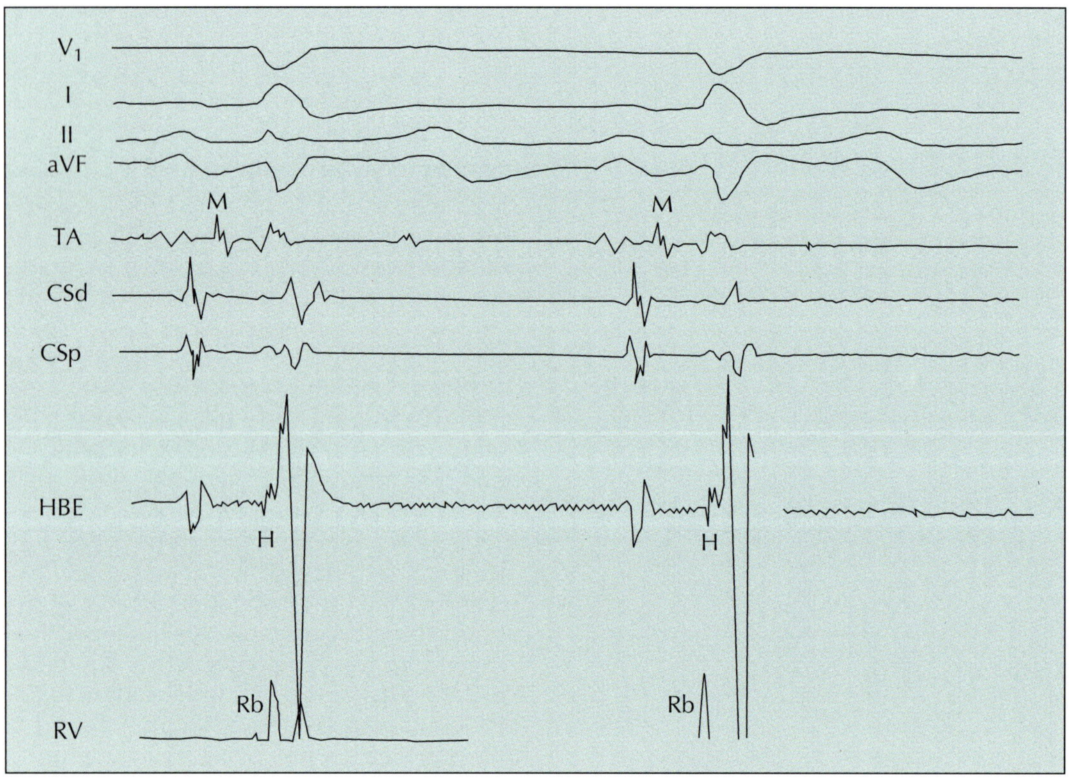

FIGURE 5-17. Sinus rhythm in a patient with a Mahaim fiber. There is a baseline left bundle branch block (LBBB) pattern in lead V_1. The tricuspid annulus (TA) catheter lies along the right posterolateral atrioventricular groove. The right bundle (*Rb*) is activated before the His bundle due to preexcitation over the Mahaim fiber. As compared with a regular accessory pathway, there is a long atrioventricular interval at the site of the Mahaim fiber as a result of its slow, decremental conduction. Surface leads V_1, I, II, and aVF are shown. Intracardiac leads: CSd—distal coronary sinus; CSp—proximal coronary sinus; H—His electrogram; HBE—His bundle electrogram; M—Mahaim potential; RV—right ventricle.

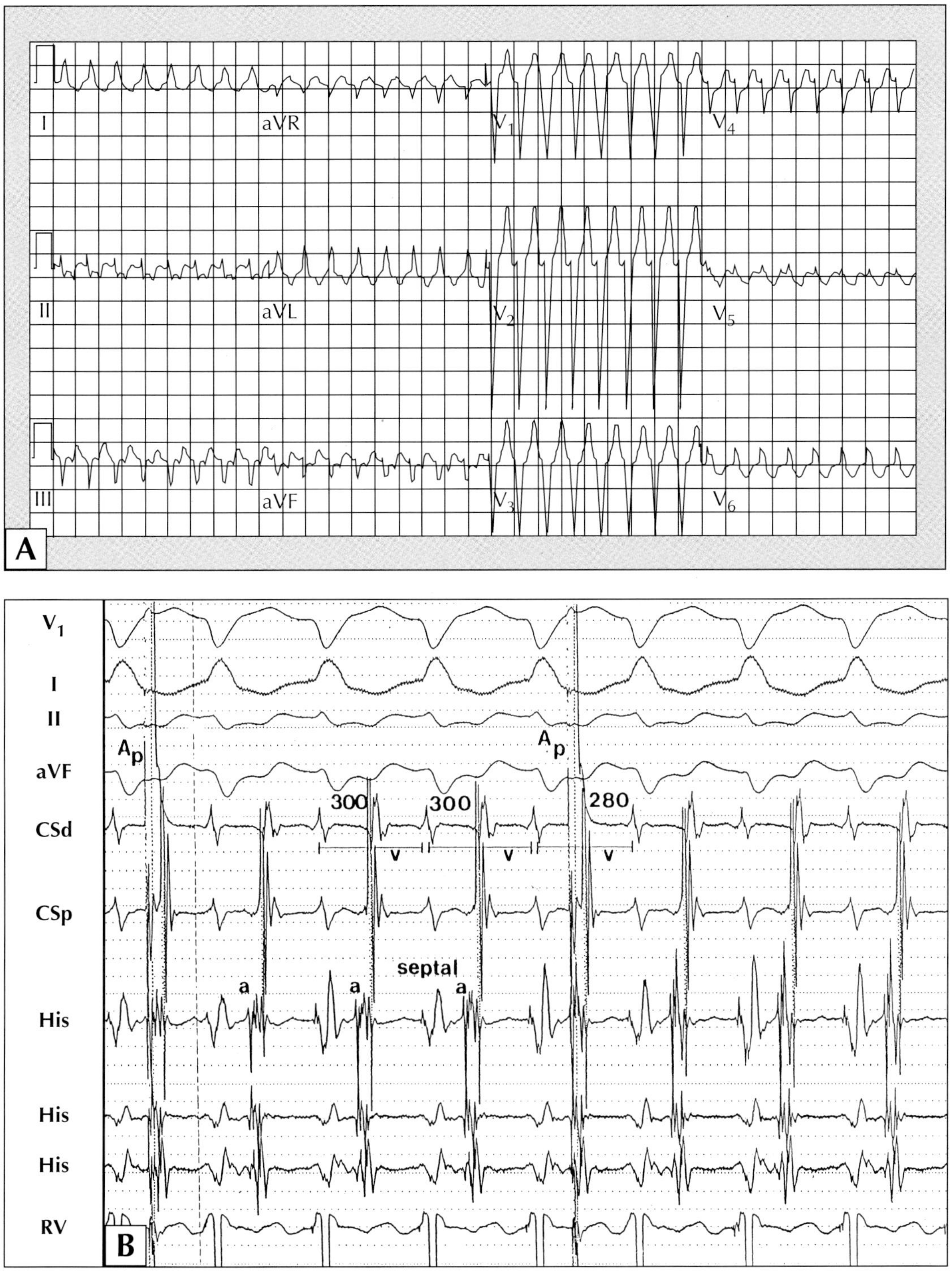

FIGURE 5-18. Electrocardiogram (ECG) of a tachycardia utilizing a Mahaim fiber. In **A**, the tachycardia has a wide complex left bundle branch block (LBBB) morphology with a late precordial transition. The tachycardia uses the Mahaim fiber in the antegrade direction and the atrioventricular (AV) node in the retrograde direction (antidromic tachycardia). The axis is leftward, because the Mahaim fiber joins the peripheral right bundle in the inferior portion of the right ventricle. **B**, The intracardiac recordings are shown. An atrial premature complex (APC) occurs when the septal atrial electrogram is depolarized. In this fashion, the APC cannot travel antegradely to the ventricle via the AV node because it is refractory. However, the ventricular electrogram following the APC is advanced and of the same preexcited configuration as during the tachycardia. This proves that the Mahaim fiber likely participates in the tachycardia circuit. An APC during septal atrial refractoriness during a wide complex tachycardia is analogous to a premature ventricular complex (PVC) during His bundle refractoriness during a narrow complex tachycardia. Tachycardia termination with an atrial extrastimulus when the septal a is refractory proves that the Mahaim fiber is part of the circuit. (Surface leads V_1, I, II, and aVF are shown.) Intracardiac leads: a—atrial ECG on the His catheter, which is septal; A_p—atrial pacing; CSd—distal coronary sinus signal; CSp—proximal coronary sinus signal; His—His bundle signal; RV—right ventricular signal.

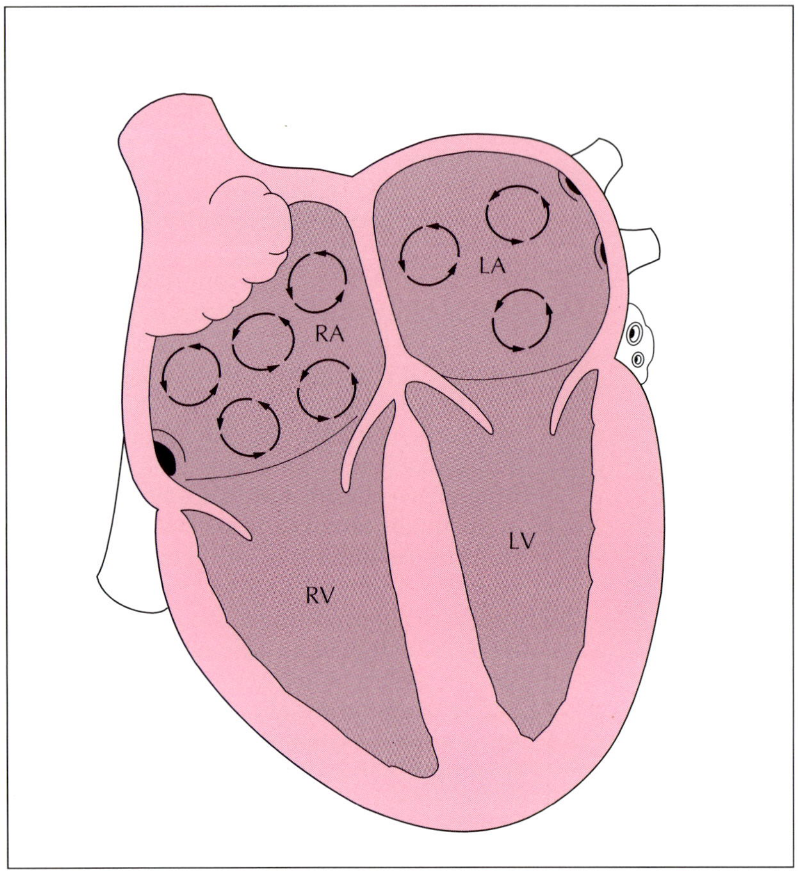

FIGURE 5-19. Atrial fibrillation. Based on the work of Allessie *et al.* [7], atrial fibrillation (AF) is thought to be due to multiple wavelets of conduction produced by reentry. Perpetuation of AF depends on the relative dimensions of the atria and the size of the reentrant circuit. Compared with atrial flutter, in which there is one reentrant circuit and organized atrial activity, atrial fibrillation demonstrates no organized atrial contraction. This leads to blood stasis, the formation of clots, and the possibility of embolic events. Thus, most patients with chronic atrial fibrillation are given anticoagulants to reduce the risk of embolic events such as strokes. LA—left atrium; LV—left ventricle; RA—right atrium; RV—right ventricle.

STROKE AND EFFECTS OF ANTICOAGULATION

STUDY	PATIENTS, *n*	THERAPY
SPAF I	1330	Coumadin v. placebo, aspirin, 325 mg
BAATAF	420	Coumadin v. placebo
AFASAK	1007	Coumadin v. placebo, aspirin, 75 mg

FIGURE 5-20. Effect of anticoagulation on the risk of stroke in atrial fibrillation. Coumadin decreases the risk of embolic stroke and TIAs, while the advantages of aspirin are less clear. In the SPAF trial, investigators evaluated both Coumadin and aspirin among patients with nonrheumatic atrial fibrillation. Group I patients were randomized to Coumadin therapy, aspirin, or placebo. They were all thought to be eligible for Coumadin. Group II patients, thought to be ineligible for Coumadin were randomized to aspirin or placebo. They were followed for a mean of 1.3 years. In the Group I patients, by comparision with placebo, Coumadin decreased the risk of stroke or embolism from 7.4% to 2.3%. Among the Group I and Group II patients, by comparison with placebo, those treated with aspirin had a reduction of primary outcomes from 6.3% to 3.6%. The differences in outcome data between patients assigned to Coumadin verses those assigned to aspirin were unavailable.

In the BAATAF trial, 420 patients received Coumadin or placebo. Mean follow-up was 2.2 years. The reduction in the risk for ischemic stroke resulting from Coumadin was 86%. Major bleeding plus transfusion was increased by an absolute amount of 0.4% per year among Coumadin patients.

The Copenhagen AFASAK study followed 1007 patients with chronic nonrheumatic atrial fibrillation—335 given Coumadin, 336 given aspirin, and 336 given placebo. Endpoints included stroke, transient cerebral attacks, embolic events, and death. The incidence of embolic complications was lower in the Coumadin group than in the aspirin or placebo groups. In summary, these trials show that the risk of stroke in atrial fibrillation patients is decreased with Coumadin with little increase in the frequency of bleeding. The role of aspirin is still being investigated. Other studies also verify the efficacy of anticoagulation in atrial fibrillation [8]. AFASAK—Atrial Fibrillation, Aspirin, Anticoagulation Study (Denmark); BAATAF—Boston Area Anticoagulation trial in Atrial Fibrillation; SPAF—Stroke Prevention in Atrial Fibrillation Study. (*Adapted from* Laupacis and coworkers [8]; with permission.)

TREATMENT MODALITIES FOR ATRIAL FIBRILLATION

Pharmacologic therapy: goal is to restore sinus rhythm or rate control
- AV nodal blocking agents: Digoxin, β blockers, calcium channel blockers
- Type IA: procainamide, quinidine, disopyramide
- Type IC: flecanide, propafenone
- Type III: amiodarone, sotalol

Surgery
- Maze procedure

Catheter ablation
- Complete AV node ablation + pacemaker
- AV node modification for rate control
- Catheter maze procedure (investigational)

FIGURE 5-21. Treatment of atrial fibrillation. Many drugs are available for rate control of atrial fibrillation. However, studies show that antiarrhythmic agents can be toxic and are associated with an increased risk of sudden death or proarrhythmia, especially in patients with congestive heart failure. The risk/benefit ratio of proarrhythmia from drugs for conversion and maintenance of sinus rhythm must be compared with allowing the patient to remain in atrial fibrillation and maintaining rate control and anticoagulation. Catheter ablation techniques include complete atrial ventricular (AV) node ablation and placement of a permanent pacemaker or modifying the slow zone (posteroseptal region) for rate control without placing a permanent pacemaker. Anticoagulation is still mandatory. Currently, there is investigation into using a catheter approach for reproducing the Maze procedure. The Maze procedure is a surgical procedure that makes use of precisely placed incisions in the right atrium that restore normal sinus rhythm.

REFERENCES

1. Mahaim I, Winston MR: Recherches d'lanatomic comparee et du pathologic experimentale sur les connexions hautes du faisceau de His-Tawara. *Cardiologia* 1941, 5:189–260.
2. Klein L, Hackett FK, Zipes DP, Miles WM: Radiofrequency catheter ablation of Mahaim fibers at the tricuspid annulus. *Circulation* 1993, 87:738.
3. McClelland J, Jackman W, Beckman K, *et al.*: Direct recordings of right atriofascicular accessory pathway (Mahaim) potentials at the tricuspid annulus (abstract). *PACE* 1992, 15:547.
4. Tchou PT, Lehmann MH, Jazayeri M, Akhtar M: Atriofascicular connection or a nodoventricular Mahaim fiber? Electrophysiologic elucidation of the pathway and associated reentrant circuit. *Circulation* 1988, 77:837–848.
5. Murdock CJ, Leitch JW, Klein GJ, *et al.*: Epicardial mapping in patients with nodoventricular accessory pathways. *Am J Cardiol* 1991, 68:208.
6. Grogin HR, Lee RJ, Kwasman M: Radiofrequency catheter ablation of atriofascicular and nodoventricular Mahaim tracts. *Circulation* 1994, 90:272–281.
7. Allessie MA, Lammers WJEP, Bonke FIM, Hollen J: Experimental evaluation of Moe's multiple wavelet hypothesis of atrial fibrillation. In *Cardiac Electrophysiology and Arrhythmias.* Edited by Zipes DP, Jalife J. Orlando: Grune and Stratton; 1985:265–275.
8. Laupacis A, *et al.*: Risk factors for stroke and efficacy of antithrombotic therapy in atrial fibrillation. *Arch Intern Med* 1994, 154:1449-1457.

VENTRICULAR TACHYCARDIA: MECHANISMS, DIAGNOSIS, AND TREATMENT

6

CHAPTER

Michael D. Lesh

Ventricular arrhythmias have become increasingly important to the clinical cardiologist because of the increasing number of patients surviving sudden cardiac death, the sophisticated diagnostic modalities that are now available, a large range of treatment options, and the recognition that some treatments may actually be more harmful than helpful. Ventricular tachyarrhythmias comprise a spectrum of mechanisms and clinical presentations. Therefore, rational therapy must be based on an understanding of the likely mechanism of each patient's arrhythmias, with a clearly defined goal of such therapy. Ventricular arrhythmias span a range from completely benign to life threatening. For example, simple premature ventricular beats are found in most normal persons on 24-hour ambulatory electrocardiographic (ECG) recordings. On the other hand, it is now believed that at least 90% of the 300,000 to 400,000 cases of sudden cardiac death that occur each year in the United States are the result of ventricular tachycardia (VT) or ventricular fibrillation (VF). In only 15% to 20% of these cases is an acute myocardial infarction (MI) present, although coronary artery disease (CAD) and old infarction are present in most.

To determine the mechanism of ventricular arrhythmias, it is important to document the ECG manifestation of the arrhythmia, *ie*, whether it is monomorphic, pleomorphic (a few changing morphologies), or polymorphic. One should also know whether the arrhythmia is nonsustained or sustained, whether it is associated with symptoms, and what precipitating factors, if any, are present. However, there is not necessarily a direct relationship between these findings. For example, some sustained ventricular arrhythmias may be only mildly symptomatic or asymptomatic. A common misconception is that a patient presenting with a wide complex tachycardia that does *not* result in syncope or cardiac death must have supraventricular tachycardia with aberration; a better rule is that any patient with coronary or structural heart disease presenting with a wide complex tachycardia has VT until proven otherwise, regardless of symptoms.

Ventricular tachycardia may occur as the result of normal or abnormal automaticity, triggered activity, or reentry. Requirements for reentry include unidirectional block of a premature beat that initiates tachycardia, slowed conduction, a functional or anatomically determined circuit, and adequate recovery of excitability at the site of initial block that allows tachycardia to continue. In the setting of chronic healed MI, reentry occurs at the border zone of the infarct where normal muscle interdigitates with scar.

It is important to divide any sustained, wide complex tachycardia into either supraventricular tachycardia with aberrant conduction or VT, and several criteria are available for utilizing the 12-lead ECG to do so. However, invasive electrophysiologic (EP) testing ultimately may be required to confirm the diagnosis and guide therapy. Along with the ECG or EP diagnosis of VT, each patient must be evaluated for reversible causes, such as ischemia or electrolyte disturbances. In addition, the cardiac substrate, such as CAD with healed infarction, dilated cardiomyopathy, or long QT syndrome, must be defined.

After determining the likely mechanism and substrate of the ventricular arrhythmias and the presence or absence of reversible causes, it is important to define the goals of therapy. Therapeutic endpoints might include reducing the risk of sudden death, relieving symptoms, or preventing recurrent syncope. No therapy is indicated for asymptomatic premature ventricular contractions in the absence of structural heart disease because they have no prognostic significance. Even after myocardial infarction, when patients with complex ventricular ectopy may have an increased risk of dying, antiarrhythmic drugs (other than β blockers) may not reduce the risk of fatal VT or VF without a larger increase in drug-related proarrhythmia. For those patients in whom therapy is indicated, options include antiarrhythmic drugs, surgery, catheter ablation, and implanted devices with antitachycardia pacing/cardioversion/defibrillation capabilities. Whereas benign arrhythmias require no therapy, malignant arrhythmias mandate an aggressive approach guided by careful methods, such as invasive EP testing, rather than empirically administered drugs of undefined efficacy or proarrhythmic potential.

Mechanisms of Ventricular Tachycardia

CATEGORIZATION OF VENTRICULAR ARRHYTHMIAS

ECG TYPE	CARDIAC SUBSTRATE	DURATION AND TIMING
Monomorphic VT	Normal heart	Isolated beats
Pleomorphic VT	Cardiomyopathy	Couplets or triplets
Torsades de pointes	Coronary artery disease without infarct	Parasystole
Polymorphic VT	Coronary artery disease with acute infarct	Nonsustained VT (<30 bpm)
Ventricular flutter	Coronary artery disease with healed infarct	Sustained, self-terminating VT
Ventricular fibrillation	Valvular or other structural heart disease	Sustained VT
	Functional electrical disorder (*eg*, long QT syndrome)	Incessant VT
	Exercise-induced arrhythmia	
	Reversible/metabolic disorder (*eg*, electrolyte disorder or ischemia)	
	Drug-induced proarrhythmia	

CLINICAL PRESENTATION	PROGNOSTIC SIGNIFICANCE	ELECTROPHYSIOLOGIC MECHANISM
No symptoms	Benign	Normal or abnormal automaticity
Palpitations	Increased risk for sudden death but no intervention identified to reduce risk	Triggered activity
Pre-syncope	Increased risk for sudden death and intervention known to reduce risk	Reentrant
Syncope	Malignant	Combined disorder
Chest pain/heart failure/fatigue/other cardiac symptoms		
Aborted sudden death		

FIGURE 6-1. Categorization of ventricular arrhythmias.

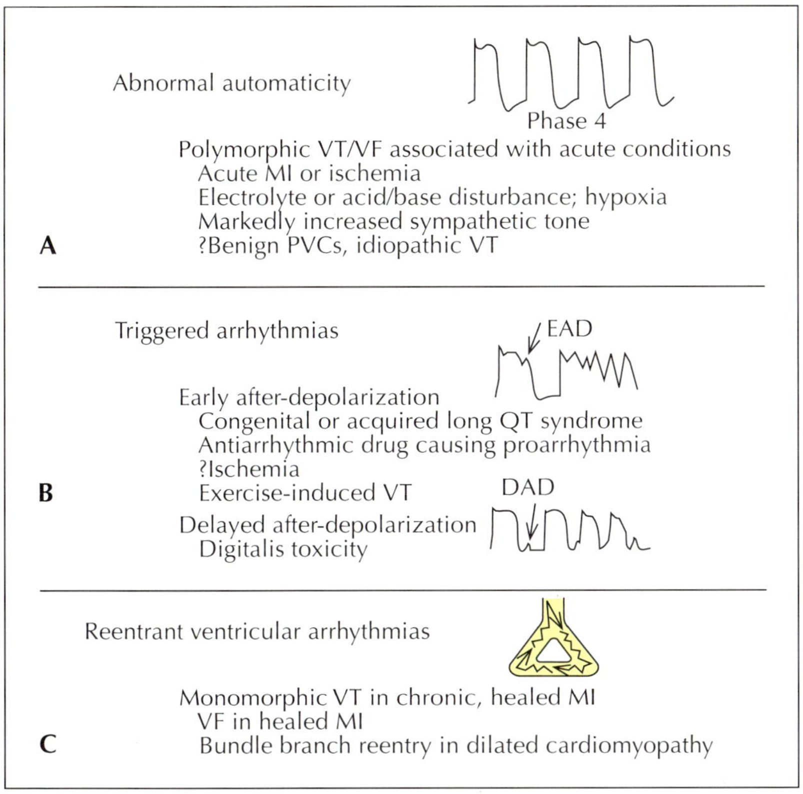

FIGURE 6-2. Mechanisms of ventricular arrhythmias, with clinical arrhythmias occurring as a likely consequence of those mechanisms. **A,** Abnormal automaticity. **B,** Triggered arrhythmias. **C,** Reentrant ventricular arrhythmias. DAD—delayed after-depolarization; EAD—early after-depolarization; MI—myocardial infarction; PVC—premature ventricular contraction; VF—ventricular fibrillation; VT—ventricular tachycardia.

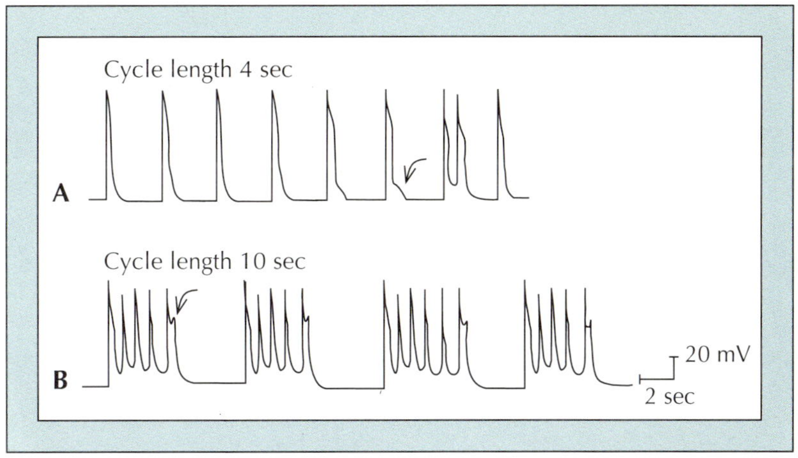

FIGURE 6-3. Electrocardiographic pattern of early after-depolarizations (EAD) from a cesium-treated Purkinje fiber in a tissue bath preparation. **A,** At a 4-second pacing cycle length, progressive development of a hump during the repolarization phase of the action potential (*arrow*) eventually results in a single, triggered (*ie*, nonpaced) action potential on the subsequent beat. **B,** At slower pacing rates, a series of triggered action potentials follows each paced beat, with EADs (*arrow*) appearing as a sequence of oscillations at plateau membrane potential. (*Adapted from* Binah and Rosen [1]; with permission.)

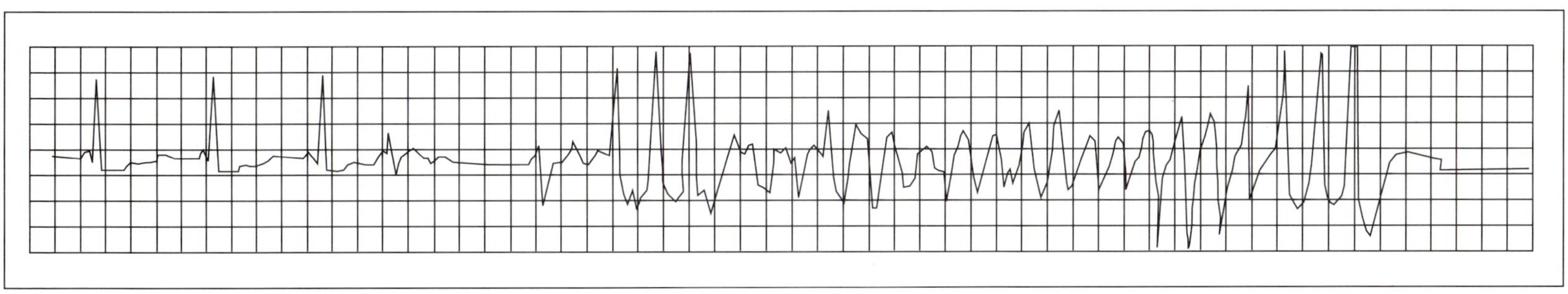

FIGURE 6-4. Rhythm strip (lead II) from a patient with recurrent syncope following initiation of quinidine therapy for benign premature ventricular contractions (PVC). Classic torsades de pointes is present, which may be a clinical manifestation of a triggered arrhythmia. Three typical features appear with this arrhythmia: During sinus beats the QT interval is prolonged and the T-wave morphology is multiphasic and bizarre; a PVC that occurs immediately at the end of a large U wave starts a short/long/short sequence; this sequence then initiates a run of polymorphic ventricular tachycardia that also seems to start immediately at the end of a large U wave. Such giant slow waves may represent the surface electrocardiographic manifestation of an early after-depolarization, adding evidence to the hypothesis that this is a triggered arrhythmia.

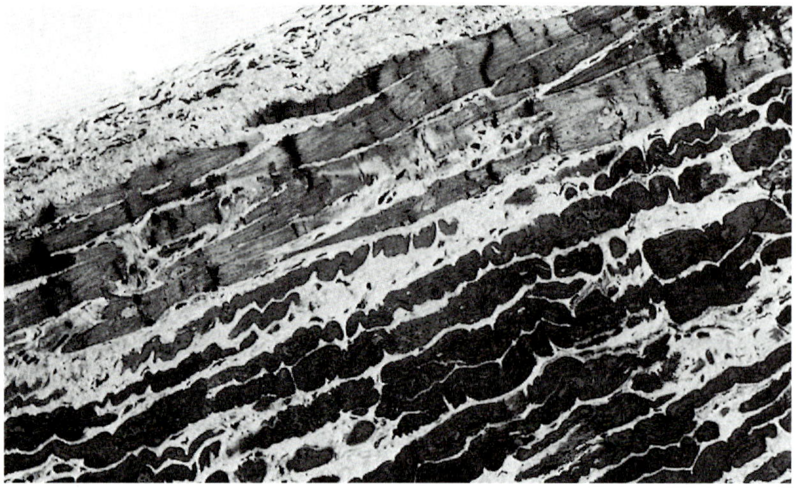

FIGURE 6-5. The histologic substrate for sustained, monomorphic ventricular tachycardia (VT) in the setting of chronic healed myocardial infarction. This section is from a patient who underwent surgery to remove that portion of the endomyocardium responsible for his VT. Note the interdigitation of scar and relatively normal surviving muscle bundles. Microelectrode experiments indicate that the surviving muscle cells have relatively normal action potential characteristics, with normal resting membrane potential and action potential upstroke. Therefore, VT does not result from any abnormality of the cellular electrophysiologic properties themselves; rather, patchy scarring results in uncoupling of the normal cell-to-cell pathway for current spread, resulting in serpiginous, slow conduction. This nonuniformly anisotropic substrate has the characteristics required for sustained reentrant tachycardia. (*Adapted from* Wit and Josephson [2]; with permission.)

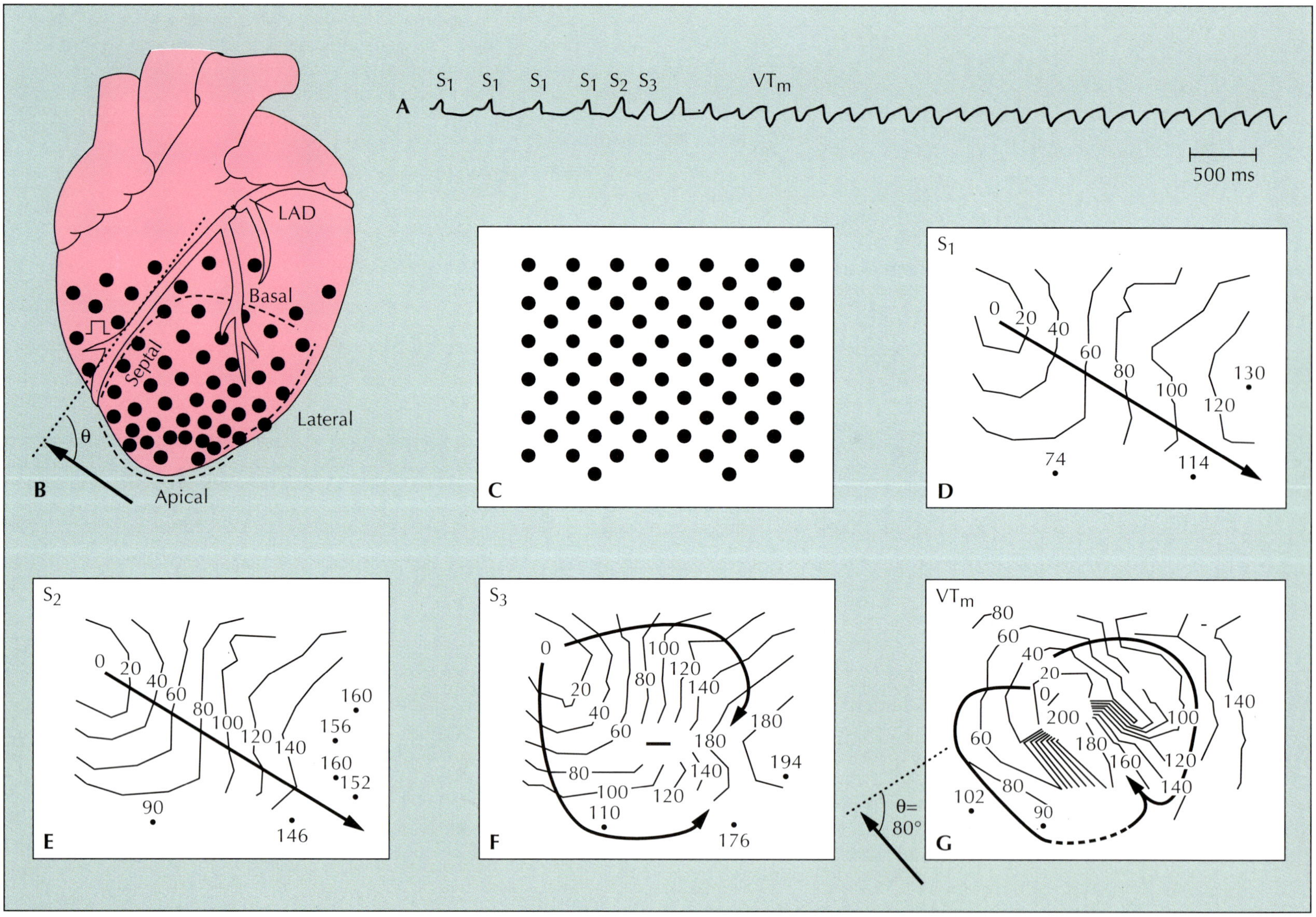

FIGURE 6-6. Mechanism of sustained monomorphic ventricular tachycardia (VT). Shown in this figure is a canine model of healing myocardial infarction produced by occlusion and reperfusion of the left anterior descending coronary artery (LAD). **A,** The electrocardiogram shows basic beats (S_1) followed by the premature beats (S_2, S_3) that initiate sustained VT (VT_m). **B,** Recording electrode sites on the anterior aspect of the heart (*dots*), along with the occluded LAD. The pacing site is also shown near the apical septum. **C,** The recording electrode array. **D,** The basic drive beat passes through the anterior left ventricle relatively undisturbed, as shown in the map of isochromal activation lines drawn at 20-ms intervals. **E,** The first premature beat (S_2) conducts with some slowing. **F,** The second premature beat (S_3) blocks along the septal margin of the anterior left ventricle and conducts slowly around the lines of block, leading to sustained reentry, with a "figure 8" pattern, as shown in **G.** Note that the common reentrant wave front is conducted longitudinally to the myocardial fiber axis, and that the arcs of block occur transverse to the fiber axis, implying the importance of anisotropic tissue structure in reentrant VT. (*Adapted from* Cardinal and coworkers [3]; with permission.)

Diagnosis of Ventricular Tachycardia

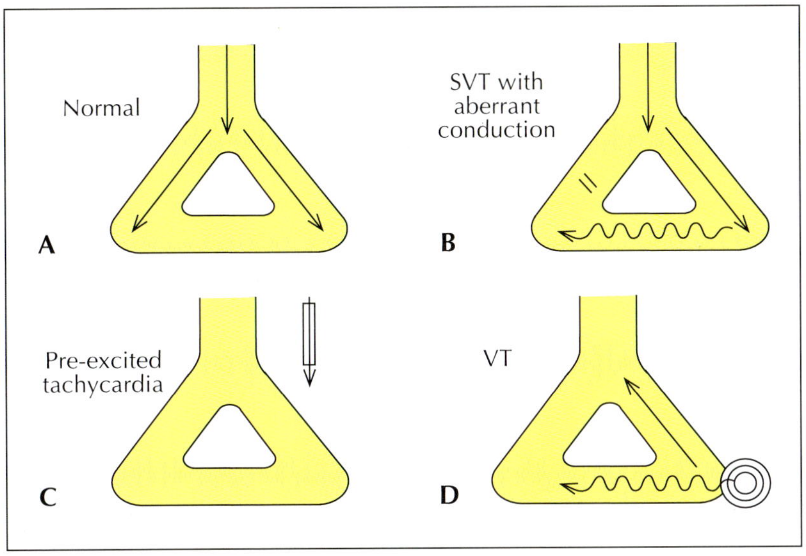

Figure 6-7. Differential diagnosis of wide complex tachycardia (WCT). Normal QRS complexes are narrow because conduction proceeds over the His Purkinje system to rapidly activate the ventricles (**A**). A WCT can result from supraventricular tachycardia (SVT) with aberrant conduction (**B**), from an atrial or other supraventricular arrhythmia with rapid conduction over an accessory atrioventricular connection in a patient with Wolff-Parkinson-White syndrome (**C**), or from an origin in the ventricle itself (**D**). VT—ventricular tachycardia.

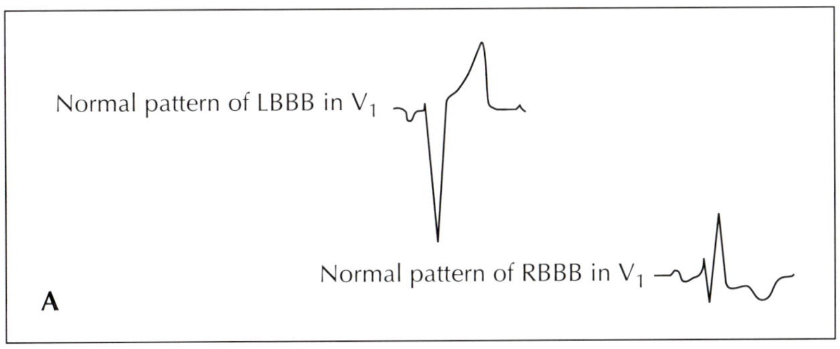

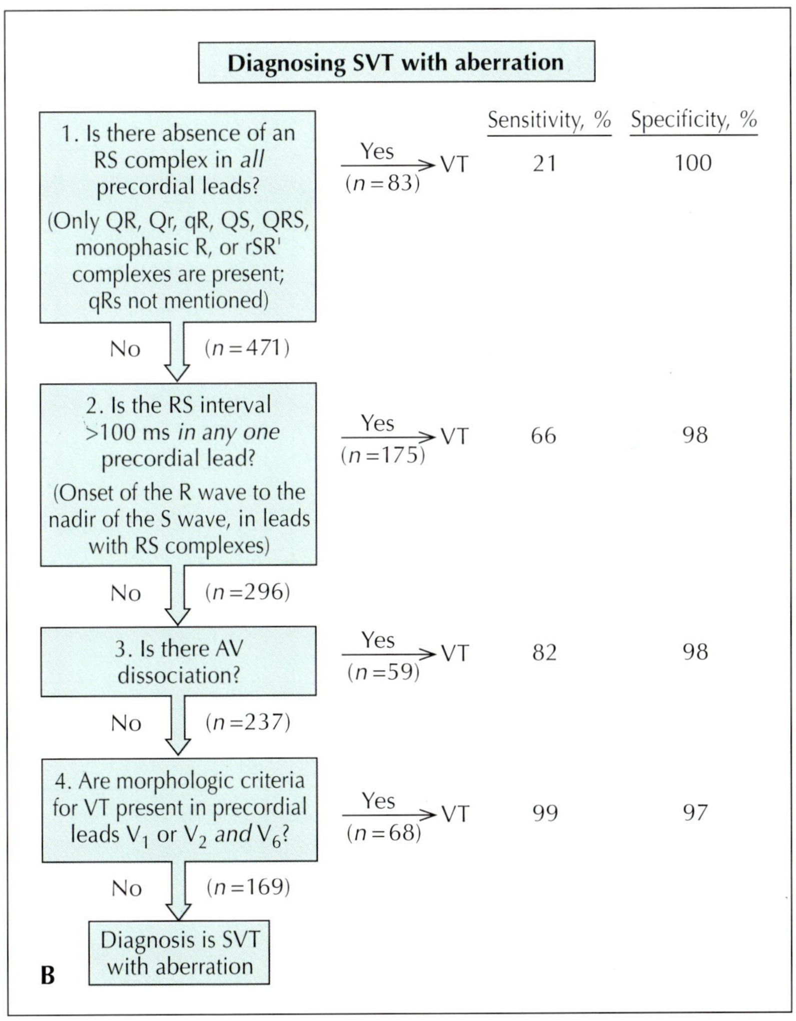

Figure 6-8. The 12-lead electrocardiogram in the differential diagnosis of wide complex tachycardia. Brugada *el al.* [4] analyzed 384 cases of ventricular tachycardia (VT) and 170 cases of supraventricular tachycardia (SVT) with aberrancy, representing 554 patients with tachycardia (those taking antiarrhythmic medications were excluded). They then devised a systematic approach for diagnosing wide QRS complex tachycardia with regular rhythmicity. **A,** The first step is to exclude sinus tachycardia or atrial tachycardia with right bundle branch block (RBBB) or left bundle branch block (LBBB). This can usually be done by finding P waves in lead V_1: the ST segment and T wave are always smooth, unless distorted by a P wave. However, missing this diagnosis should not affect the ability to diagnose VT or SVT, unless the patient is taking QRS-lengthening drugs. **B,** Steps in diagnosis of SVT with aberration. A *yes* answer at any point indicates that no further steps need to be taken. When the answer is *no*, proceed to the next step. The cumulative sensitivity using this method is 97% and specificity is 99%. (*continued*)

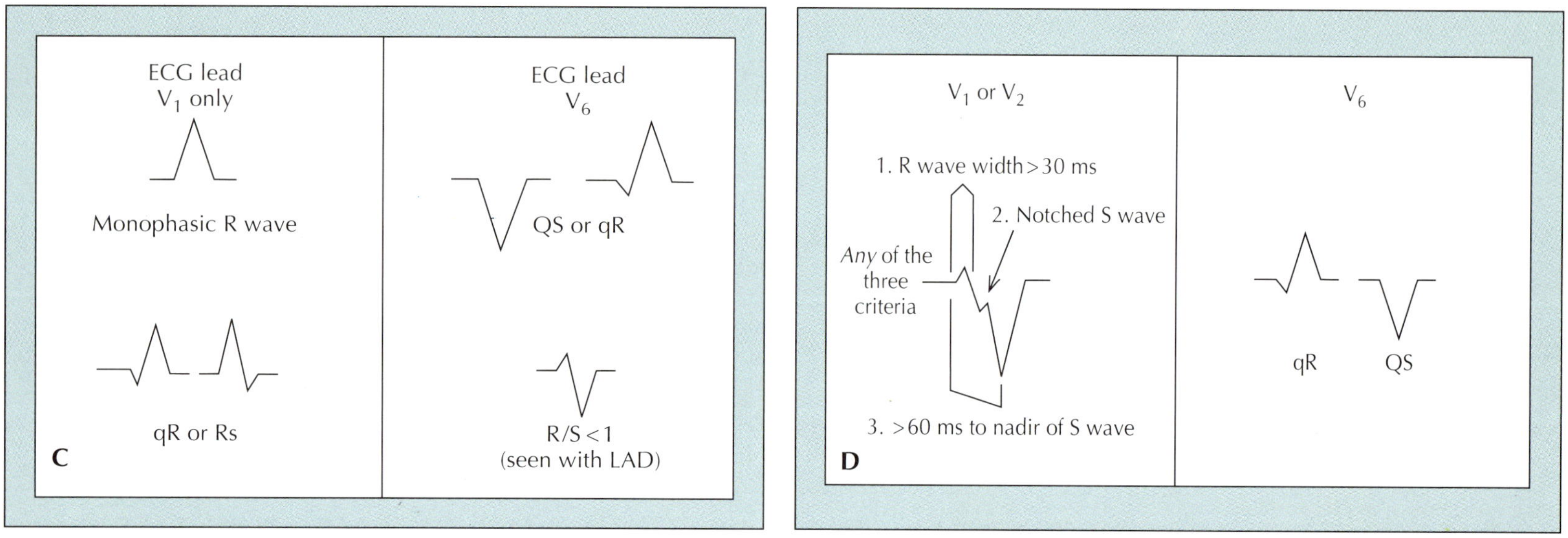

FIGURE 6-8. *(continued)* **C,** Morphologic criteria favoring diagnosis of VT in the presence of RBBB-type QRS complexes (dominant *positive* in V_1). Both leads must meet these criteria in order to diagnose VT. **D,** Morphologic criteria used to diagnose VT in the presence of LBBB-type QRS complexes (dominant *negative* in V_1). Both leads must meet these criteria to diagnose VT. (*Adapted from* Brugada and coworkers [4]; with permission.)

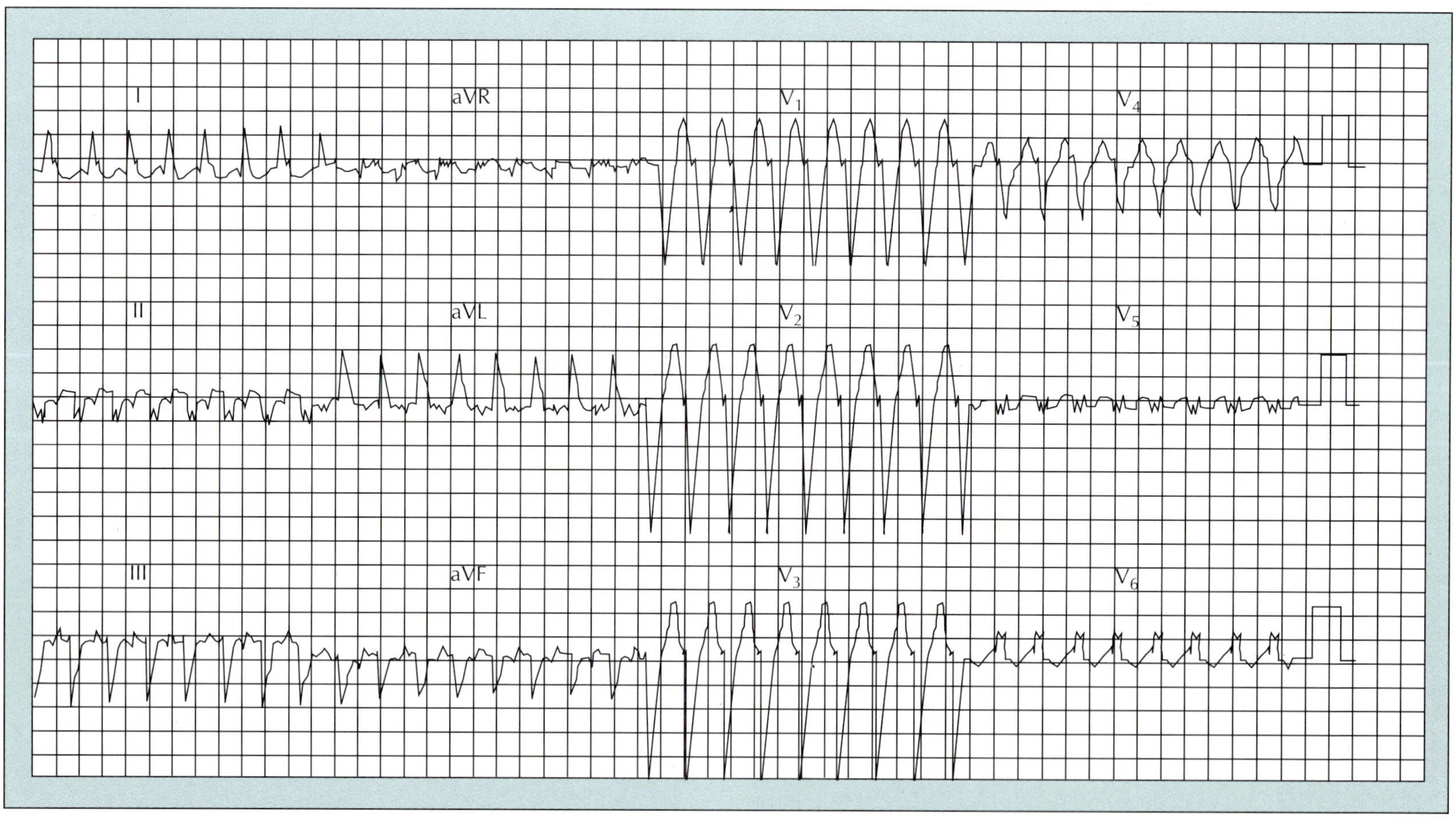

FIGURE 6-9. A 12-lead electrocardiogram from a 30-year-old man with multiple episodes of presyncope with wide complex tachycardia and left bundle branch morphology. Criteria for supraventricular tachycardia with aberrant conduction are present, including no atrioventricular dissociation, rapid initial deflection in V_1 and V_2, and upright complex in V_6.

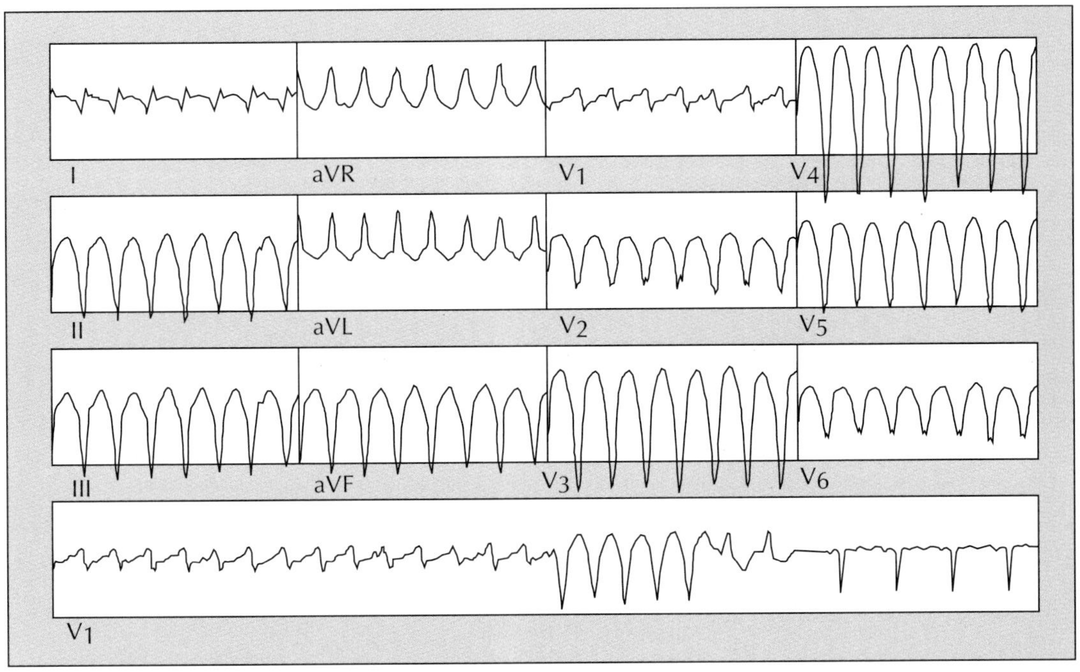

FIGURE 6-10. A 12-lead electrocardiogram (ECG) from a 60-year-old woman with an inferior wall myocardial infarction from 10 years earlier. The patient presented with mild shortness of breath but denied palpitations or chest pain. The ECG shows a wide complex tachycardia (WCT) with left bundle branch morphology. Morphologic criteria for monomorphic ventricular tachycardia are met. The rate is slower and symptoms are less prominent than in Fig. 6-9. Neither the presence of tachycardia nor the degree of symptoms is reliable in determining the mechanism of WCT.

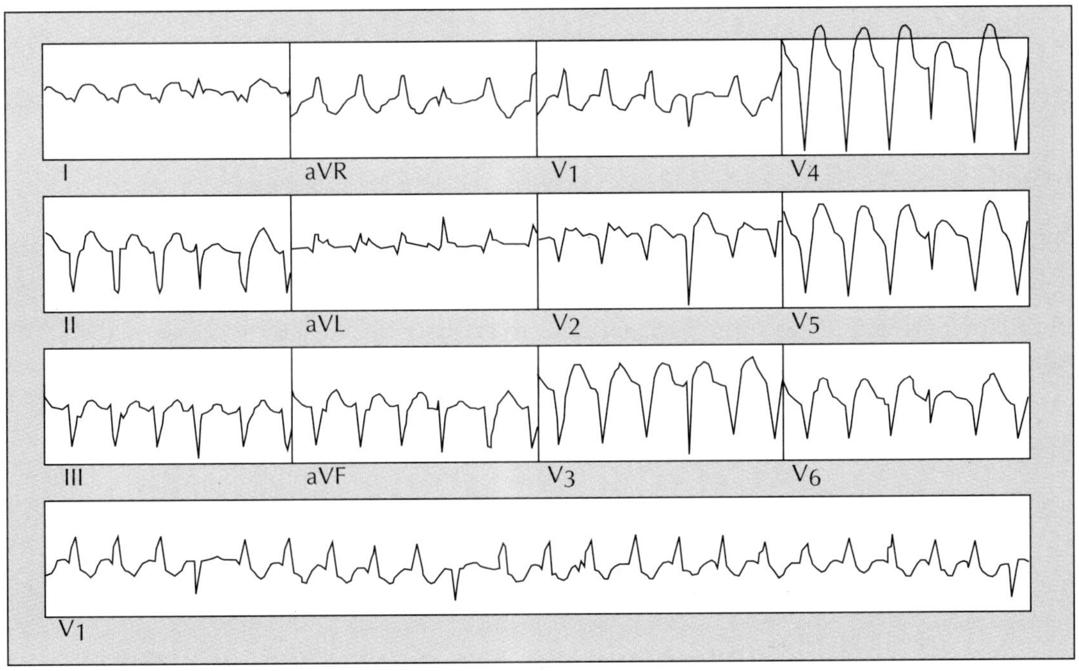

FIGURE 6-11. A 12-lead electrocardiogram showing a wide complex tachycardia at 140 bpm in a 65-year-old man with prior myocardial infarction. Note the presence of several narrow complex beats (*eg,* the fourth and tenth beats on the bottom strip). These sinus capture beats make the diagnosis of ventricular tachycardia very likely.

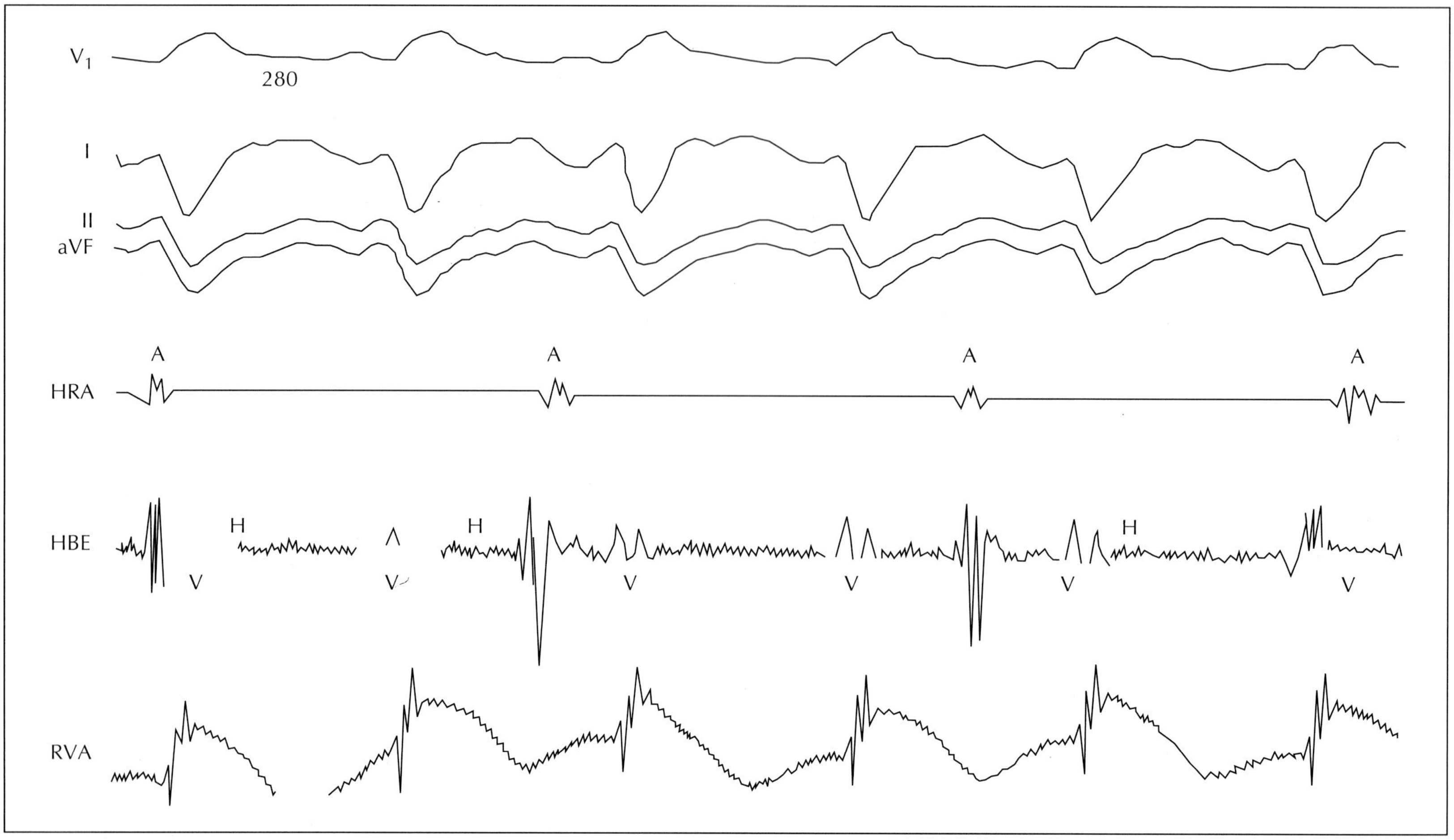

FIGURE 6-12. Electrophysiologic study confirming a diagnosis of ventricular tachycardia in a patient presenting with wide complex tachycardia of unclear mechanism. Shown are surface leads V_1, I, II, and aVF, along with intracardiac recordings from the high right atrium (HRA), His bundle (HBE), and right ventricular apex (RVA). During tachycardia at cycle length 280 ms (214 bpm), the signal from the HRA is dissociated from the tachycardia and occurs at a much slower rate (labeled *A*). Thus, the possibility of supraventricular tachycardia with aberration is essentially eliminated. H—His bundle; V—ventricle.

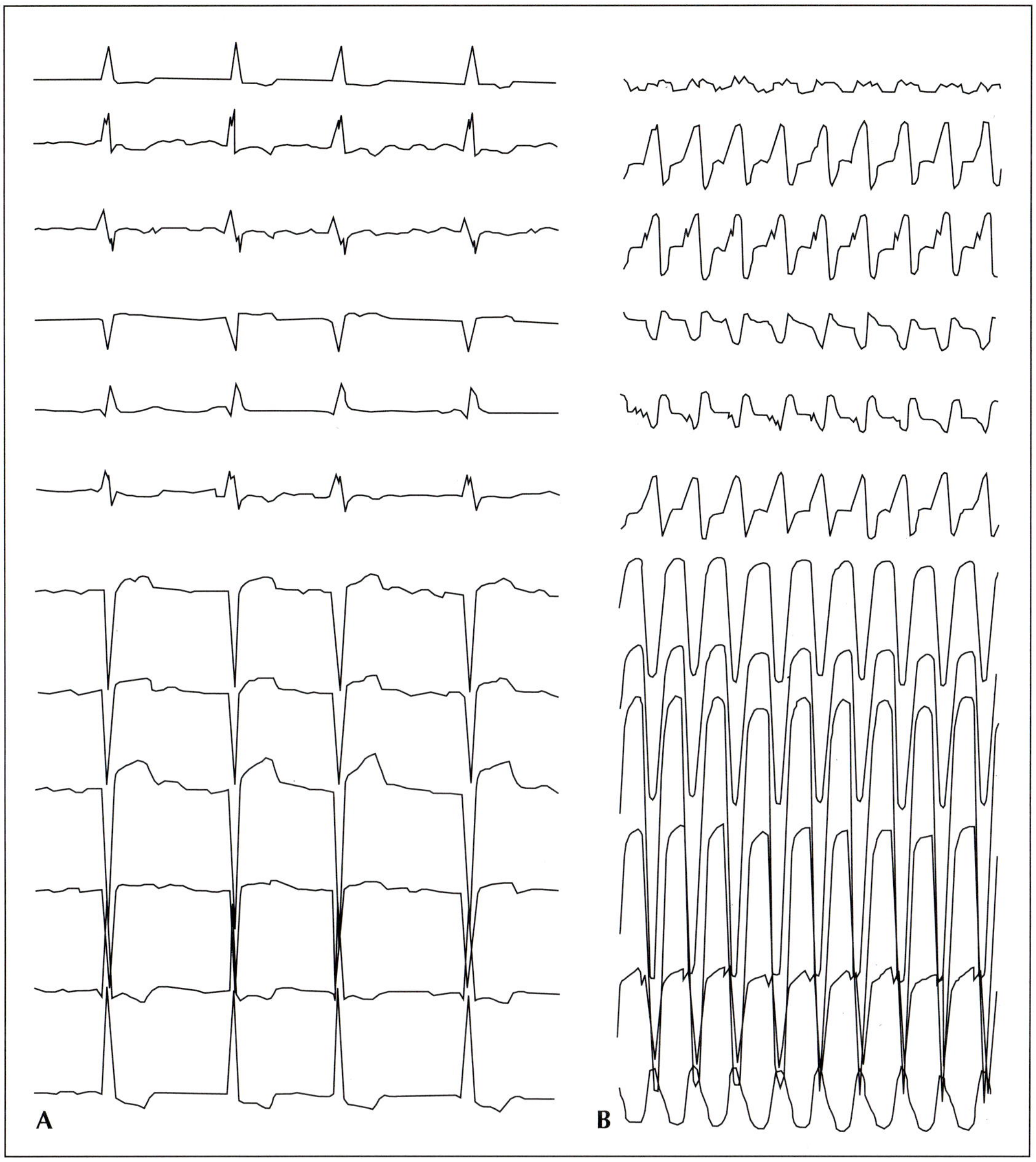

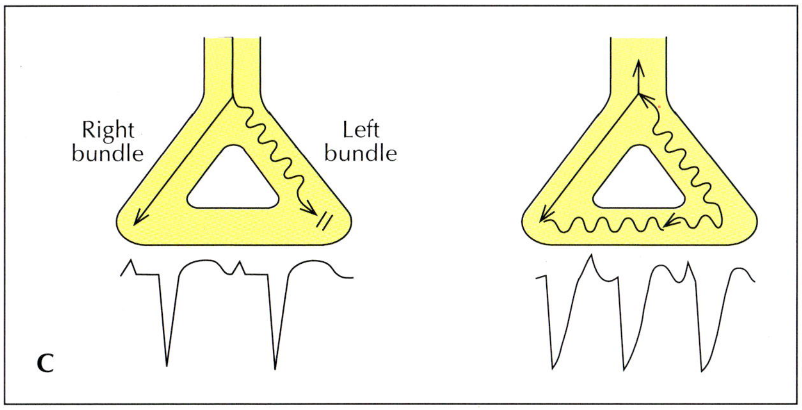

FIGURE 6-13. Aborted sudden death in a 65-year-old man. The patient had an ischemic cardiomyopathy with a left ventricular ejection fraction of 20%, although myocardial infarction was ruled out and he had no current signs of ischemia. **A,** The 12-lead electrocardiogram (ECG) shows sinus rhythm with an incomplete left bundle branch block.

B, At electrophysiologic (EP) testing, a wide complex tachycardia was induced at the rate of 250 bpm, which was accompanied by almost immediate loss of consciousness requiring cardioversion. The QRS morphology of the tachycardia is similar to, although slightly wider than, sinus rhythm, so a diagnosis of supraventricular tachycardia with aberration might be considered. However, ECG analysis confirmed a diagnosis of bundle branch (so-called macro reentrant) ventricular tachycardia (BBR-VT).

C, Pathophysiology includes a diseased left bundle (LB) and ventricular muscle. During tachycardia, an impulse proceeds down the right bundle (RB; hence the left bundle morphology), across the diseased intraventricular system, and up the LB. Because the His-Purkinje system is involved, these tachycardias are almost always quite rapid (> 200 bpm) and patients with BBR-VT present with syncope or aborted sudden death. Hallmarks include LB intraventricular conduction defect in sinus, LB morphology in VT, idiopathic or ischemic dilated cardiomyopathy, long His to ventricle (HV) interval at EP study, and importantly, BBR-VT that can be cured with radiofrequency catheter ablation of the RB. A pacemaker usually is not required.

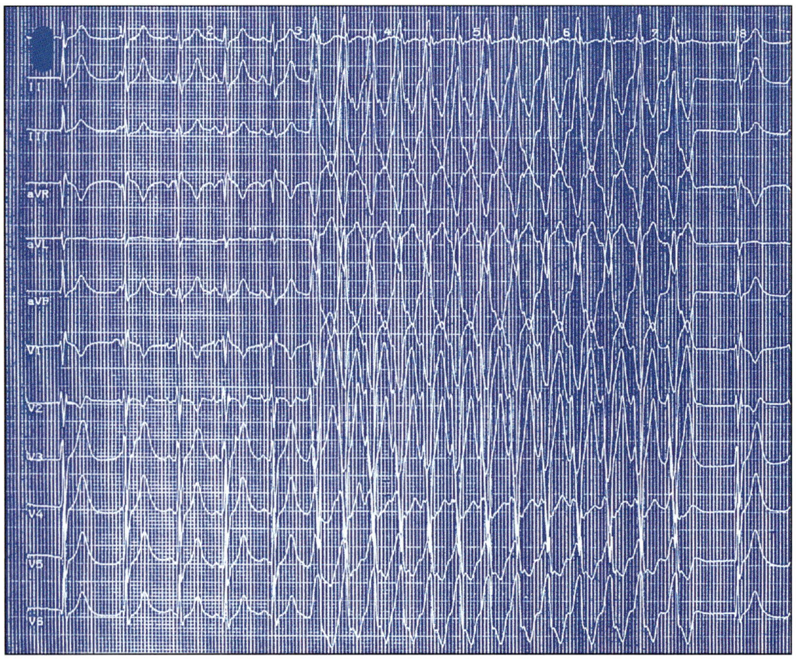

FIGURE 6-14. A 12-lead electrocardiogram from a 26-year-old woman with exercise-induced palpitations. She has paroxysmal wide complex tachycardia of left bundle morphology. Evaluation showed no evidence of structural heart disease. The diagnosis is idiopathic ventricular tachycardia (VT), or so-called benign, repetitive monomorphic VT. The origin is generally in the right ventricular outflow tract. Although the exact mechanism is unknown, there is evidence for a focal site of abnormal automaticity or triggered activity. These tachycardias sometimes respond to β- or calcium-channel–blocking drugs. In refractory cases, catheter ablation (*see* Fig. 6-15) can be considered.

THERAPY FOR VENTRICULAR TACHYCARDIA

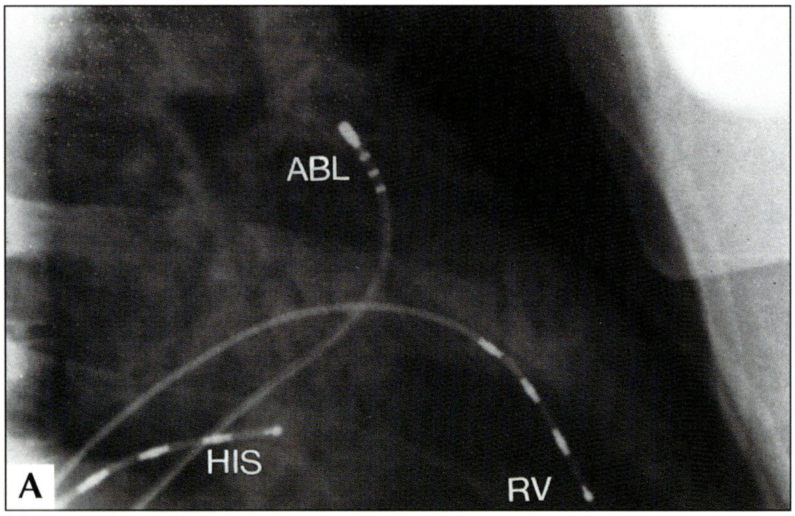

FIGURE 6-15. Catheter ablation in a patient with idiopathic right ventricular outflow tract (RVOT) ventricular tachycardia (VT). **A,** A right anterior oblique radiograph of catheters in position during electrophysiologic testing and ablation. A catheter is positioned in the RVOT just below the pulmonic valve at the site of ablation. **B,**Twelve-lead electrocardiogram. Ablation is targeted at the site where pacing produces a morphology (*right*) identical to that during spontaneous VT (*left*). (*continued*)

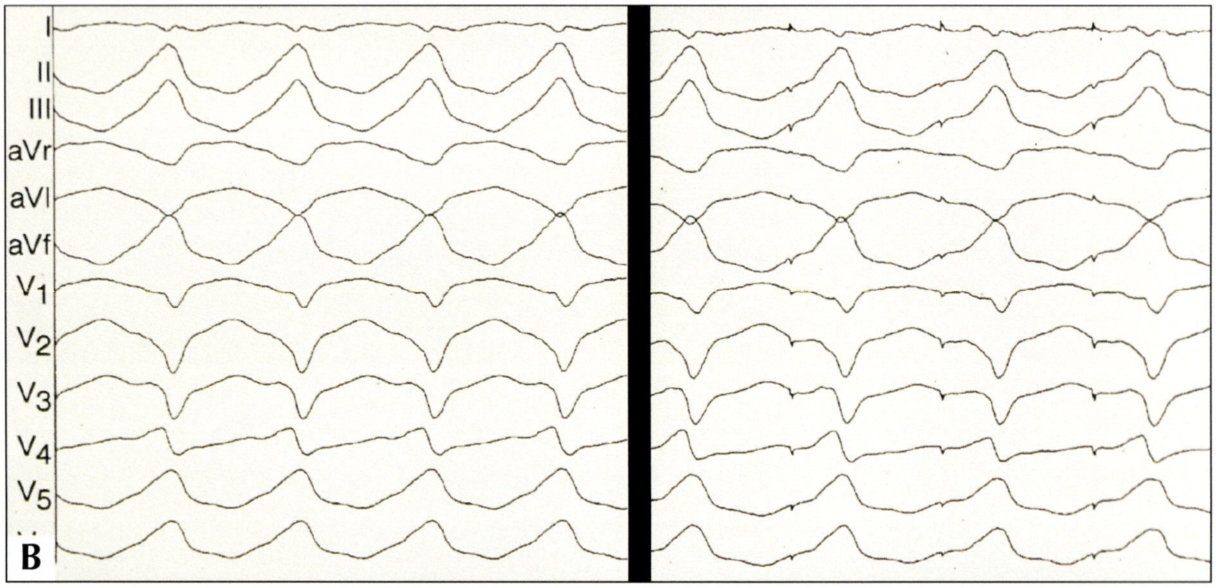

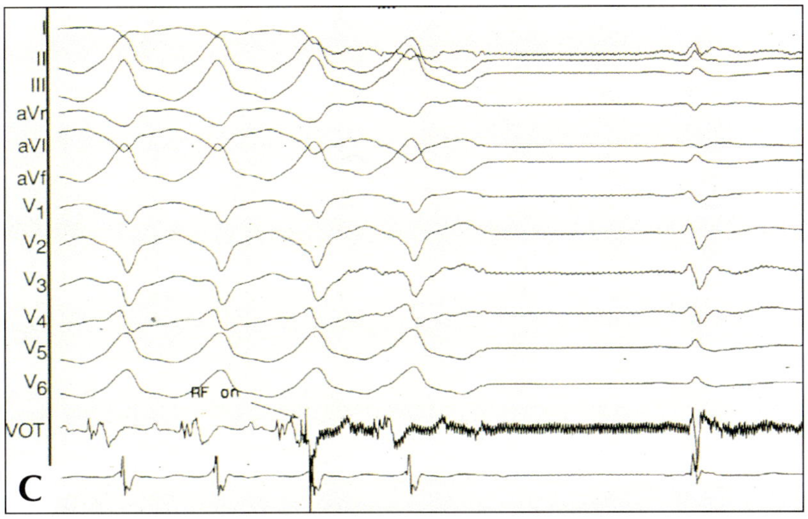

FIGURE 6-15. (*continued*) **C,** Shortly after radiofrequency energy is delivered to the RVOT, there is abrupt termination of tachycardia, and long-term resolution without medication has been achieved. ABL—tip-deflectable catheter, HIS—His bundle catheter; RV—right ventricular apex catheter.

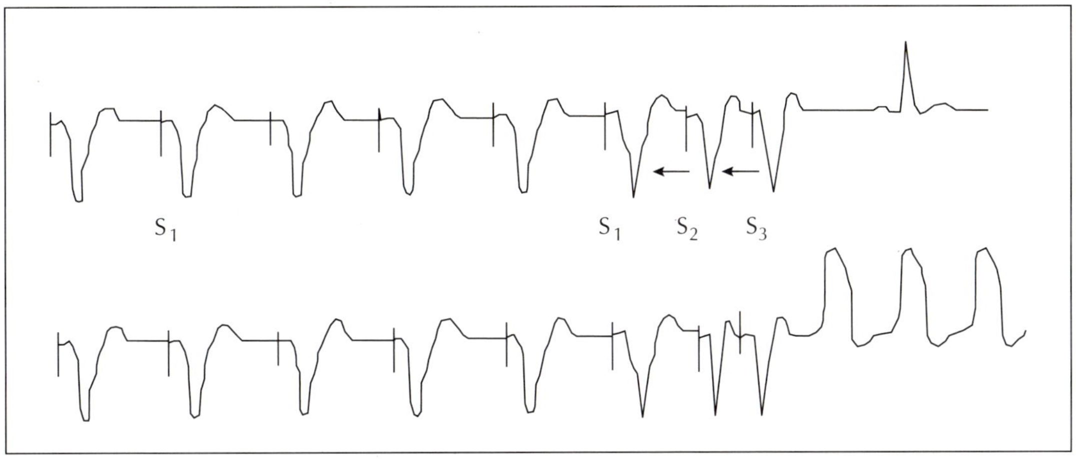

FIGURE 6-16. Programmed electrical stimulation (PES). PES can be used in the diagnosis and management of ventricular tachycardia (VT) by inserting a catheter into the right ventricle. Although this is the typical application, the left ventricle can also be used. Eight or more beats at a basic drive rate (S_1) are introduced, followed by one, two, or three premature extra beats (S_2,S_3,S_4). These extra beats are placed at programmed intervals, and the intervals are shortened by scanning diastole until refractoriness. This technique has a sensitivity and specificity of over 90% for the induction of reentrant sustained monomorphic VT in patients with healed myocardial infarction (MI). However, it is not sensitive in patients whose VT is due to acute MI, reversible ischemia, electrolyte disturbances, or other etiologies. The induction of nonsustained VT, polymorphic VT, or ventricular fibrillation has reduced specificity, especially if induced with aggressive stimulation with very early premature beats. Repeat PES following drug administration in patients with inducible sustained VT may be used to help predict drug efficacy.

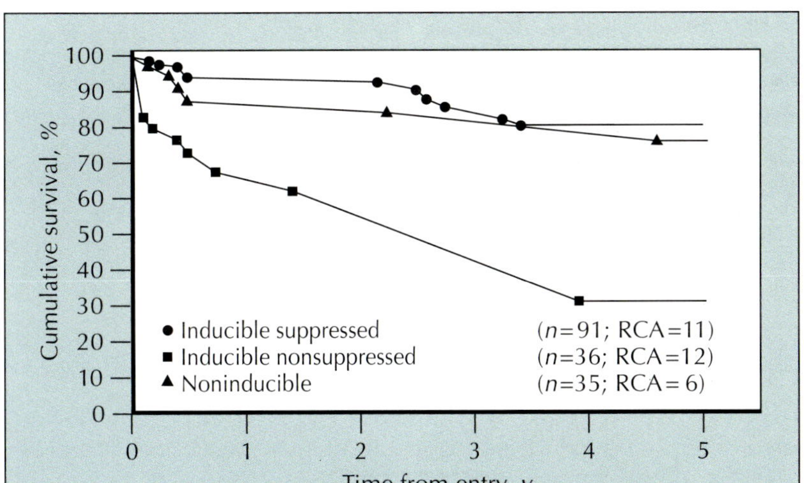

FIGURE 6-17. Cumulative survival free of cardiac arrest in 166 patients with aborted sudden death based on the results of electrophysiology (EP)-guided drug therapy. The group who had inducible ventricular tachycardia (VT) or ventricular fibrillation (VF) at baseline and whose VT was rendered noninducible by drug therapy at repeat EP testing had the best outcome. Those with VT or VF in whom no drug could suppress inducibility had a poor outcome in this study, which was done before the use of implantable defibrillators became widespread. Even in those treated with a drug predicted to be effective, the actual sudden death rate at 5 years was 15%, prompting the search for better antiarrhythmic drugs and the widespread use of nonpharmacologic therapy, especially implantable defibrillators. RCA—number of patients with recurrent cardiac arrest in each group. (*Adapted from* Wilber and coworkers [5]; with permission.)

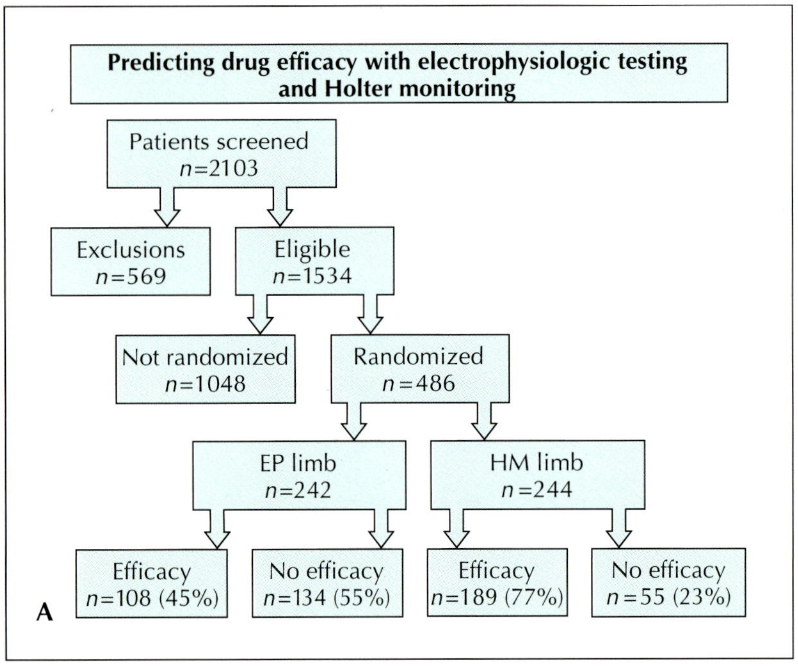

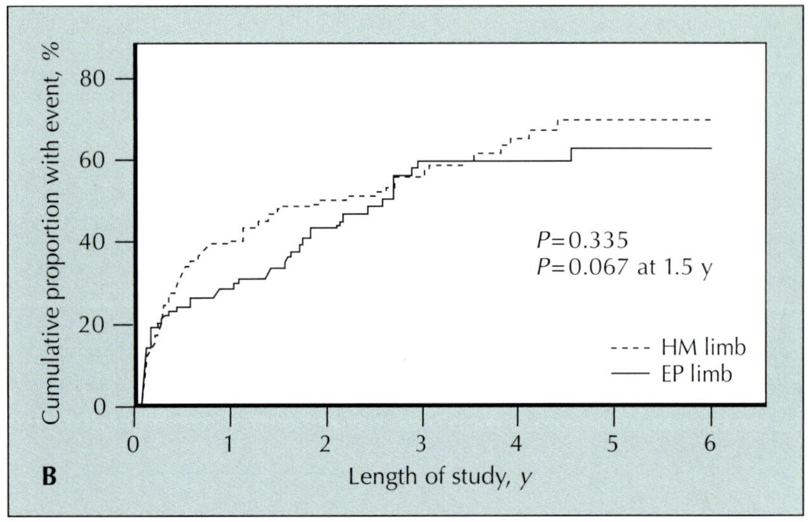

C. SUMMARY OF EVENT RATES FOR SUBJECTS WITH PREDICTED DRUG EFFICACY

ENDPOINT, %	YEAR 1	YEAR 3	YEAR 6
Recurrence of arrhythmia	36±3	59±4	68±4
Sudden death	7±2	13±3	18±4
Cardiac death	10±2	16±3	24±5
Death	12±2	24±4	35±6

FIGURE 6-18. A, The Electrophysiologic Study Versus Electrocardiographic Monitoring (ESVEM) trial. The recently completed ESVEM trial attempted to determine whether electrophysiologic (EP) testing or Holter monitoring (HM) was best in predicting drug efficacy in patients with sustained ventricular tachycardia (VT) or those surviving cardiac arrest [6,7]. Of 2103 patients screened, 486 were randomized to HM or EP testing to guide antiarrhythmic drug therapy. HM had a greater chance of predicting antiarrhythmic drug efficacy, defined as 100% suppression of runs of VT greater than 15 beats, 90% reduction of shorter runs, 80% of pairs, and 70% of ventricular ectopic beats and absence of exercise-induced VT ($P < 0.0001$).

B, In 297 subjects for whom drug efficacy was predicted and who were censored on drug discontinuation, the rate of arrhythmia recurrence was the same, regardless of the method of guiding therapy. In both cases the risk of recurrent VT was approximately 70% at 6 years. **C**, The actuarial rates for arrhythmia recurrence and sudden, cardiac, and total death are shown for those patients treated with a drug predicted to be effective by EP study or HM. Treatment with amiodarone or nonpharmacologic therapy (surgery, ablation, or implanted devices) was not an option in the ESVEM trial. The ESVEM trial has taught us that serial drug testing may not be the best approach for patients with aborted sudden death. Standard current practice for patients with sudden death or sustained VT not due to a reversible cause is EP testing to confirm the diagnosis, followed by a single-drug trial with sotalol or amiodarone, then nonpharmacologic therapy if drug treatment fails. The results of a randomized trial (*see* Fig. 6-24*B*) will be required to determine the most effective and cost-effective way to manage sudden death survivors and VT patients.

TREATMENT OPTIONS FOR SYMPTOMATIC SUSTAINED VT OR VF NOT DUE TO A REVERSIBLE CAUSE

NO STRUCTURAL HEART DISEASE
Drugs
Calcium-channel blockers
β-blockers
Class I or III agents
RF catheter ablation

IDIOPATHIC CARDIOMYOPATHY
Drugs (especially amiodarone)
Implanted ATP/defibrillator
Catheter ablation for bundle branch reentrant VT, if present

PRIOR MYOCARDIAL INFARCTION
Drugs
Class I or III, guided by electrophysiologic testing or Holter monitor
Nonpharmacologic
Map-guided surgery
Catheter ablation
Implanted antitachycardic pacer/defibrillator

LONG QT SYNDROME
β-blockers and dual-chamber pacing to shorten QT interval
Stellate ganglionectomy
Implanted defibrillator and pacing

FIGURE 6-19. Treatment options for patients with ventricular tachycardia (VT) or ventricualr fibrillation (VF). The therapy recommended depends on presentation and substrate. ATP—antitachycardia pacing; RF—radiofrequency.

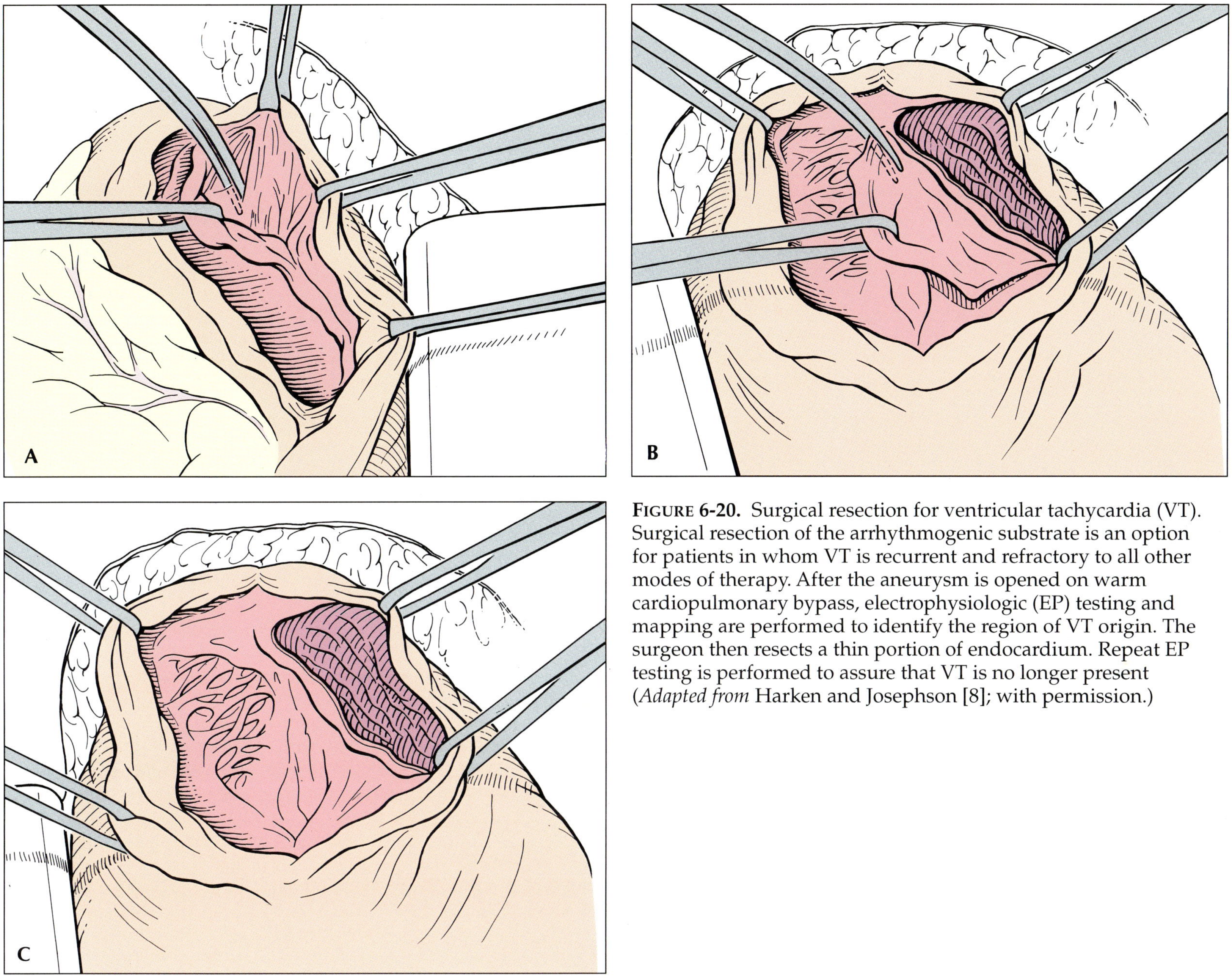

Figure 6-20. Surgical resection for ventricular tachycardia (VT). Surgical resection of the arrhythmogenic substrate is an option for patients in whom VT is recurrent and refractory to all other modes of therapy. After the aneurysm is opened on warm cardiopulmonary bypass, electrophysiologic (EP) testing and mapping are performed to identify the region of VT origin. The surgeon then resects a thin portion of endocardium. Repeat EP testing is performed to assure that VT is no longer present (*Adapted from* Harken and Josephson [8]; with permission.)

RESULTS OF SURGERY FOR VT

STUDY	PROCEDURES	PATIENTS, *n*	HOSPITAL MORTALITY, %	SURVIVORS, *n* (NO INDUCIBLE OR SPONTANEOUS VT)	TOTAL	SUCCESS RATE, %	ESTIMATED SURVIVAL, %(Y)
Borggrefe *et al.* [9]	SER, EEM, Cryoablation	665	12	244	330	74	57(5)
Miller *et al.* [10]; Hargrove and Miller [11]	SER, Cryoablation	269	15	156	229	68	60(5)
McGiffin *et al.* [12]	EEM, SER, Cryoablation	123	23	54	87	62	33(5)
Swerdlow *et al.* [13]	SER, Cryoablation, EEM	105	16	54	79	68	60(4)
Ostermeyer *et al.* [14]	EEM, SER	93	6	50	84	59	70(5)
Haines *et al.* [15]; Hobson *et al.* [16]	SER, Cryoablation	92	6	75	86	87	70(5)
Cox [17]	SER, Cryoablation	65	14	55	56	98	68(5)
Willems [18]	SER, Cryoablation	64	18	NR	NR	NR	67(2)
Lawrie *et al.* [19]	SER, Cryoablation	80	13	60	70	85	58(3)

FIGURE 6-21. Results of surgery for ventricular tachycardia (VT). From the results of selected reported series consisting of more than 50 patients being treated for VT, perioperative mortality is approximately 15%, and the success rate is 70% to 90% in those surviving hospitalization [9–19]. EEM—encircling endocardial myotomy; NR—not reported; SER—subendocardial resection; VT—ventricular tachycardia. (*Adapted from* DiMarco [20]; with permission.)

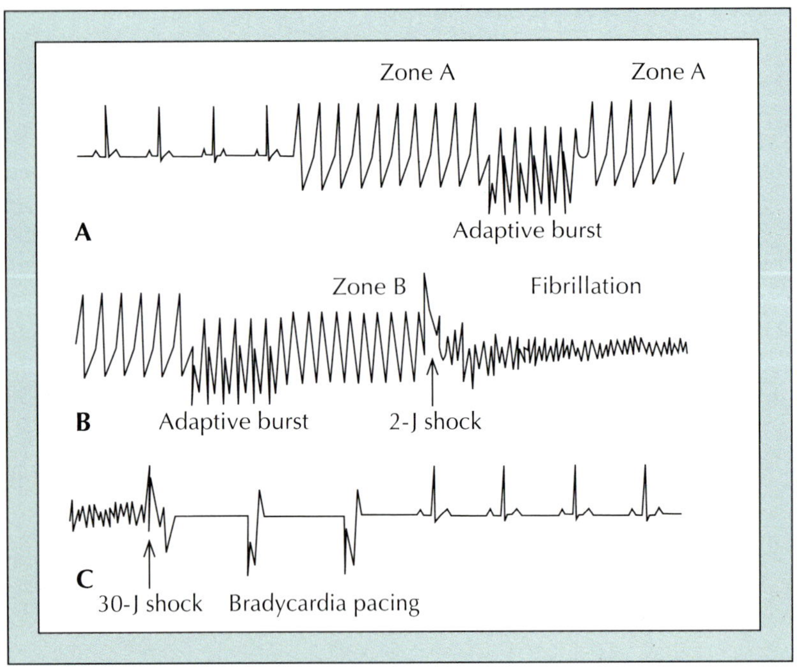

FIGURE 6-22. Incorporation of tiered or *zone* therapy in newer implantable devices for selective antitachycardia pacing, lower energy cardioversion, or high-energy defibrillation. Recordings show idealized tiered antitachycardia therapy. **A,** Onset of ventricular tachycardia (VT) with slower rate (zone A). Overdrive pacing is initiated with an adaptive burst, but tachycardia resumes with the same rate. **B,** Repeat burst pacing leads to acceleration of VT rate (zone B), and a low-energy (2 J) cardioversion shock leads to ventricular fibrillation (VF). **C,** VF is effectively terminated with 30-J shock delivery. (*Adapted from* Akhtar and coworkers [21]; with permission.)

DEVICES FOR TACHYCARDIA: INDICATIONS FOR AICD

Failure of diagnosis
- Sudden death, noninducible, negative Holter monitor recording

Failure of therapy
- Clinical recurrence on a drug predicted effective by electrophysiologic testing
- Clinical recurrence on amiodarone
- Clinical recurrence after surgery or ablation

Predicted failure of therapy
- Still inducible on type I drug
- Amiodarone with multiple risk factors
- Inducible after surgery or ablation

FIGURE 6-23. Indications for using automatic implantable cardioverter/defibrillator (AICD).

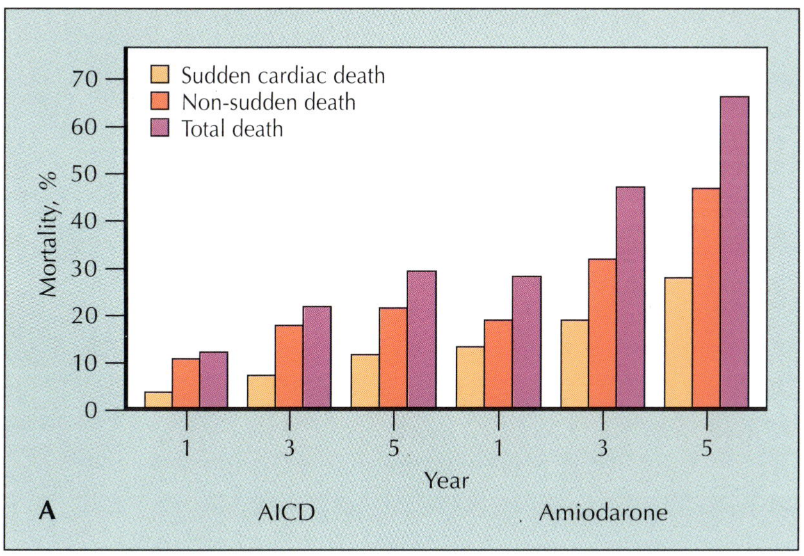

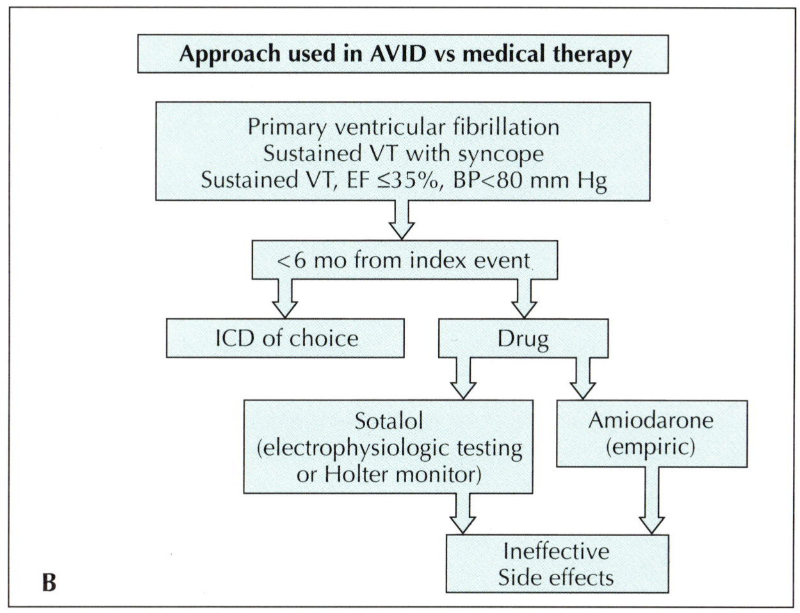

FIGURE 6-24. Automatic implantable cardioverter/defibrillator (AICD) versus drug therapy. The results of studies shown in **A** indicate that AICD therapy is associated with a lower incidence of sudden and nonsudden death compared with treatment with amiodarone, which is probably the most effective antiarrhythmic drug available. Caution must be exercised, however, in comparing studies that probably did not enroll comparable patient groups. It is still unknown whether amiodarone (or sotalol, another effective class III drug) or AICD is best in a matched cohort of patients with sustained ventricular tachycardia (VT) or ventricular fibrillation (VF). **B,** The Antiarrhythmic Drug Versus Implanted Defribrillator (AVID) trial, sponsored by the National Institutes of Health (NIH), is underway to evaluate this issue. Patients are randomized to an implanted cardioverter device (ICD; using thoracotomy or nonthoracotomy, tiered therapy or not, at the investigators' discretion) versus medical therapy, either amiodarone or sotalol. Both efficacy and cost data will be acquired. The results of this study may have profound implications for the way VT and VF are managed in the next decade. BP—blood pressure; EF—ejection fraction. (Part A *adapted from* Winkle [22] and Herre [23]; with permission.)

References

1. Binah O, Rosen MR: Mechanisms of ventricular arrhythmias. *Circulation* 1992, 85(suppl I): I-25–I-31.
2. Wit AW, Josephson ME: Fractionated electrograms and continuous electrical activity: fact or artefact? In *Cardiac Electrophysiology and Arrhythmias.* Edited by Zipes DP, Jalife J. New York: Grune and Stratton; 1985:350–361.
3. Cardinal R, Vermeulen M, Shenasa M, *et al.*: Anisotropic conduction and functional dissociation of ischemic tissue during reentrant ventricular tachycardia in canine myocardial infarction. *Circulation* 1988, 77:1162–1176.
4. Brugada P, Brugada J, Mont L, *et al.*: A new approach to the differential diagnosis of a regular tachycardia with a wide QRS complex. *Circulation* 1991, 83:1649–1659.
5. Wilber DJ, Garan H, Kelly E, *et al.*: Out-of-hospital cardiac arrest: role of electrophysiologic testing in the prediction of long-term outcome. *N Engl J Med* 1988, 318:19–24.
6. Mason JW: A comparison of electrophysiologic testing with Holter monitoring to predict antiarrhythimic-drug efficacy for ventricular tachyarrhythmias. Electrophysiologic Study Versus Electrocardiographic Monitoring (ESVEM) Investigators. *N Engl J Med* 1993, 329:445–451.
7. Mason JW: A comparison of seven antiarrhythmic drugs in patients with ventricular tachyarrhythmias. Electrophysiologic Study Versus Electrocardiographic Monitoring (ESVEM) Investigators. *N Engl J Med* 1993, 329:452–458.
8. Harken AH, Josephson ME: Surgical management of ventricular tachycardia. In *Tachycardias: Mechanisms, Diagnosis, and Treatment.* Edited by Josephson ME and Wellens HJ. Philadelphia: Lea & Febiger; 1982: 475.
9. Borggrefe M, Podczek A, Ostermeyer J, *et al.*: Long-term results of electrophysiologically guided antitachycardia surgery in ventricular arrhythmias: a collaborative report on 665 patients. In *Nonpharmacological Therapy of Tachyarrhythmias.* Edited by Breithardt G, Borggrefe M, Zipes DP. Mount Kisco, New York: Futura Publishing Co., Inc; 1987:109–132.
10. Miller JM, Keinzle MG, Harken AH, *et al.*: Subendocardial resection for ventricular tachycardia: predictors of surgical success. *Circulation* 1984, 70:624–631.
11. Hargrove WC, Miller JM: Risk stratification and management of patients with recurrent ventricular tachycardia and other malignant ventricular arrhythmias. *Circulation* 1989, 79(suppl I): I-178–I-181.
12. McGiffin DC, Kirklin JK, Plumb VJ, *et al.*: Relief of life-threatening ventricular tachycardia and survival after direct operation. *Circulation* 1987, 76(suppl V): V-93–V-103.
13. Swerdlow CD, Mason JW, Stinson EB, *et al.*: Results of operations for ventricular tachycardia in 105 patients. *J Thorac Cardiovasc Surg* 1986, 92:105–113.
14. Ostermeyer J, Borggrefe M, Breithardt G, *et al.*: Direct operations for the management of life-threatening ischemic ventricular tachycardia. *J Thorac Cardiovasc Surg* 1987, 94:848–865.
15. Haines DE, Lerman BB, Kron IL, DiMarco JP: Surgical ablation of ventricular tachycardia with sequential map-guided subendocardial resection: electrophysiological assessment and long-term follow-up. *Circulation* 1988, 77:131–141.
16. Hobson CE, DiMarco JP, Haines DE, *et al.*: The influence of cardiogenic shock on outcome in directed resection for ventricular tachycardia. *J Thorac Cardiovasc Surg* 1991, 102:348–354.
17. Cox JL: Patient selection criteria and results of surgery for refractory ischemic ventricular tachycardia. *Circulation* 1989, 79(suppl I):I-163–I-177.
18. Willems AR: Ventricular tachycardia or ventricular fibrillation late after myocardial infarction [Dissertation]. Dordrecht, The Netherlands: University of Amsterdam; 1990:145.
19. Lawrie GM, Pacifico A, Kaushik R, *et al.*: Factors predictive of results of direct ablative operations for drug-refractory ventricular tachycardia: analysis of 80 patients. *J Thorac Cardiovasc Surg* 1991, 101:44–55.
20. DiMarco JP: Management of sudden cardiac death survivors: role of surgical and catheter ablation. *Circulation* 1992, 85(suppl I): I-125–I-130.
21. Akhtar M, Garan H, Lehmann H, Troup PJ: Sudden cardiac death: management of high-risk patients. *Ann Intern Med* 1991, 114:499–512.
22. Winkle RA, Mead RH, Ruder, *et al.*: Long-term outcome with the automatic implantable cardioverter-defibrillator. *J Am Coll Cardiol* 1989, 13:1353–1361.
23. Herre JM, Sauve MJ, Malone P, *et al.*: Long-term results of amiodarone therapy in patients with recurrent sustained ventricular tachycardia or ventricular fibrillation. *J Am Coll Cardiol* 1989, 13:442–449.

THE LONG QT SYNDROME

7

CHAPTER

Harlan R. Grogin

A long QT interval or prolonged QTU interval is responsible for polymorphic ventricular tachycardia (PMVT) in patients with the congenital or acquired long QT syndromes (LQTS). The QT interval is an electrocardiographic measurement of the time between the earliest ventricular activation and termination of ventricular recovery. It is influenced by adrenergic stimuli, heart rate, and drugs. Because it includes ventricular depolarization, the QT interval is limited at times as a measurement for ventricular repolarization. It also may be difficult to distinguish the terminal portion of the T waves from U waves. Another limitation is that a single ECG lead may not be sensitive to nonuniform recovery of excitation in local cardiac regions. In this chapter, we review congenital and acquired LQTS.

Congenital LQTS was first reported by Jervell and Lange Nielson [1] who described a syndrome of sudden death in deaf children. A similar syndrome without deafness was reported by Romano *et al.* [2]. Patients may be completely asymptomatic, with the only abnormality being prolongation of the QT interval. Symptoms may include palpitations, syncope, and sudden death. The mechanism for the long QT interval includes two major theories. One hypothesis is that there is cardiac sympathetic imbalance, an explanation based on experimental observations [3–5]. The other mechanism is a primary cell membrane defect involving defective control of cardiac ion channels.

Future research on the genetic mechanism and its effect on channel expression may become the way to identify these patients as well as provide a target for therapeutic interventions. Therapy ranges from implantation of the cardioverter defibrillator in very high-risk patients to using dual chamber pacing in combination with β-blocking drugs.

Compared with congenital LQTS, acquired LQTS is usually due to drugs but may result from electrolyte imbalances or intrinsic heart disease. In contrast to PMVT associated with congenital LQTS, in which there may be no pause prior to the episode, in acquired LQTS, PMVT is usually preceded by a pause, thus the designation "pause dependent." The mechanism for PMVT associated with the acquired LQTS is thought to be related to after-depolarizations. Therapy is focused on reducing the QT interval by pacing and, most importantly, by withholding the offending agents. Intravenous magnesium also may be effective in some of these patients [6].

Mechanisms and Manifestations

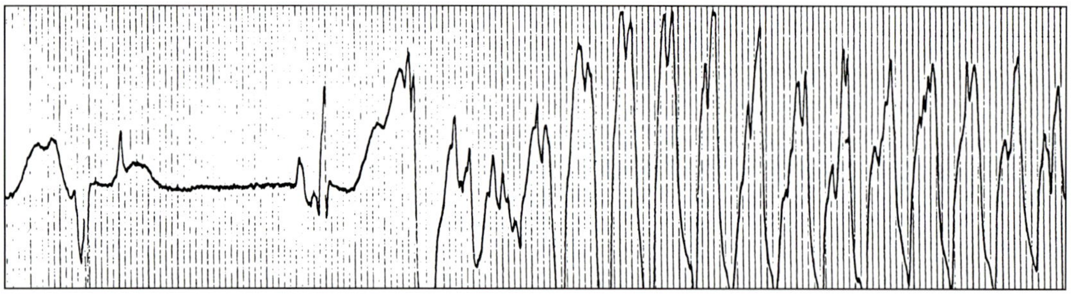

Figure 7-1. Polymorphic ventricular tachycardia. Polymorphic ventricular tachycardia (PMVT), as depicted in this electrocardiogram, presents with consecutive complexes of more than one morphology. PMVT is frequently initiated by a premature ventricular complex following a pause. The pause generally follows late cycle premature complexes. The T wave of the beat following the pause may exhibit bizarre changes in amplitude and morphology. Torsades de pointes is a specific form of PMVT associated with a prolonged QT interval and characteristic cyclic changes in amplitude and polarity of the QRS complex. Whereas torsades de pointes implies an associated long QT interval, PMVT may still occur in the setting of a normal QT interval. PMVT with a normal QT interval is found in patients with coronary artery disease and ischemia or in patients with normal hearts (exercise induced, with coronary spasm, or pause dependent).

CAUSES OF PMVT WITH LONG QT INTERVAL

ACQUIRED

Drugs
- Antiarrhythmic drugs (quinidine, procainamide, disopyramide, amiodarone, sotalol, bepridil)
- Psychotropic drugs (phenothiazine, tricyclic antidepressants)
- Antimicrobial drugs (amantadine, chloroquine, pentamidine, erythromycin)

Organophosphorous insecticide poisoning

Liquid protein diets

Electrolyte imbalances
- Hypokalemia
- Hypomagnesemia
- Hypocalcemia

Antihistamines
- terfenadine
- astemizole

Intrinsic heart disease
- Mitral valve prolapse
- Myocarditis
- Myocardial ischemia (coronary induced or spasm)
- Severe congestive heart failure

Polymorphic VT in normal hearts with normal QT intervals
- Exercise induced
- Spasm induced
- Idiopathic

IDIOPATHIC LONG QT SYNDROME

Lange-Jervell-Nielson Syndrome

Romano-Ward Syndrome

Sporadic

Figure 7-2. Polymorphic ventricular tachycardia (PMVT) associated with a long QT interval can be separated into idiopathic (congenital or sporadic) and acquired forms. The hereditary forms are known as the long QT syndrome (LQTS). LQTS consists of patients at great risk after sudden cardiac death associated with prolonged QT intervals and may be inherited as an autosomal dominant trait without hearing loss (Romano-Ward syndrome) or an autosomal recessive trait with hearing loss (Jervell-Lange-Nielson syndrome). The syndrome should be suspected in children or young adults presenting with seizures, syncope, or aborted sudden death. Untreated patients face a very high risk for sudden cardiac death due to PMVT, which degenerates into ventricular fibrillation. A voluntary worldwide registry suggests that 75% of untreated patients will die suddenly. In contrast, those treated with β-blockers have a much improved prognosis but still face a 6% risk of sudden cardiac death. VT in the congenital form is frequently precipitated by sudden changes in sympathetic activity (adrenergic dependent) and is generally suppressed by β-adrenergic blockade. Acquired forms are much more common and are usually associated with precipitating factors such as drugs that prolong repolarization. The most common offenders are antiarrythmic agents, particularly those that prolong the action potential duration. The chief offenders appear to be the class IA drugs (quinidine, procainamide, disopyramide) or sotalol. Each of these agents prolongs the action potential duration by blocking the delayed rectifier potassium channels. These agents are usually, but not always, associated with QT prolongation, and the PMVT is almost always provoked by a preceding pause. Other drugs incriminated in the induction of PMVT include the tricyclic antidepressants as well as phenothiazine derivatives (i.e., thorazine or Mellaril). More recently, PMVT has been found to be associated with the use of terfenadine (Seldane) or astemizole (Hismanal). The parent compounds are associated with prolongation of the QT interval, but the metabolites are harmless. In patients with severe liver disease or in those with normal liver function exposed to drugs that impair the metabolism of these agents, resulting high levels of the parent compound may provoke PMVT. Common drugs that impair the metabolic breakdown of terfenadine include erythromycin or ketoconazole, and the latter drugs should not be used in combination with terfanedine.

The most important aspect of treatment of drug-induced PMVT depends on a proper diagnosis with prompt cessation of the offending drug. The diagnosis should be suspected if a patient treated with the above-mentioned drugs presents with syncope, seizures, or palpitations. Electrolyte abnormalities should be sought and corrected. If PMVT recurs, then use of a bolus infusion of magnesium (1 to 2 g over 10 min followed by continuous infusions) are indicated. The most effective acute therapy is use of a temporary transvenous cardiac pacemaker. The cardiac rate is adjusted to mitigate the length of the pause, which appears critical for PMVT induction. As the arrhythmia is brought under control, the paced rate is gradually reduced and the pacemaker ultimately removed.

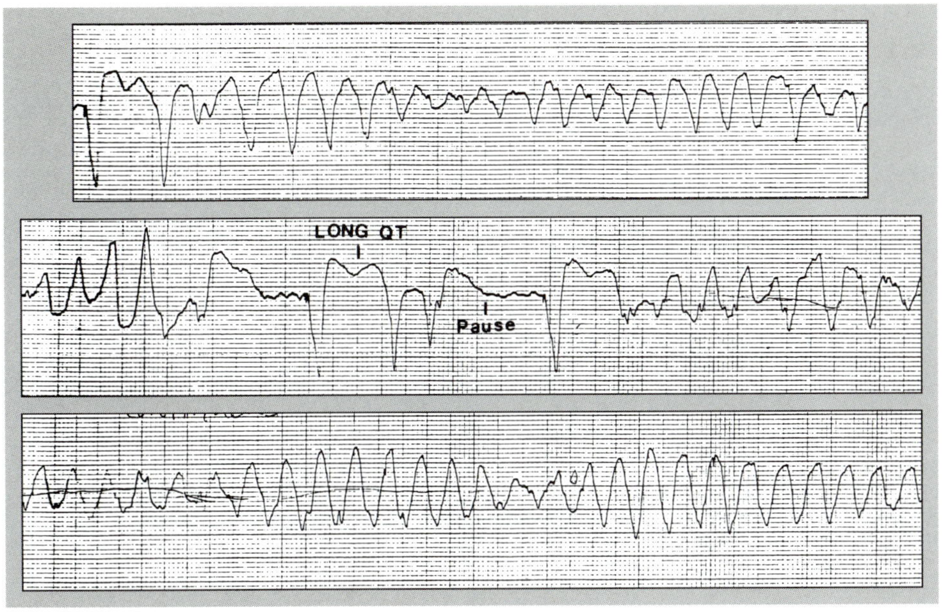

FIGURE 7-3. Torsades de pointes. When viewed in a single lead, torsades de pointes may appear monomorphic, thus multiple simultaneous leads should be obtained. The prolonged QT or QTU interval is the common denominator and may be congenital or acquired. In the top strip there is a polymorphic ventricular tachycardia that seems to undulate around a fixed baseline. The continuation of this strip is seen in the middle strip. Note that the arrhythmia self-terminates, a frequent characteristic of torsades de pointes. However, it is reinitiated after a characteristic pause followed by a shortly coupled premature ventricular complex. The arrythmia continues in the bottom strip with its undulating nature.

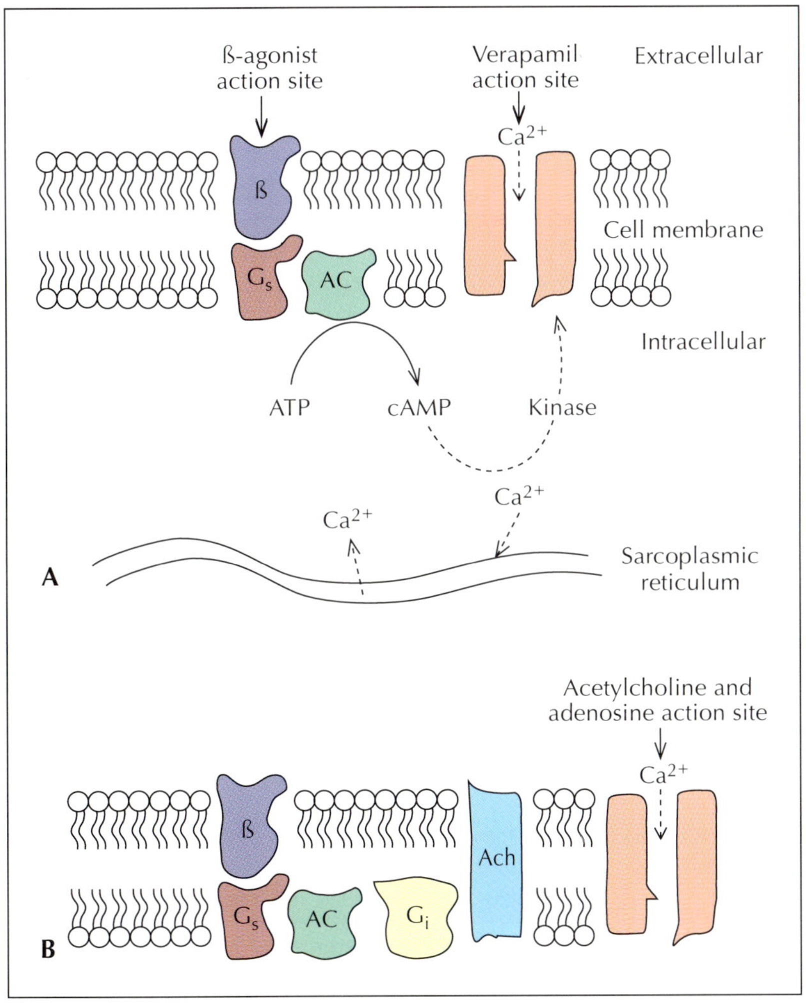

FIGURE 7-4. The mechanism for polymorphic ventricular tachycardia (PMVT) associated with the acquired long QT syndrome (LQTS). It is thought that the mechanism involved in PMVT associated with LQTS is related to after-depolarizations that cause triggered activity. Arrhythmias due to triggered activity may be related to intracellular calcium (Ca^{2+}). **A**, Catecholamines initiate triggered activity by stimulating β-receptors (β) which in turn increase cAMP through a stimulatory G protein (Gs) on adenylate cyclase (AC). The increased cAMP leads to an increase in the activation of a protein kinase, which phosphorylates the calcium channel. This results in an increase of calcium entering the cell. In turn, increased calcium concentration increases release of calcium from the sarcoplasmic reticulum. β-blockers inhibit this process by blocking the receptor. Verapamil blocks inward Ca^{2+} current, reducing intracellular Ca^{2+} and in turn triggered arrhythmias from after-depolarizations.

B, Adenosine and acetylcholine inhibit the formation of cAMP. This explains why adenosine may aid in abolishing arrhythmias due to triggered activity. Gi—inhibitory proteins. (Note: Similar Fig. 2-23 is used in the discussion of the action of Class II antiarrhythmics.) Ach—acetylcholine.

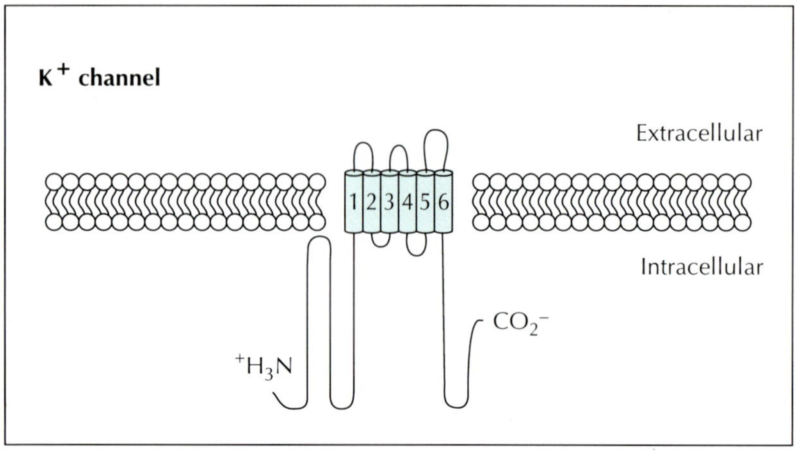

FIGURE 7-5. Potassium ion channels as related to long QT. Insights into the molecular basis of the long QT syndrome (LQTS) have been found by genetic linkage analysis of the LQTS. In 1991, Keating *et al.* [7] discovered tight linkage between an autosomal dominant form of the LQTS and the short arm of chromosome 11 (11P15) at the Harvey-ras-I locus (LQT1). The Harvey-ras gene encodes a G protein that was initially thought to be responsible for the LQTS by its regulatory properties of potassium channels. However in 1993, several investigators determined that the LQTS was not linked to the Harvey-ras locus and that the autosomal dominant form of the LQTS is genetically heterogeneous [8-10].

In 1994, Keating *et al.* [7] identified two additional LQT loci: LQT2 was linked to chromosome 7q35 36, and LQT3 was linked to chromosome 3P21-24 [11]. These authors have subsequently found that HERG, a putative potassium channel gene related to the Drosophila gene encoding the ether-a-go-go potassium channel, is LQT2. HERG has been characterized as an outwardly rectifying, rapidly activating delayed-rectifier potassium channel found in cardiac myocytes [12]. Delay in the opening of the outward rectifier potassium channel would prolong the action potential, thus resulting in the phenotype of the LQTS. The gene for LQT3 was found to be a sodium channel (SCN5A) [13]. A mutation causing a delay in the inactivation of the sodium ion channel would also result in the phenotype of the LQTS. Although different ion channel abnormalities have been found for LQT2 and LQT3, the resultant phenotype is similar, thus providing a unifying explanation of the disorder. Since there are other forms of the autosomal dominant and autosomal recessive LQTS that have not been genetically linked to a gene, one can speculate that the remaining defective genes encode for other ion channels such as calcium or chloride channels or regulators of ion channels. (Note: Similar Figure 2-2 is used in the discussion of cardiac ion channels.)

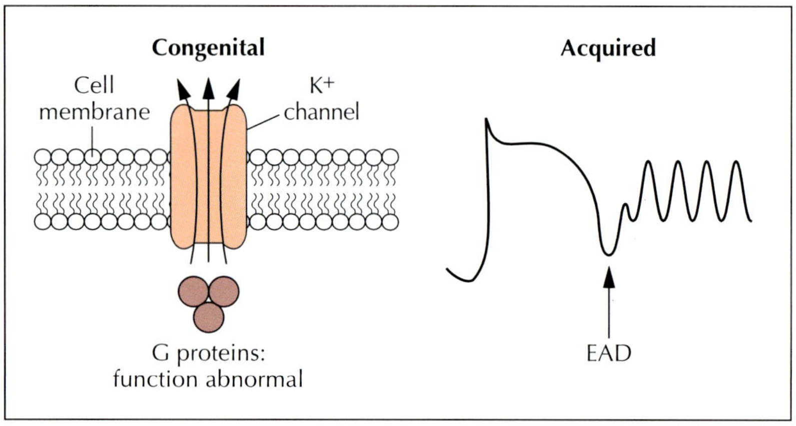

FIGURE 7-6. Mechanisms for polymorphic ventricular tachycardia (PMVT). The unifying link between PMVT in congenital and acquired long QT syndromes (LQTS) is a membrane defect with diminished repolarizing currents in both syndromes. Because these repolarization currents are severely depressed in congenital LQTS, enhancement of depolarizing currents by sympathetic stimulation leads to triggered arrhythmias. With pause-dependent LQTS (acquired forms), abnormal outward repolarizing currents lead to the genesis of early after-depolarizations (EAD), which are exacerbated by pauses.

CONGENITAL VERSUS ACQUIRED LONG QT SYNDROME (LQTS)

SYNDROME VARIABLES	CONGENITAL LQTS	ACQUIRED LQTS
Presentation	Asymptomatic; presyncope; syncope or cardiac arrest; provoked by sympathetic stimulation or stress	PMVT with symptoms; Torsades de pointes
Findings	Normal or long QT interval; low resting heart rate; sinus pauses; impaired chronotropic response; abnormal TU and T waves; high-degree AV block	Onset preceded by pauses; normal to marked prolongation of QT interval; abnormal U waves
Diagnosis	Long QT interval; body surface mapping; MIBG imaging; echocardiographic findings; genetic markers	Associated with an underlying cause
Mechanisms	Sympathetic imbalance creates increased dispersion of refractoriness; membrane abnormality involves K^+ and/or Na^+ channels	Triggered activity due to after-depolarizations
Modulating Factors		
Increased sympathetic tone	+++	+
Pause induced	+	+++
Electrolyte abnormality	?	++
Ischemia	?	++
β agonists	+++	N
β antagonists	N	?
Treatment	β antagonists + chronic pacing; left cervicothoracic sympathectomy; implantable defibrillator	Discontinue precipitating agents; isoproterenol; overdrive pacing; magnesium IV; amiodarone IV

FIGURE 7-7. Congenital versus acquired long QT syndrome. +—weak relationship; ++—stronger relationship; +++—strongest relationship; ?—unknown; N—no relationship; MIBG—metaiodobenzylguanidine imaging.

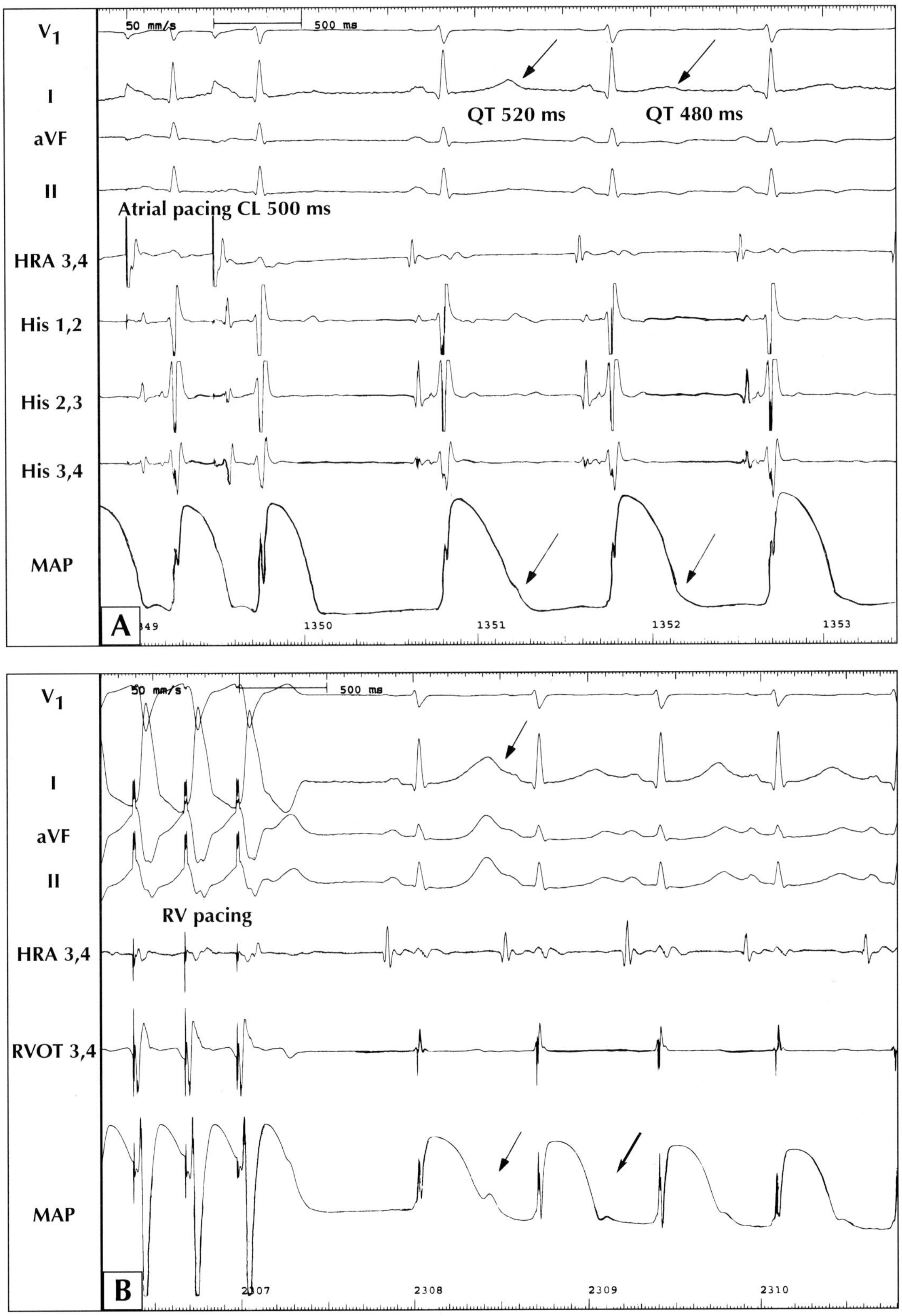

FIGURE 7-8. Post pause T-wave changes. The electrocardiogram in **A** is from a patient with the long QT syndrome. Shown are surface leads (V1, I, II, and aVF) and intracardiac leads from the high right atrium (HRA), His bundle position (HIS), and monophasic action potential (MAP) catheter in the right ventricle. The MAP catheter is an extracellular endocardial recording that resembles transmembrane action potentials in morphology and duration. The first two beats are atrially paced at a cycle length of 500 ms. There is a pause prior to a sinus beat with a QT interval of 520 ms, followed by another sinus beat with a QT interval of 480 ms. Note, the T wave of the first sinus beat after the pause is slightly accentuated (*upper left arrow*) compared with the next beat (*upper right arrow*). On the MAP catheter this is related to "hump" at the end of depolarization, an after-depolarization (*lower left arrow*). It is not seen in the following beat (*lower right arrow*). However, this after-depolarization does not lead to ventricular arrhythmias.

B, Post-pause T-wave changes are more prominent, which begin after three ventricular paced beats. The post pause sinus beat has a prominent T wave (QT interval 550 ms) compared with the next sinus beat (QT interval 450 ms). On the MAP catheter a delayed after-depolarization (*lower left arrow*) is clearly seen that is absent in the next beat (*lower right arrow*).

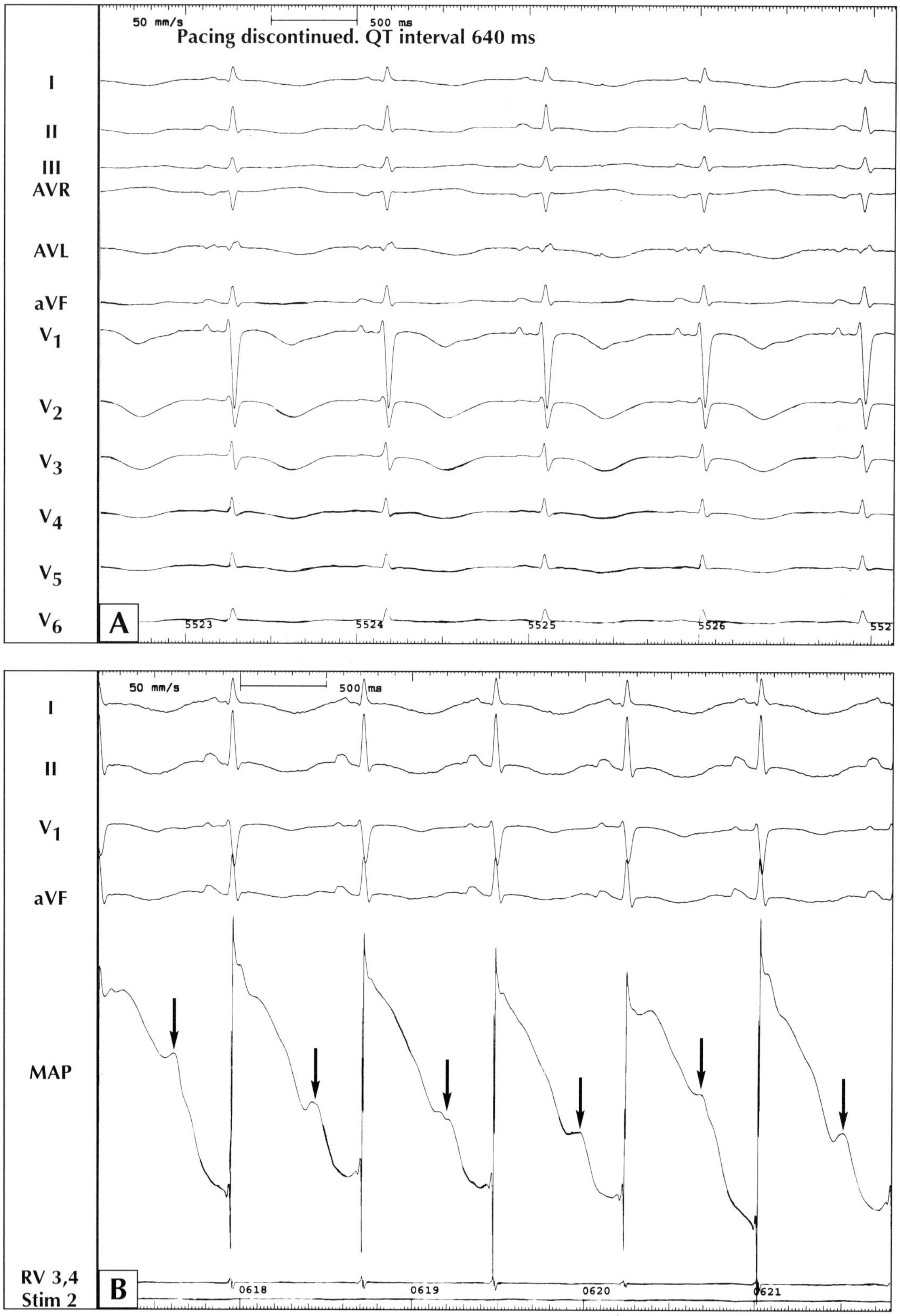

FIGURE 7-9. After-depolarizations related to a long QT. **A**, Baseline 12-lead ECG from a 33-year-old woman with metastatic cancer, presenting with torsades de pointes and syncope. The QT interval is markedly prolonged at 640 ms. **B** shows four surface leads (I,II, V1, and aVF) and two intracardiac leads from the right ventricle, including a monophasic action potential (MAP) electrocardiogram. Note that all the sinus beats that have a long-QT interval have after-depolarizations. (*Arrows* indicate after-depolarizations.)

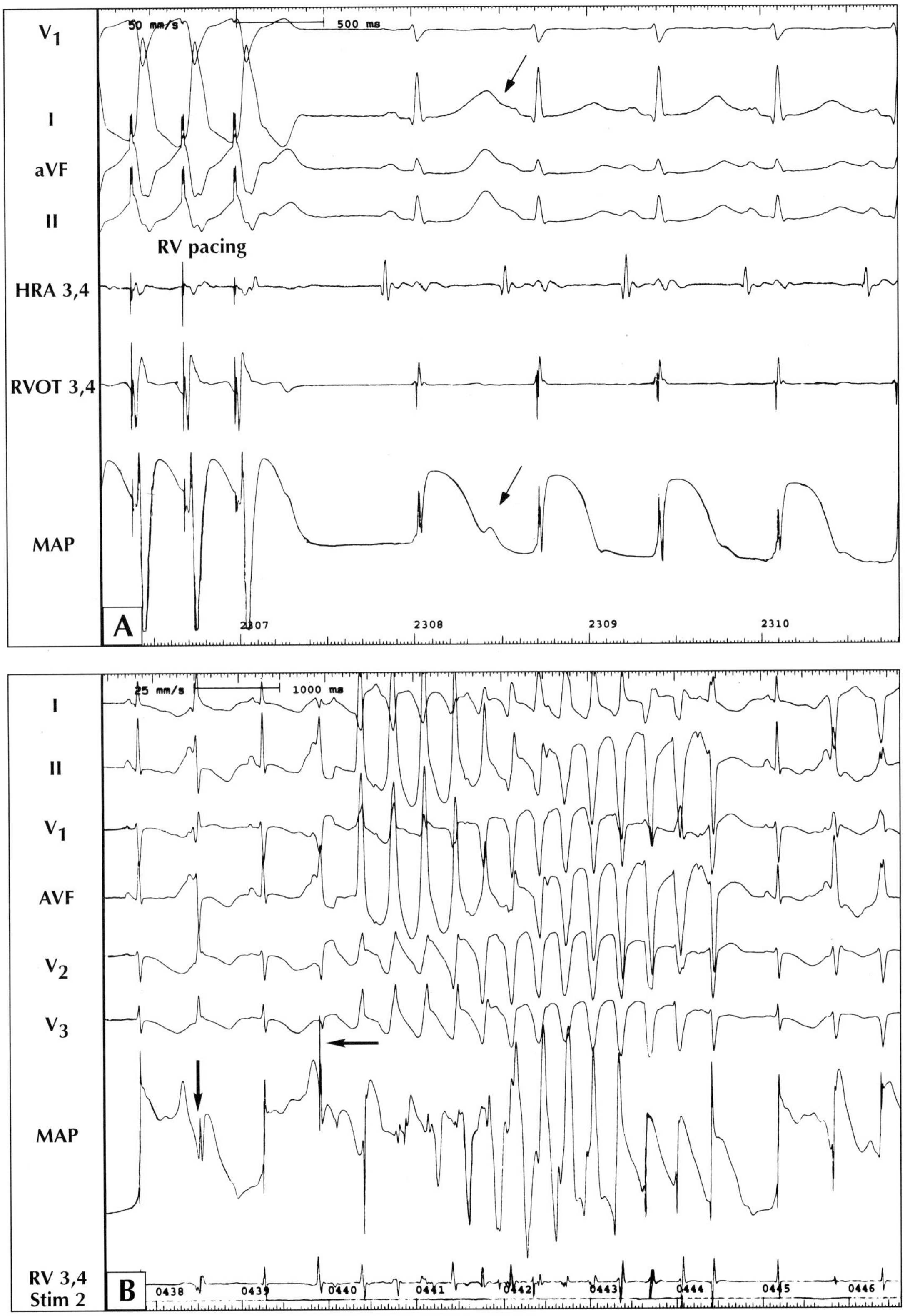

FIGURE 7-10. Post-pause T-wave changes. In **A**, three ventricular paced beats are followed by a pause. The first beat after the pause has an abnormal T wave (*top arrow*) compared with subsequent T waves and is associated with an after-depolarization on the monophasic action potential (MAP) catheter (*arrow at bottom*). There is no arrhythmia.

B, Spontaneous initiation of polymorphic ventricular tachycardia (PMVT) is seen in the same patient. In the surface leads (I, II, V1, aVF, V2, and V3), the morphology is clearly polymorphic. On the MAP catheter, the first ventricular beat that starts the arrhythmia (*right arrow*) is from an after-depolarization. Note, the second beat (*left arrow*) is also a ventricular complex from an after-depolarization. It is followed by a pause prior to the initiation of the PMVT. The PMVT was decreased but not abolished by esmolol or intravenous diltiazem, but with the addition of ventricular pacing, the patient had no further ventricular arrhythmias.

Treatment

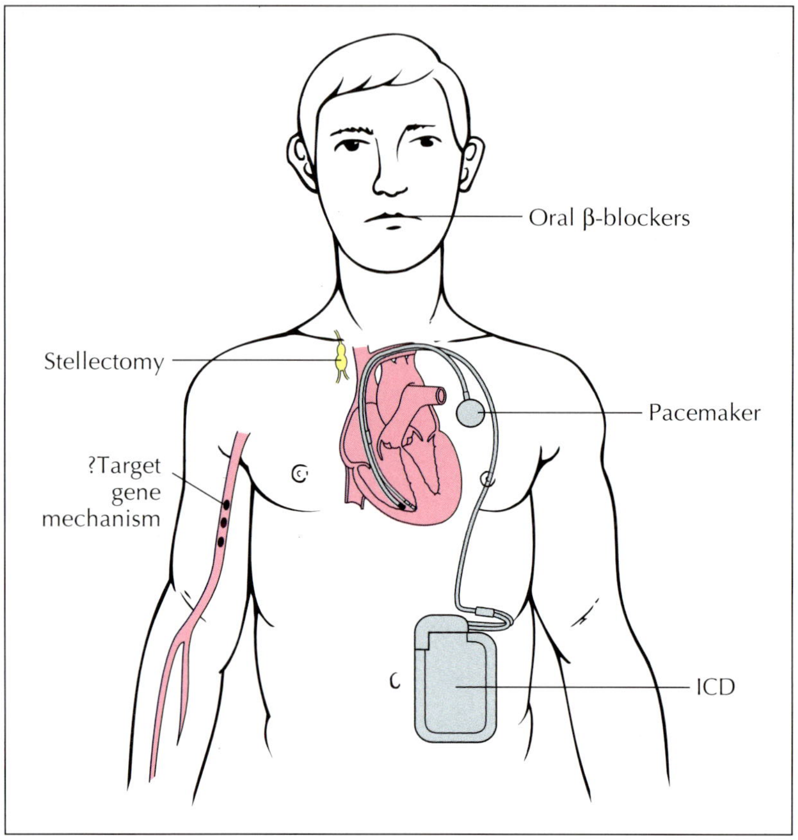

Figure 7-11. Treatment of congenital long QT syndrome (LQTS). Treatment for the LQTS has evolved and changed as our understanding of the mechanism for the arrhythmia increases. Left cervico ganglion stellectomy was used early on, but this has been replaced by more effective methods of treatment, including implantable cardioverter defibrillators (ICDs) and the use of the combination of β blockade and permanent pacing [14,15]. The efficacy of β-blocker therapy has been demonstrated and remains the drug of first choice for patient management. Failing this therapy, other available options include a left cervico-sympathectomy, cardiac pacing with full doses of β-blockers, or use of a defibrillator. The available data suggest that although symptoms are reduced, there is, nevertheless, a significant incidence of recurrent syncope (40%) or sudden cardiac death (8%) in patients undergoing cervico-thoracic sympathectomy. The rationale for use of chronic cardiac pacing rests on the observations that in some patients with LQTS, polymorphic ventricular tachycardia may be triggered by pauses. The recurrence rate of syncope or torsade de pointes in patients treated with combined therapy is less than 10%. There is a growing experience in the use of defibrillator therapy for these patients, especially with the availability of smaller generators and transvenous insertions. Even in patients undergoing defibrillator treatment, adjunctive therapy with β-blockers and possibly cardiac pacing may be required to decrease the incidence of device discharges. As our understanding of genetic mechanisms for genes coding for abnormal proteins or receptors increases, it may be possible to prophylactically direct therapy at the underlying etiology rather than treating the resultant arrhythmia.

References

1. Jervell A, Lange-Nielsen F: Congenital deaf mutism, functional heart disease with prolongation of the QT interval and sudden death. *Am Heart J* 1957, 54:59.
2. Romano C, Gemme G, Pongiglione R: Aritmie cardiache rare in eta' pediatrica. *Clin Ped* 1963, 45:656.
3. Abildskov JA: The sympathetic imbalance hypothesis of QT interval prolongation. *J Cardiovasc Electrophysiol* 1991, 2:355.
4. Schwartz PJ, Locati EH, Moss AJ, *et al.*: Left cardiac sympathetic denervation in the therapy of congenital long QT syndrome. A worlwide report. *Circulation* 1991, 84:503.
5. Schwartz PJ, Locati E, Priori SG, Zaza A.: The long QT syndrome. In: *Cardiac Electrophysiology: From cell to bedside.* Zipes DP, Jalife J, eds. Philadelphia, WB Saunders 1990; 589.
6. Tzivoni D, Banai S, Schugar C, *et al.*: Treatment of torsades de pointes with magnesium sulfate. *Circulation* 1988, 77:392.
7. Keating M, Atkinson D, Dunn C, *et al.*: Linkage of a cardiac arrhythmia, the long QT syndrome, and the Harvey ras-1 gene. *Science* 1991a, 252:704–706.
8. Benhorin J, Kalman YM, Madina A, *et al.*: Evidence of genetic heterogeneity in the long QT syndrome. *Science* 1993, 260:1960–1962.
9. Curran ME, Atkinson D, Timothy K, *et al.*: Locus heterogeneity of autosomal dominant long QT syndrome. *J Clin Invest* 1993, 92:799–803.
10. Towbin JA, Li H, Taggart T, *et al.*: Evidence of genetic heterogeneity in Romano-Ward long QT syndrome (LQTS): analysis of 23 families. *Circulation* 1994, 90:2635–2644.
11. Jiang C, Atkinson D, Towbin JA, *et al.*: Two long QT syndrome loci map to chromasomes 3 and 7 with evidence for further heterogeneity. *Nature Genet* 1994, 8:141–147.
12. Sanguinetti MC, Jiang C, Curran MB, Keating MT: A mechanistic link between an inherited and an acquired cardiac arrhythmia: HERG encodes the IKr potassium channel. *Cell* 1995, 81(2):299–307.
13. Wang Q, Shen J, Splawski I, *et al.*: SCN5A mutations associated with an inherited cardiac arrhythmia, long QT syndrome. *Cell* 1995, 80(5):805–811.
14. Eldar M, Griffin JC, Abbott JA, Scheinman MM: Permanent cardiac pacing in patients with the long QT syndrome. *J Am Coll Cardiol* 1987, 10:600.
15. Moss AJ, Liu JE, Gottlieb S, *et al.*: Efficacy of permanent pacing in the management of high-risk patients with long QT syndrome. *Circulation* 1991, 84:1524.

Implantable Pacemakers For the Management of Cardiac Rhythm Disorders

8

CHAPTER

James L. Cockrell
and Andreana Siu

Implantable devices for the management of cardiac rhythm disorders have been in clinical use since 1958 when Elmquist and Senning [1] implanted the first pulse generator in a patient with atrioventricular heart block. Since this time enormous advances in design, particularly the development of integrated electronics and microprocessor technology, have allowed ever increasing memory and computing capability within the implanted pulse generator to handle a large number of complex functions for more physiologic pacing and improved telemetry. Parallel advances in battery design and lead system development have resulted in greater pacemaker longevity.

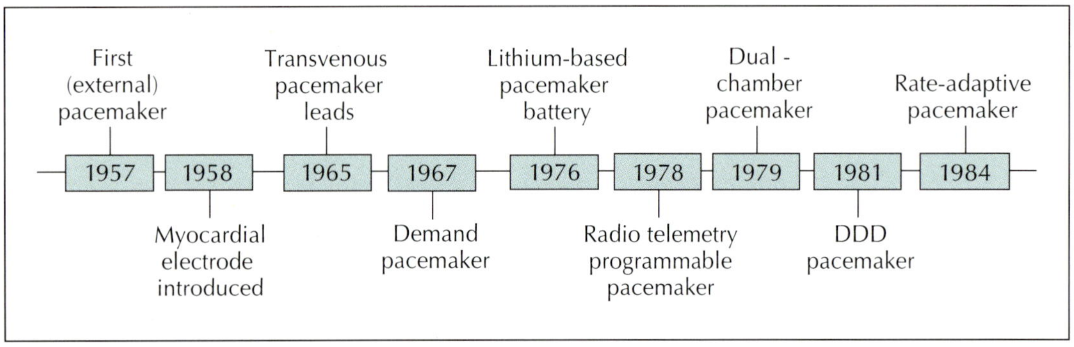

FIGURE 8-1. Milestones in cardiac pacing. The first fully implantable pacemaker was possible only after significant advances in pulse generator design and development of the Hunter-Roth myocardial electrode. The development of leads that could be positioned using the vasculature (transvenous) system in 1965 greatly simplified implantation.

The emergence of the demand pacemaker that could sense the native cardiac electrical activity, and thereby function only when needed, completed the basic pacing system and set the stage for the tremendous growth and advances to date. The introduction of the lithium-based pacemaker battery in 1976 held significant advantages in both pacemaker longevity and end-of-life reliability over its predecessor, the mercury zinc battery. This, together with the introduction of programmability by way of radiofrequency telemetry in 1978 resulted in pacemakers with extraordinary reliability that could be easily reprogrammed to meet a wider range of clinical pacing requirements.

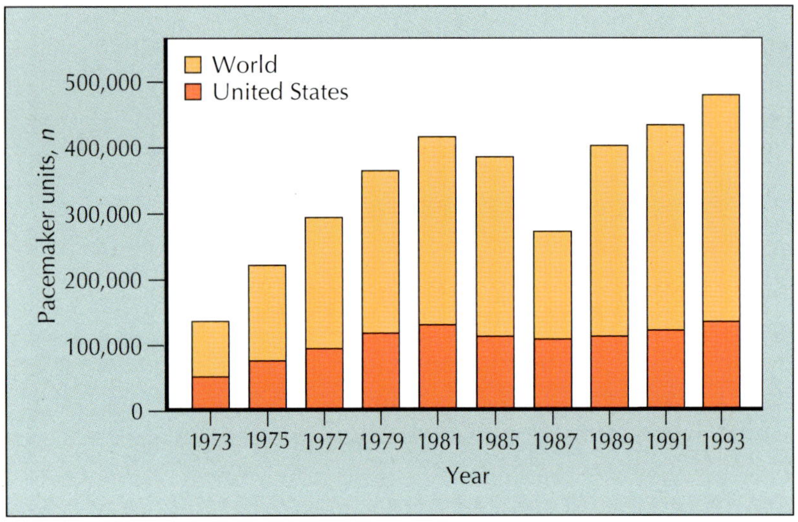

FIGURE 8-2. Growth of pacemaker implants. More recent developments, including the introduction of atrioventricular sequential pacemakers in 1979, dual chamber pacing and sensing in 1981, and pacemakers with sensor-triggered rate-adaptive capability in 1984, addressed physiologic pacing considerations to more closely approximate the normal cardiac electrophysiology.

ADVANCES IN PACING TECHNOLOGY

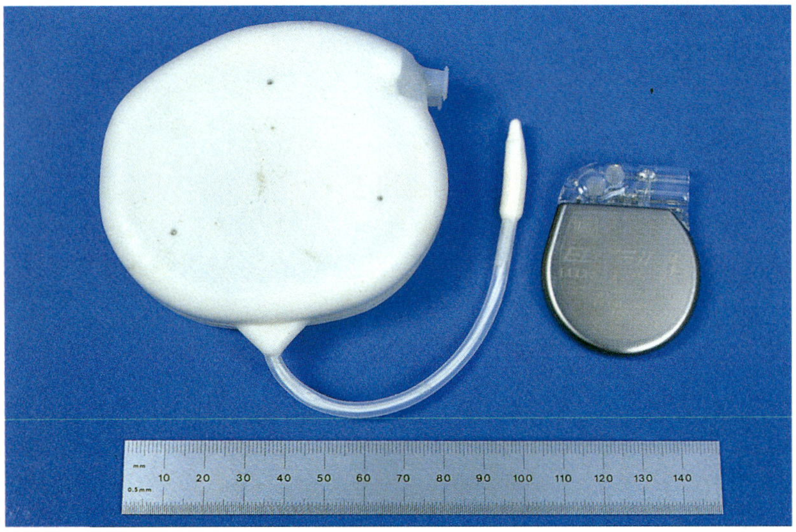

FIGURE 8-3. The early implantable cardiac pacemaker. One of the most important advances in the history of cardiac pacing has been the reduction in pulse generator size. While the first units implanted were no less than extraordinary in novelty and concept, they were bulky. This translated to significant patient discomfort and higher complication rates, including infection, migration, and skin erosion overlying the implantation site.

One of the earliest fully implantable pacemakers, representing significant technologic advances, was the Greatbatch-Chardack pulse generator (*left*) (1959) that weighed 224 g and was about 25 mm (1 in) thick. It was a single-chamber fixed-rate pulse generator without sensing (asynchronous) capability. It employed a mercury-zinc chemistry with an expected longevity of over 2 y and a capacity of 0.5 ampere-hours. Implanted in a large number of patients for an expanding number of indications, the modern pacemaker (*right*) weighs about one tenth the original (26 g), and is only 7.5 mm (just over .25 in) thick. It employs the reliable lithium iodide battery chemistry with a microprocessor and integrated circuitry. The battery has a usable capacity approaching 2.3 ampere-hours, an expected longevity of perhaps 8 y at a battery current drain of 20 μA. Available fully programmable functions include dual (atrial and ventricular) chamber pacing and sensing (demand) capability, as well as sensor-triggered rate-adaptive pacing capability. (Courtesy of Medtronic, Inc., Minneapolis, MN.)

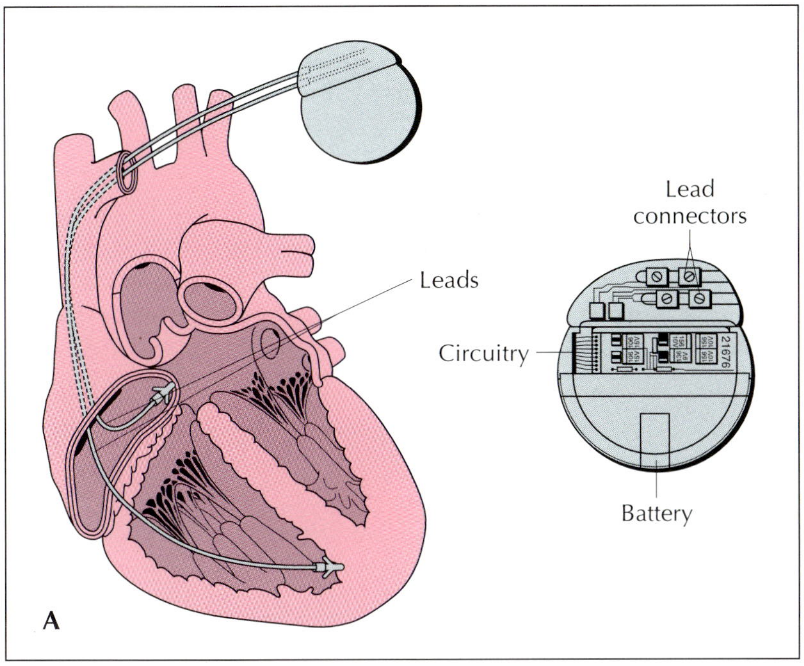

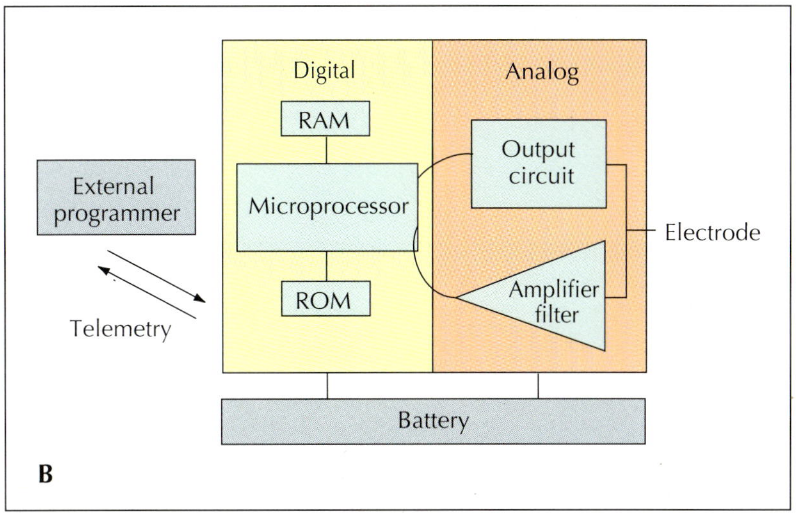

FIGURE 8-4. The pulse generator design. While early designs included a few hand-soldered transistors, resistors, and capacitors, the present devices include highly advanced, highly integrated microcircuits and microprocessors (**A**) resembling that found in personal computers. The microprocessor performs the logic chores of the pacemaker, including storage of programmable settings and interpretation and response to various sensed and paced cardiac electrical events, as well as the control of radiofrequency telemetry communications with external programmers. The microprocessor is dependent on a highly precise timer circuit based on a crystal oscillator.

Many devices (**B**) employ both "read only memory" (ROM), which contains the pacing algorithm, and "read and write memory" (RAM) for data, including programmed settings, device identification, and storage of a wide array of measured data values.

While the pacing algorithm and memory functions of the pacemaker represent the digital side of the device, certain analog elements, including filters and amplifiers for detecting intrinsic cardiac activity and controlling pacing output levels at appropriate intervals as instructed by the microprocessor, are necessary components as well.

All of these components are mounted on a circuit board and placed along with the battery within a hermetically sealed container, usually a titanium canister, for protection from the hostile environment of body fluids.

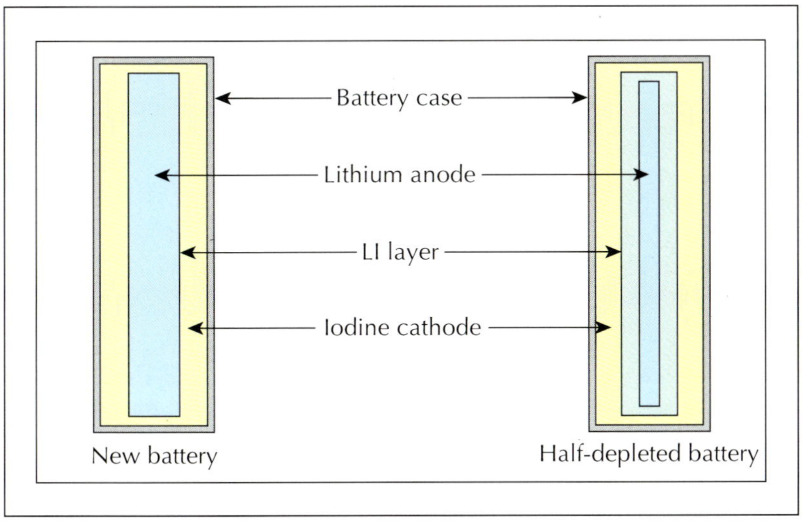

FIGURE 8-5. The pulse generator battery: cross-sections of new and partially depleted lithium/iodine pacemaker batteries. In the past, bradycardia pacemakers have employed cell chemistries, including zinc/mercuric oxide, lithium/cupric sulfide, lithium/silver chromate, and even nuclear power. The present pacing systems usually employ a lithium iodine (Li/I_2) cell. This cell's success is attributable to high reliability, *ie*, almost unknown battery failures from internal shorts, reliable depletion status, high energy-to-volume and low self-discharge loss (often less than 5% of usable energy), and good operation in hermetically sealed titanium canisters. (*Adapted from* Medtronic, Inc., Minneapolis, MN.)

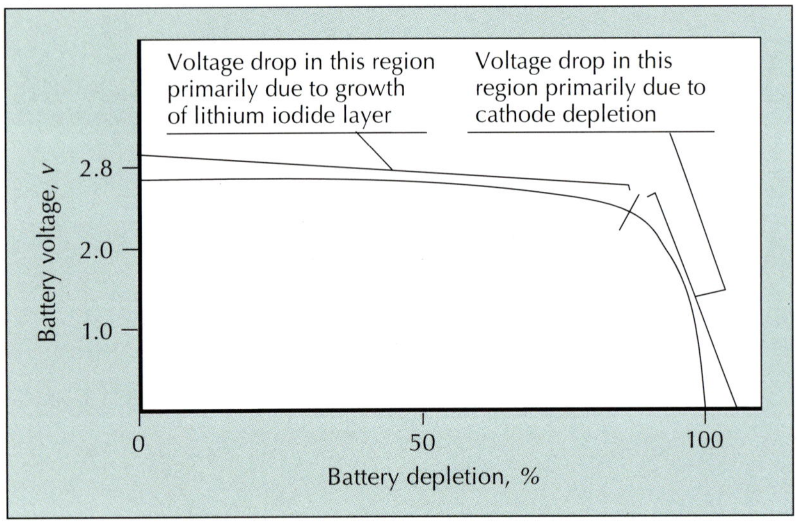

FIGURE 8-6. Typical voltage/depletion curve for cathode-limited lithium/iodine battery. This cell chemistry has a beginning voltage of 2.8 V and a usable capacity of 1 to 3 ampere hours related to the mass of cathodal iodine. Anodal lithium is in excess, resulting in safer, slower battery voltage depletion rates when the cell approaches the end of usable capacity. Typical circuitry allows normal operation down to levels of 2.3 to 2.5 V, translating into some 100,000 hours of operation at present depletion rates (usually about 20 μA). (*Adapted from* Medtronic Inc., Minneapolis, MN.)

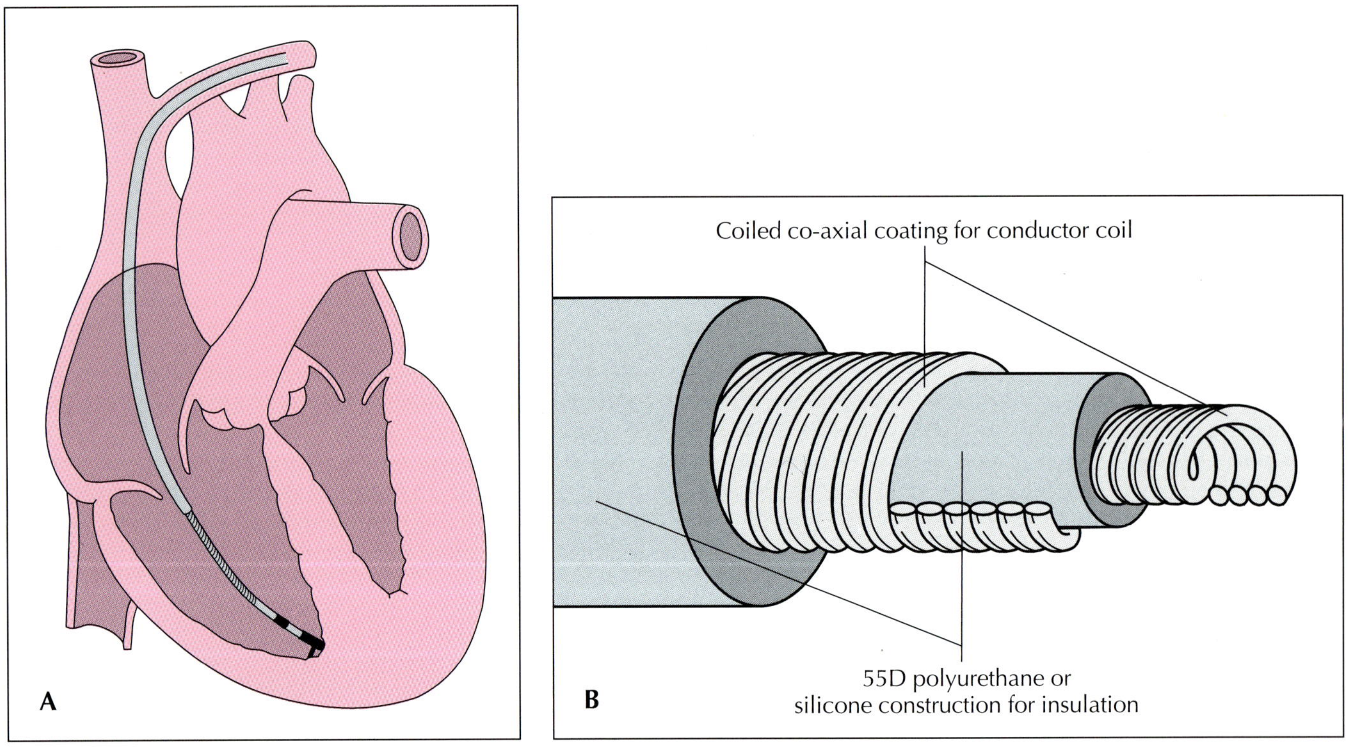

FIGURE 8-7. The pacing lead system in situ. As shown in **A**, the pacing lead must provide sufficient stimulus current with minimal current drain on the pulse generator battery, stable stimulation thresholds, and adequate sensing without sensing noncardiac electrical signals. **B,** A close-up of the coiled conductor and its casing. Earlier lead system designs were troubled by dislodgment, high thresholds, perforation, and conductor failure. Engineering innovations, including tined and screw-in lead tips; flexible, lower profile lead bodies employing a coaxial in-line design; and coiled conductors made of stronger, corrosion-resistant materials, have resulted in improved lead reliability. (Part B *adapted from* Medtronic, Inc., Minneapolis, MN.)

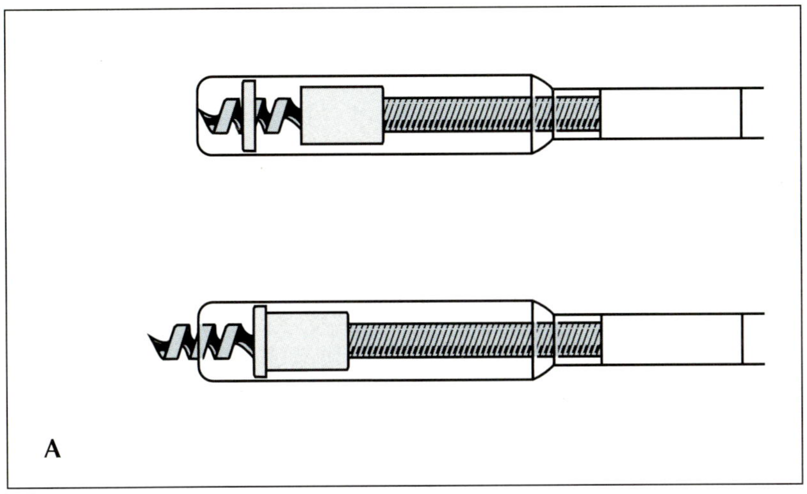

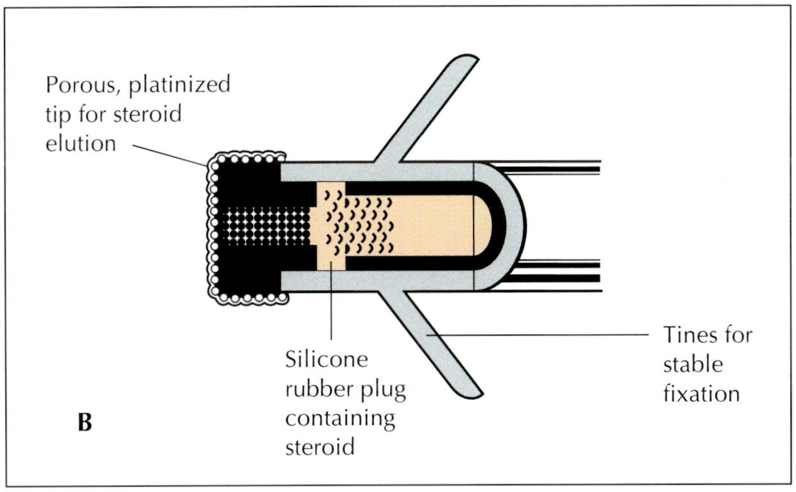

FIGURE 8-8. Close-up of porous lead tip. Additional advances, including retractable screw tip (**A**); steroid-eluting electrodes (**B**); smaller, porous electrode surface area; and improved processing techniques for lead insulation materials also have contributed to improved lead reliability. (*Adapted from* Medtronic, Inc, Minneapolis, MN.)

ELECTROPHYSIOLOGY OF PACING AND SENSING

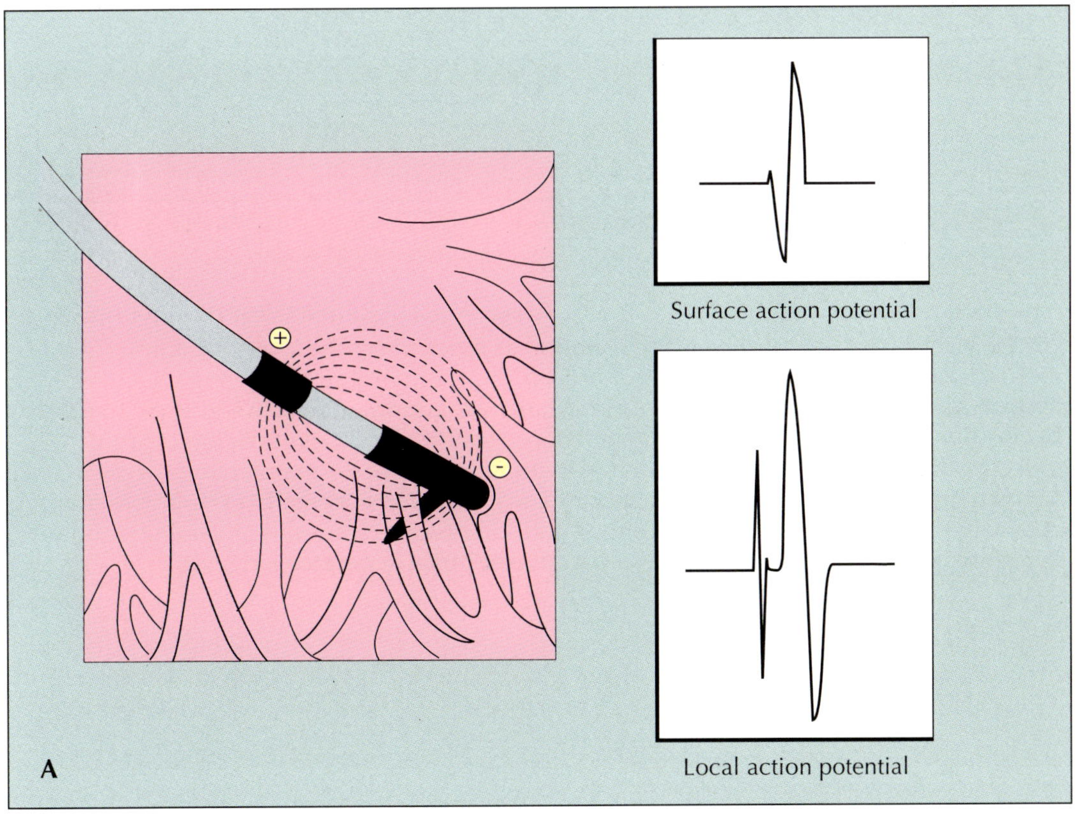

FIGURE 8-9. A, Excitation threshold. Myocardial pacing capture results when a critical mass of myocardial tissue is hyperpolarized near the anode (positive electrode) concurrent with the lowering of membrane potential in the region of the cathode (negative electrode) as a result of the passage of electrical current through viable myocardium. This results in transmembrane depolarization to excitation voltage, recorded as a local action potential, and a propagated action potential spreading throughout the myocardium as a result of its syncytial architecture, recorded as the surface action potential. The minimum stimulus necessary to produce a propagated depolarization is termed the excitation threshold. (*continued*)

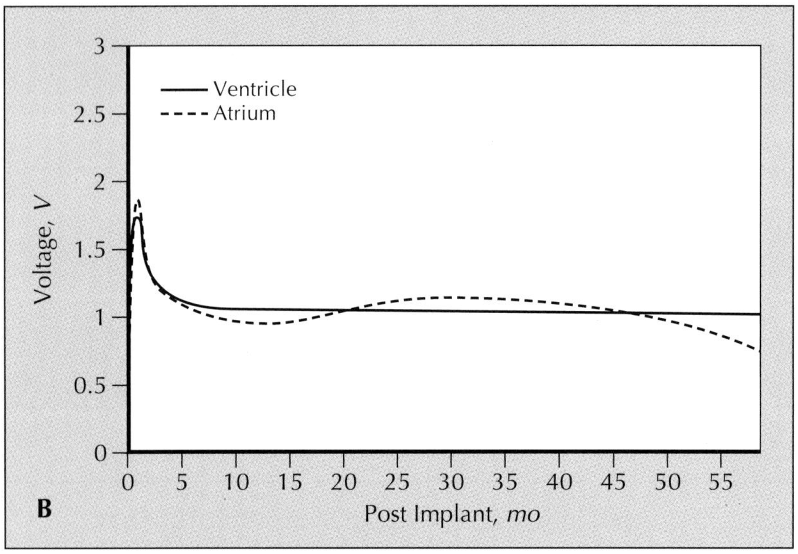

Figure 8-9. (*continued*) **B**, Excitation threshold stability. While the excitation threshold changes little over time, perhaps rising only a few percent per year, threshold changes just after implantation may peak at several times the implant value, often a few weeks after implantation. Following this relatively labile period, thresholds generally return to near implant levels in most patients by 3 months. Other factors, including certain drugs and alterations in transmembrane acid-base or electrolyte levels, may result in modest, transient increases in excitation threshold; however, such changes are generally no greater than 50%.

Capture thresholds are kept low because of smaller electrode surface areas resulting from improved lead design and because of smaller virtual electrode size (electrode and tissue scar), stemming from reduced inflammatory responses over time.

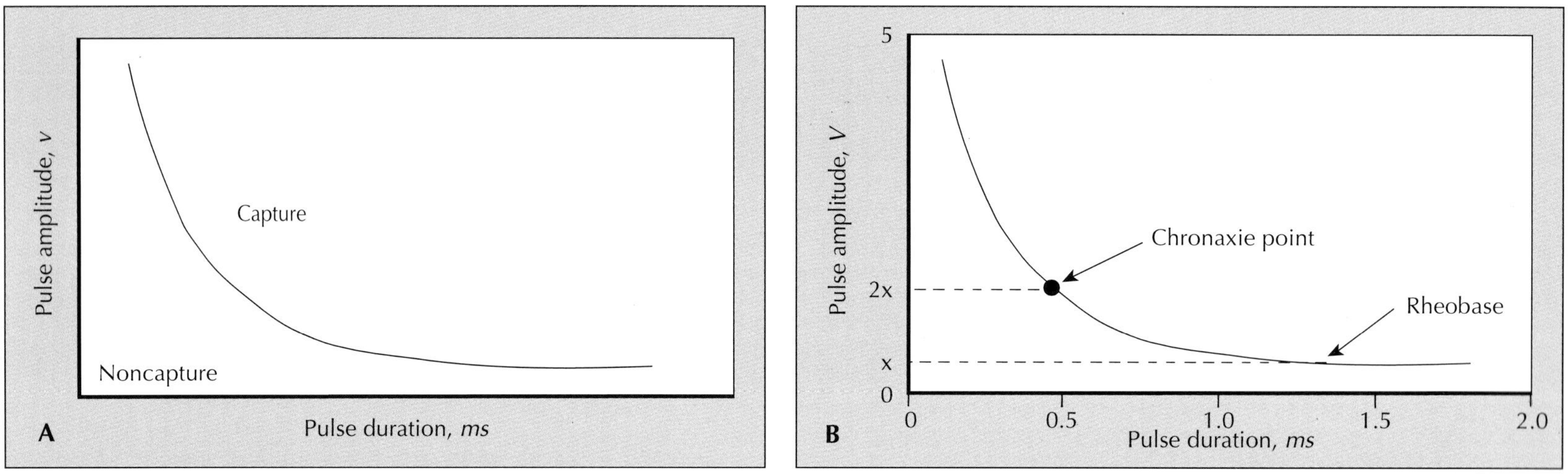

Figure 8-10. Strength-duration relationship. **A**, Successful myocardial capture is a function of the intensity of the electrical field generated by the stimulating pulse, which in turn is a result of the generated current density or amount of current passed across the electrode per unit of its surface area. In addition to the stimulating pulse amplitude, the intensity of the electrical field is influenced by impulse duration. As impulse duration increases, the stimulus amplitude required for excitation decreases in an exponential fashion. However, beyond a pulse duration of approximately 2 ms, this curve becomes essentially flat (termed rheobase) (**B**). The pulse duration at twice the reobase output amplitude (chronaxie) is at or near the energy minimum along the curve.

Pacemakers are usually programmed to provide approximately a 100% voltage or energy safety margin over pacing capture threshold. This safety margin allows for maintenance of pacing in the face of short-term fluctuations normally expected to occur as a result of short- and long-term changes in physiology, and for optimization of pacemaker pulse generator longevity.

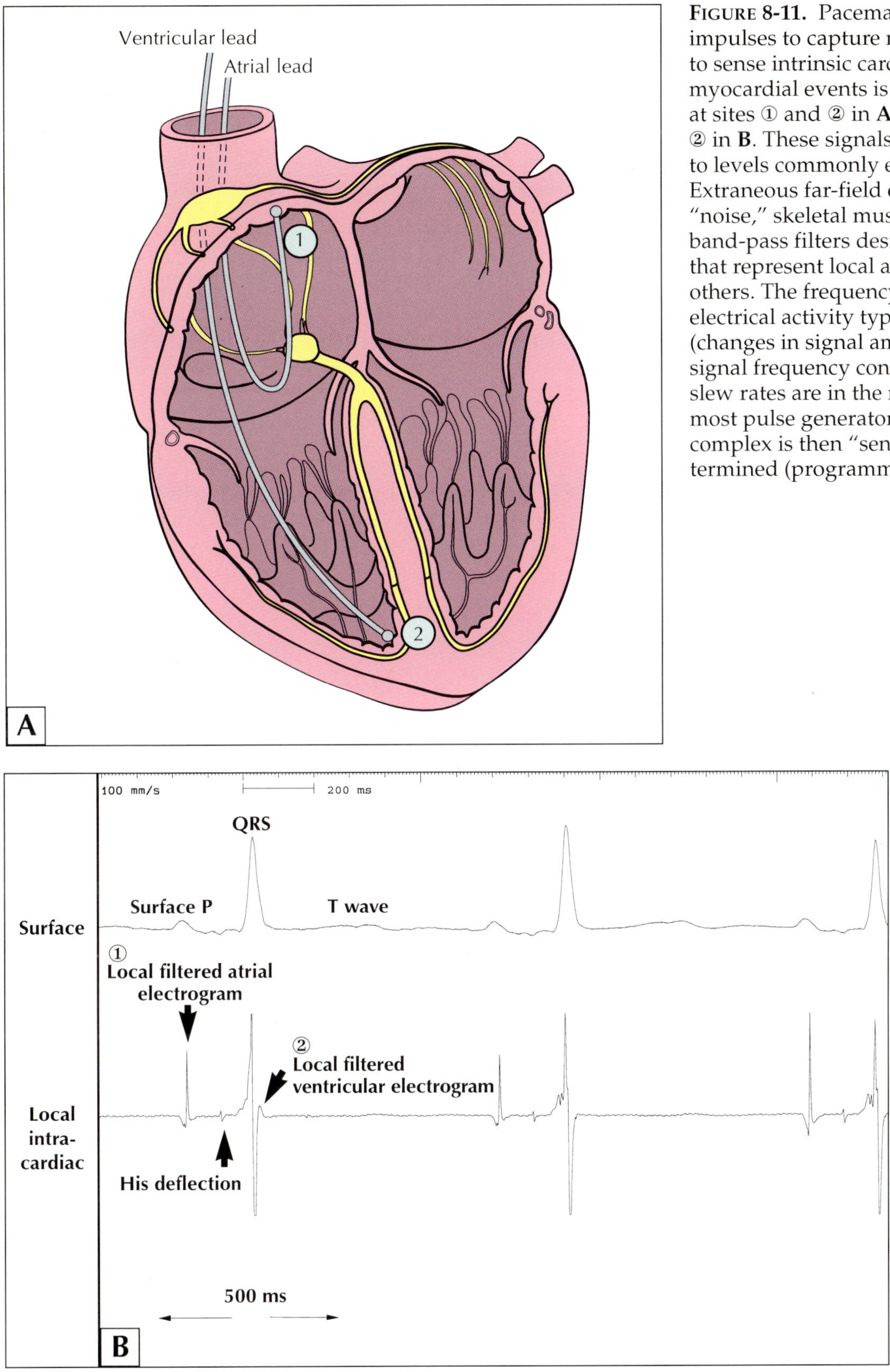

FIGURE 8-11. Pacemaker sensing. In addition to generating impulses to capture myocardium, pacemakers have the capacity to sense intrinsic cardiac activity. Electrical activity from intrinsic myocardial events is detected on the electrode lead system at sites ① and ② in **A** and is recorded as local electrogram ① and ② in **B**. These signals are amplified from biologic levels (millivolts) to levels commonly employed in electronic circuits (volts). Extraneous far-field electrical activity, including environmental "noise," skeletal muscle activity, and T waves, is filtered out by band-pass filters designed to "pass" those frequencies from signals that represent local activity and to progressively attenuate all others. The frequency band-width from signals of local myocardial electrical activity typically demonstrates associated slew rates (changes in signal amplitude with respect to time and an index of signal frequency content) that can be measured clinically. Typical slew rates are in the range of 0.5V to 3V/sec and are optimal for most pulse generator sensing systems. The amplified, filtered complex is then "sensed" by the pacing system if it is of a predetermined (programmable) amplitude.

NASPE/BPEG GENERIC (NBG) PACEMAKER CODE*

POSITION	I	II	III	IV	V
CATEGORY	CHAMBER(S) PACED	CHAMBER(S) SENSED	RESPONSE TO SENSING	PROGRAMMABILITY, RATE MODULATION	ANTITACHYARRHYTHMIA FUNCTIONS
	O=None	O=None	O=None	O=None	O=None
	A=Atrium	A=Atrium	T=Triggered	P=Simple programmable	P=Pacing (antitachyarrhythmia)
	V=Ventricle	V=Ventricle	I=Inhibited	M=Multiprogrammable	S=Shock
	D=Dual (A+V)	D=Dual (A+V)	D=Dual (T+I)	C=Communicating	D=Dual (P+S)
	S=Single (A or V)†	S=Single (A or V)†		R=Rate modulation	

*Positions I through III are used exclusively for antibradyarrhythmia functions.
†Manufacturer's designation only.

FIGURE 8-12. Modes of cardiac pacing. The mode of cardiac pacing refers to the way in which the pacemaker interacts with the underlying cardiac rhythm. The various modes may be described by the shorthand code suggested by the North American Society of Pacing and Electrophysiology (NASPE) and the British Pacing and Electrophysiology Group (BPEG) Pacemaker Code, 1987. (*Adapted from* Bernstein and coworkers [2]).

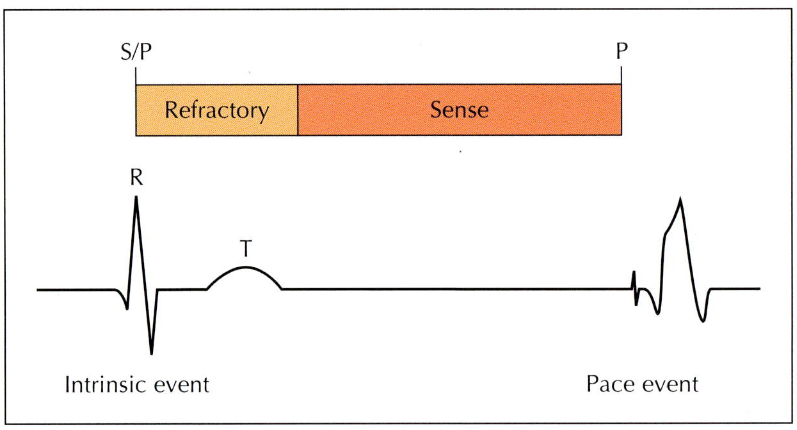

FIGURE 8-13. Single-chamber timing cycle. The basic timing cycle, that of a single-chamber fixed-rate demand pacemaker, is initiated by a stimulus or pace event immediately followed by a period (refractory period) within which all sensing ceases. The refractory period is followed by a sensing period that ends at the conclusion of the escape interval (programmed lower rate interval) with a pace event. The sense period may be interrupted at any time by an intrinsic depolarization restarting the cycle. P—pace event; S/P—sensing or pace event.

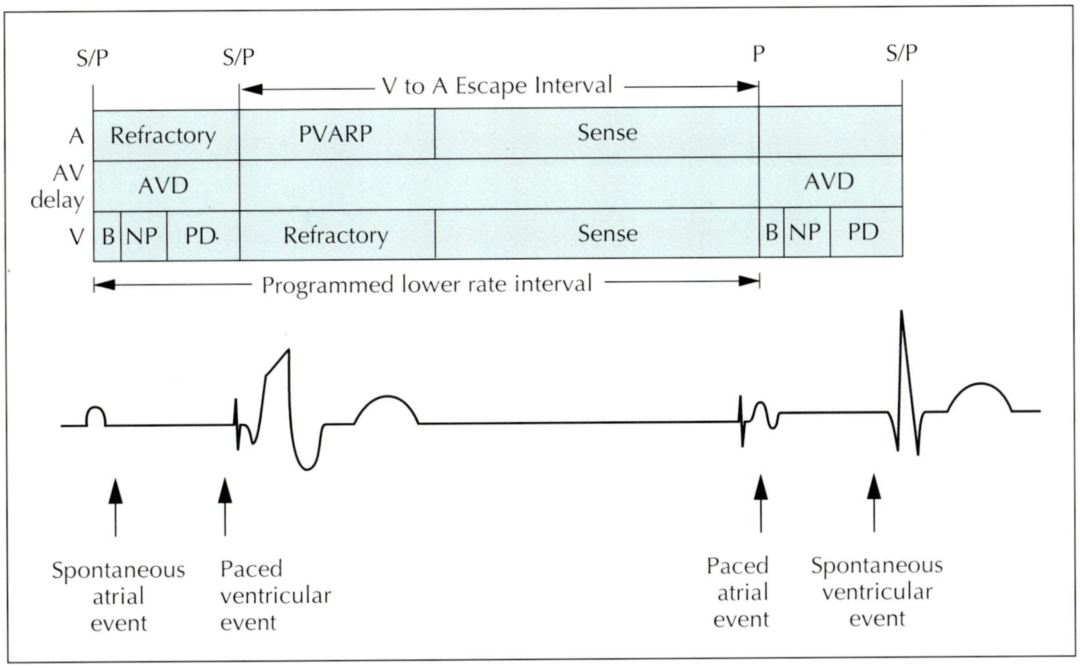

FIGURE 8-14. Dual-chamber timing cycle. Either a pace or a sense event occurring in the atrium initiates an atrioventricular (AV) delay period. This AV period is concluded by a ventricular stimulus or may be interrupted by sensing an intrinsic ventricular event. Refractory periods are initiated in both channels following either event. The refractory periods are in turn followed by sense periods in both chambers. The sense period is concluded by a pace event in the atrium or may be interrupted by sense events in either chamber. Unlike the single-chamber timing cycle, the escape interval in a dual-chamber pacemaker is shortened by the programmed AV delay period.

The ventricular channel timing system illustrated also incorporates "nonphysiologic AV delay" or "ventricular safety" pacing. The ventricular channel AV delay events (AVD) consist of three phases. First is the blanking period (B), which is a time of absolute refractoriness. The next is the nonphysiologic AV delay period (NP), ending 100 to 110 ms after an atrial event. Events sensed during this time initiate a ventricular stimulus at the conclusion of the nonphysiologic AVD phase and recycle the atrial and ventricular timing cycles. The final portion of the AVD is the physiologic period (PD). Sensed events during this period result in inhibition of ventricular channel output and initiation of a new timing cycle.

The rationale for shortened nonphysiologic AV delay ventricular safety pacing is that sensed events within the nonphysiologic AV delay are not the result of normal conduction stemming from the preceding atrial event (sensed or paced) to the ventricles. Therefore, such activity may represent either premature ventricular activity or extraneous sensed atrial activity (crosstalk). Since the system is unable to differentiate between these two possibilities, early ventricular activation "safety" pacing avoids pacing during the ventricular vulnerable period, and inappropriate ventricular channel output inhibition with crosstalk. A—atrial channel events; PVARP—post-ventricular atrial refractory period; P—pace event; S/P—sensing or pace event; V—ventricular channel events.

COMMON USES FOR PERMANENT PACEMAKER THERAPY

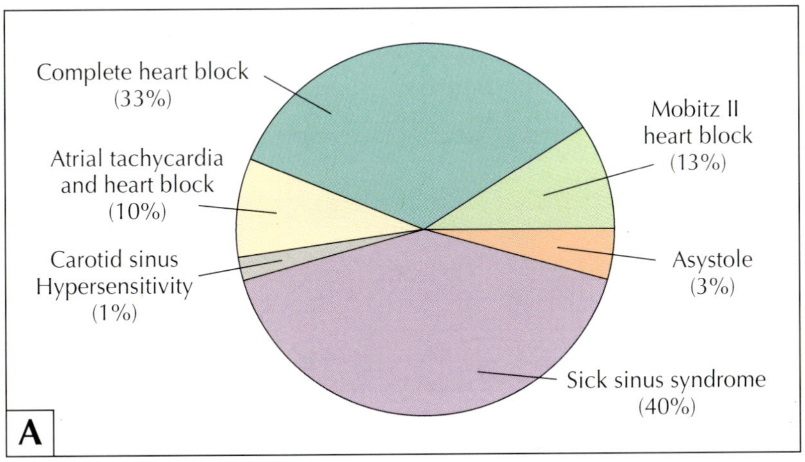

FIGURE 8-15. Indications for permanent pacemaker implantation. In **A**, the most frequent reasons for cardiac pacing at present are shown, including sinus node disease, with or without additional specialized conduction system disease, and heart block due to disease at some level along the specialized conduction system. The diagnostic ECG findings are shown in **B**, complete heart block; (*continued*)

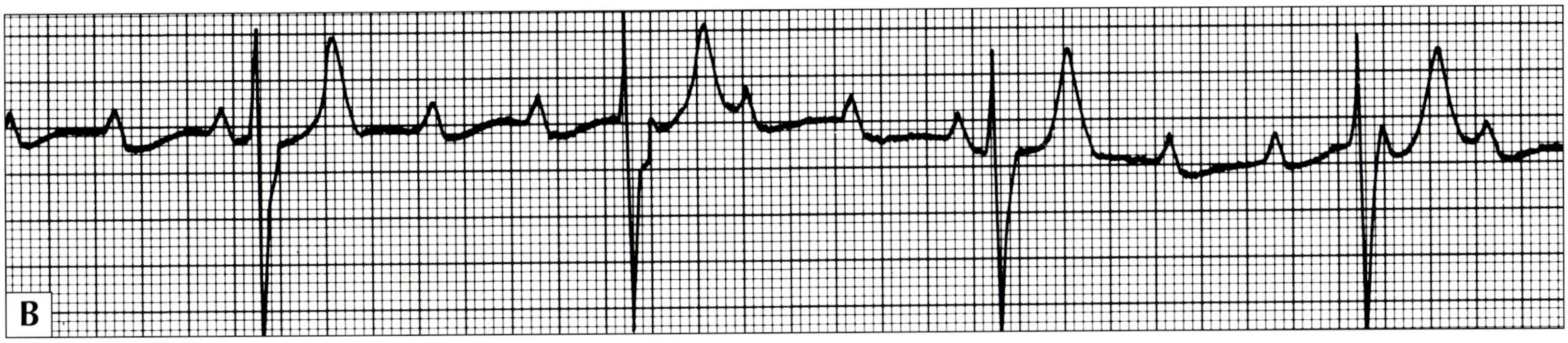

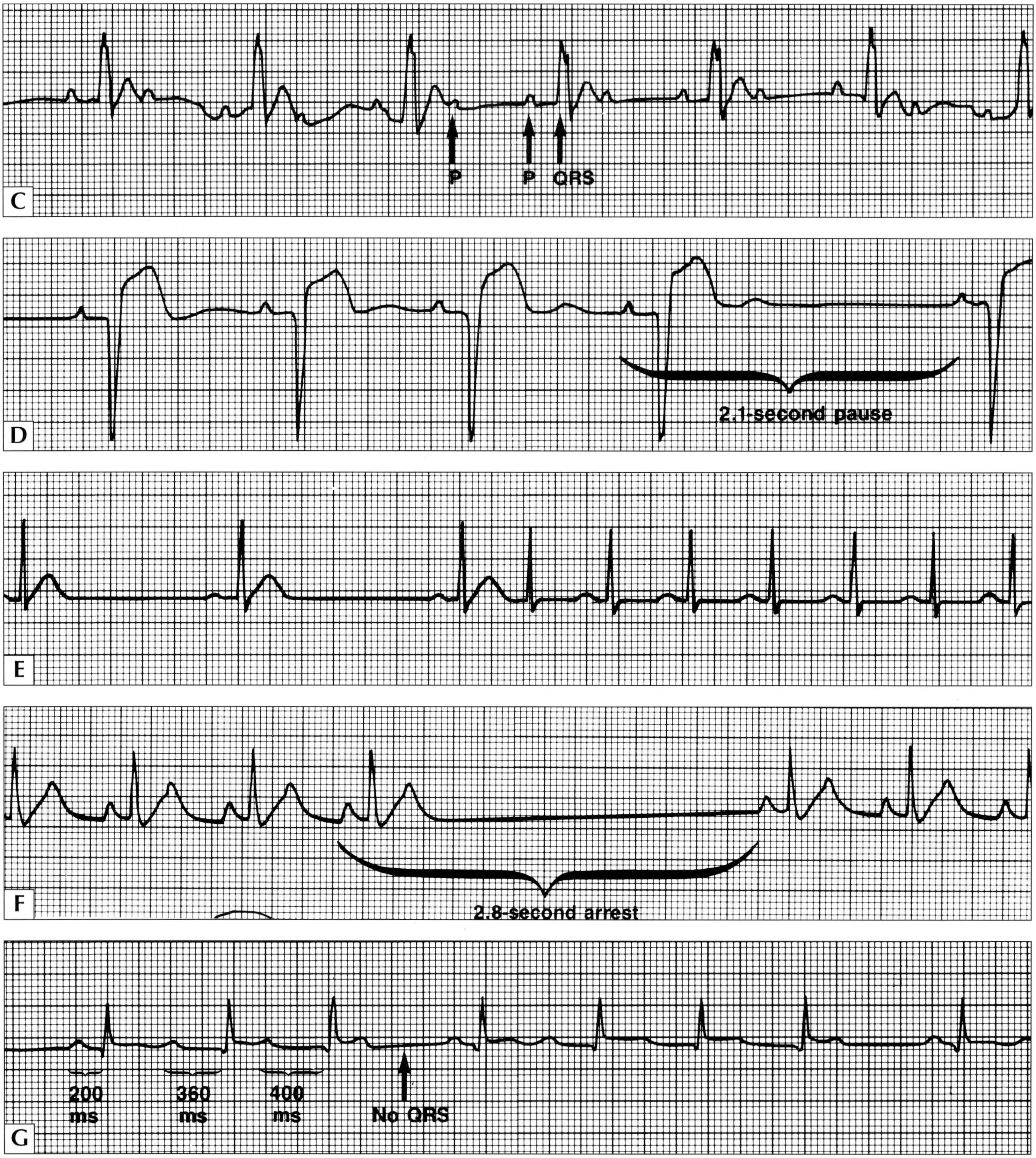

FIGURE 8-15. (*continued*) **C**, second-degree atrioventricular block with 2:1 conduction; **D**, asystole; **E**, sick sinus syndrome; **F**, carotid sinus hypersensitivity; and **G**, atrial tachycardia and atrioventricular Wenkebach conduction. (A *adapted from* VA National Registry, June 1989–June 1990 [3]; B–G *courtesy of* Ross Fletcher, MD, Washington, DC.)

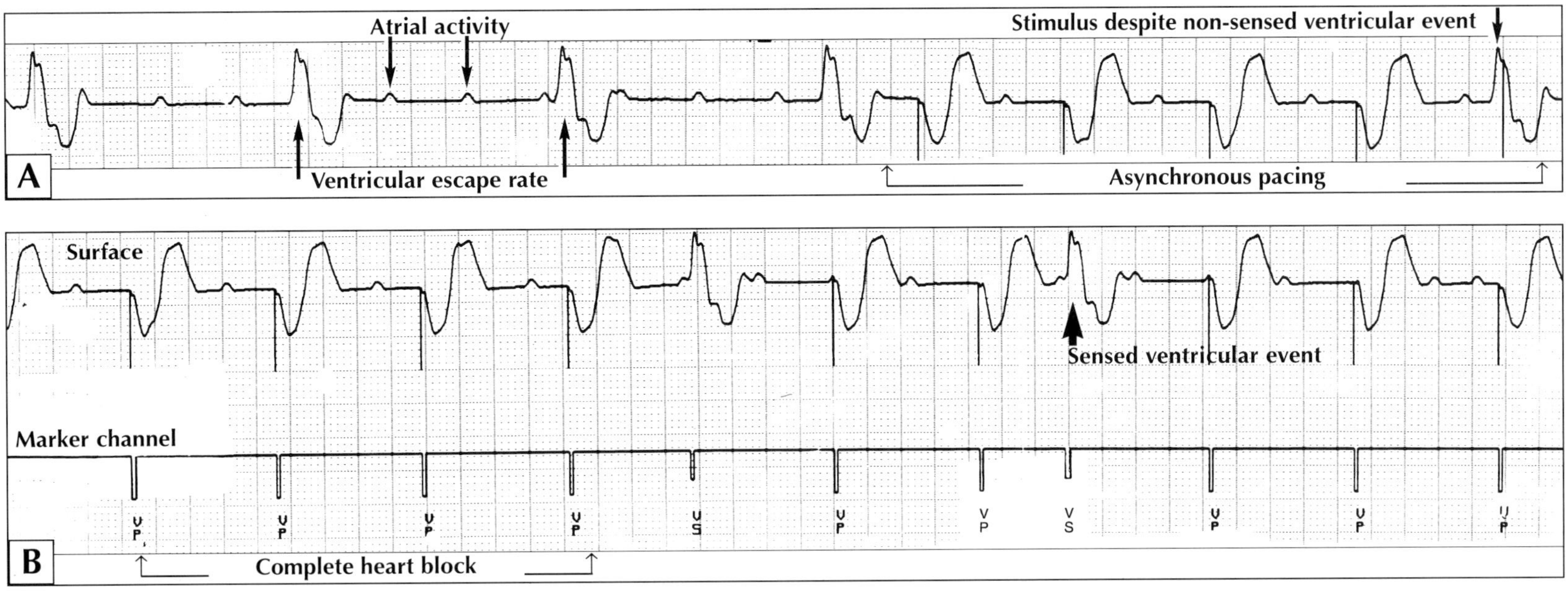

FIGURE 8-16. Asynchronous, fixed-rate pacing and demand pacing. Although the original fixed-rate ventricular pacemaker restored a stable heart rate, eliminated asystole, and represented a significant breakthrough, significant hemodynamic limitations associated with this simple pacing system remained. In **A** asynchronous pacing is demonstrated. In demand pacing, the sensing capability allows intermittent pacing when necessary and reduces competition between the native cardiac rhythm and that of the pacemaker. The demand pacemaker resulted in significant improvement in symptoms, cardiac function, and patient safety as well as battery longevity. A representative tracing using demand pacing is shown in **B**.

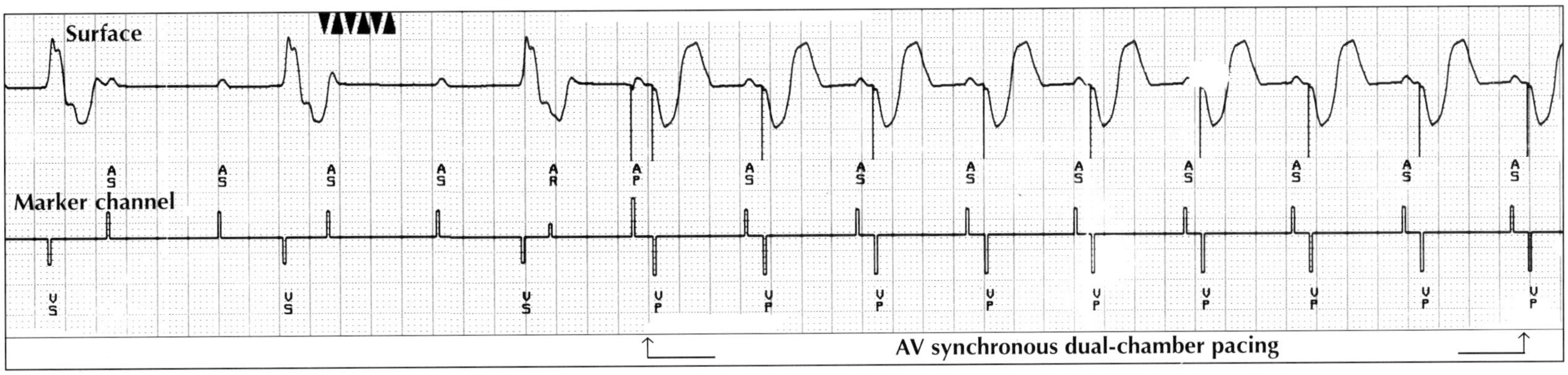

FIGURE 8-17. Atrioventricular synchrony. Atrioventricular (AV) sequential pacing, as shown in this ECG tracing, results in an improved sense of well being among patients relative to that with single chamber ventricular pacing. AV sequential pacing preserves normal atrial filling pressures and contributes some 20% (Karlof [4]) of cardiac output at rest through improved atrial transport. The benefit over single chamber pacing is perhaps most important and most evident among patients with impaired cardiac filling, including those with left ventricular hypertrophy and those with intact retrograde (ventricular-to-atrium) conduction. In addition, older patients and patients with impaired left ventricular function may particularly benefit from such AV synchrony. The advantages of AV synchronization with exercise are perhaps relatively small and harder to measure at present. Currently, research efforts are centered on more clearly defining the optimal AV delay at rest and exercise among selected patient groups with specific types of functional impairment.

A. PACEMAKER SYNDROME

Symptoms
- Fatigue, weakness, dizziness, syncope

Signs
- Hypotension, jugular venous cannon A waves

Physiology
- VA conduction, activation of arterial stretch receptors, decreased cardiac output, peripheral vascular vasodilatation

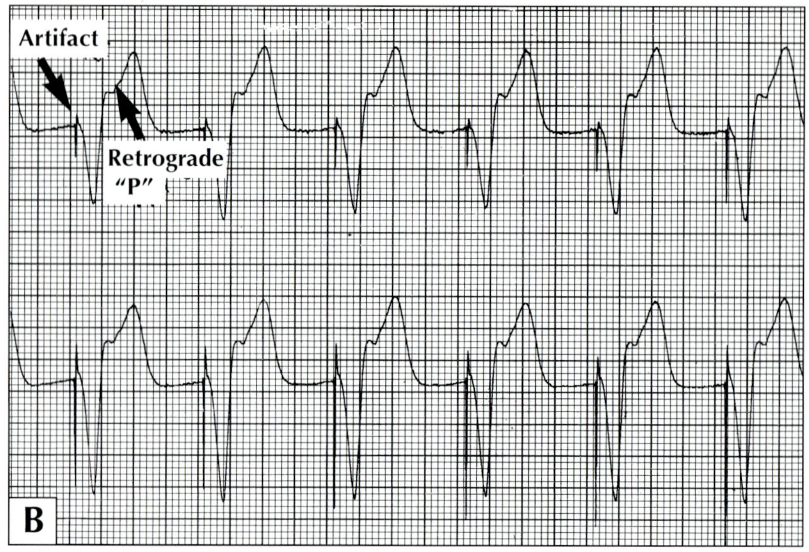

FIGURE 8-18. Pacemaker syndrome. Symptoms of syncope or dizziness (**A**) associated with hypotension following single-chamber ventricular-based (VVI) pacing are less frequent today as a result of the more widespread use of atrial-based pacing systems. When present, the syndrome occurs predominantly in the setting of intact retrograde (ventricle-to-atrium) conduction (**B**). VVI pacing may result in atrial mechanical systole at the time of closed atrioventricular valves, producing elevated atrial pressures, reduced transmitral blood flow and cardiac output, together with atrial stretch-mediated systemic and pulmonary reflexes, resulting in inappropriate peripheral vascular vasodilation.

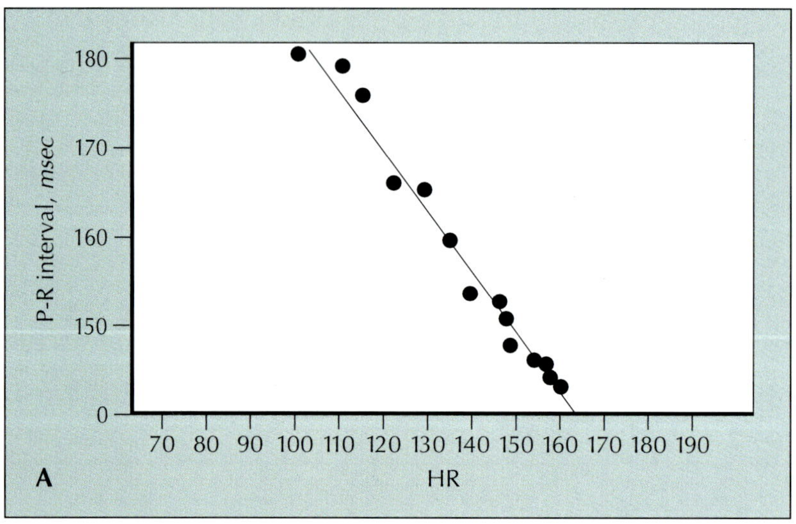

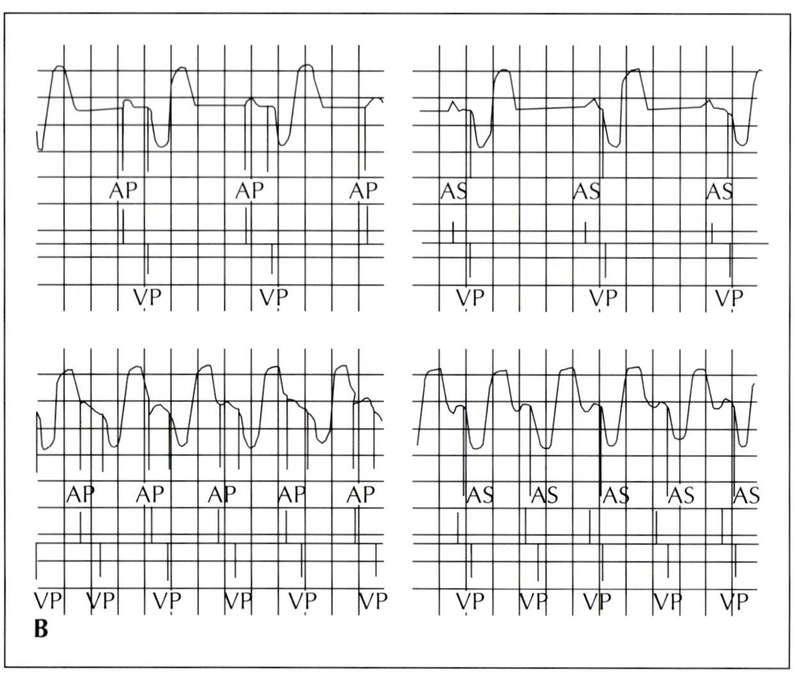

FIGURE 8-19. **A**, The native P-R interval is dynamic and shortens with exercise as shown in Figure 8-8A, along with all electrical events in response to physiologic demands with exercise. Among normal unpaced subjects this has been measured to approximate a decrease of 4 ms per 10-beat increase in heart rate per minute (Daubert, *et al.* [5]). The ECG tracings in **B** show adaptive paced atrioventricular (AV) delay shortening with increasing heart rate to approximate this relationship. AP—atrial pace; AS—atrial sense; VP—ventricular pace; VS—ventricular sense. (A *adapted from* Daubert and coworkers [5]; B *adapted from* Medtronic, Inc., Minneapolis, MN.)

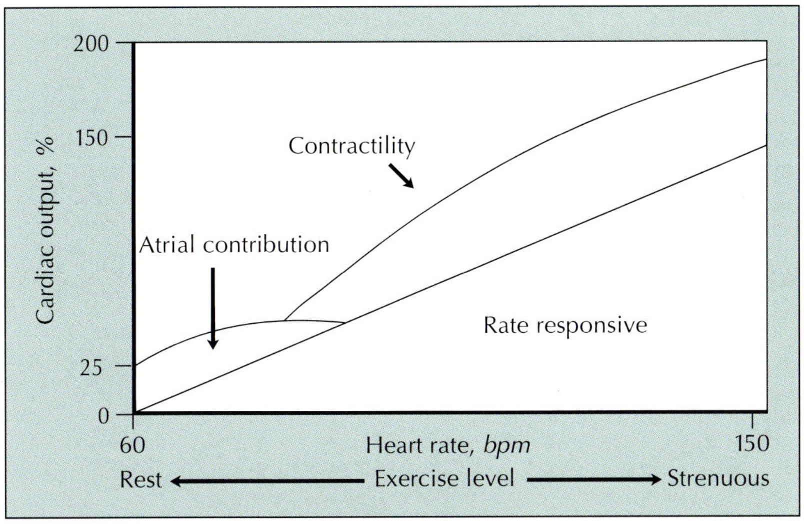

FIGURE 8–20. Heart rate. The cardiac output reserve needed to meet physiologic demands associated with peak exercise results primarily from increases in heart rate [6]. Highly trained athletes and, to a lesser degree, patients with normal cardiac function also meet these demands through significant increases in stroke volume. Patients who are not highly trained, particularly those with depressed left ventricular function, derive relatively small benefit from exercise-related increases in stroke volume.

Aging appears to result in both diminished heart rate reserve [7] and, ironically, a greater dependence upon this reserve, relative to stroke volume, to meet peak physiologic demands. These changes relate to electrical impairment within the native cardiac pacemaker (sinus node) and specialized conduction system and to mechanical changes, including impaired left ventricular filling [8] associated with reduced ventricular compliance. (*Adapted from* Benditt and coworkers [6].)

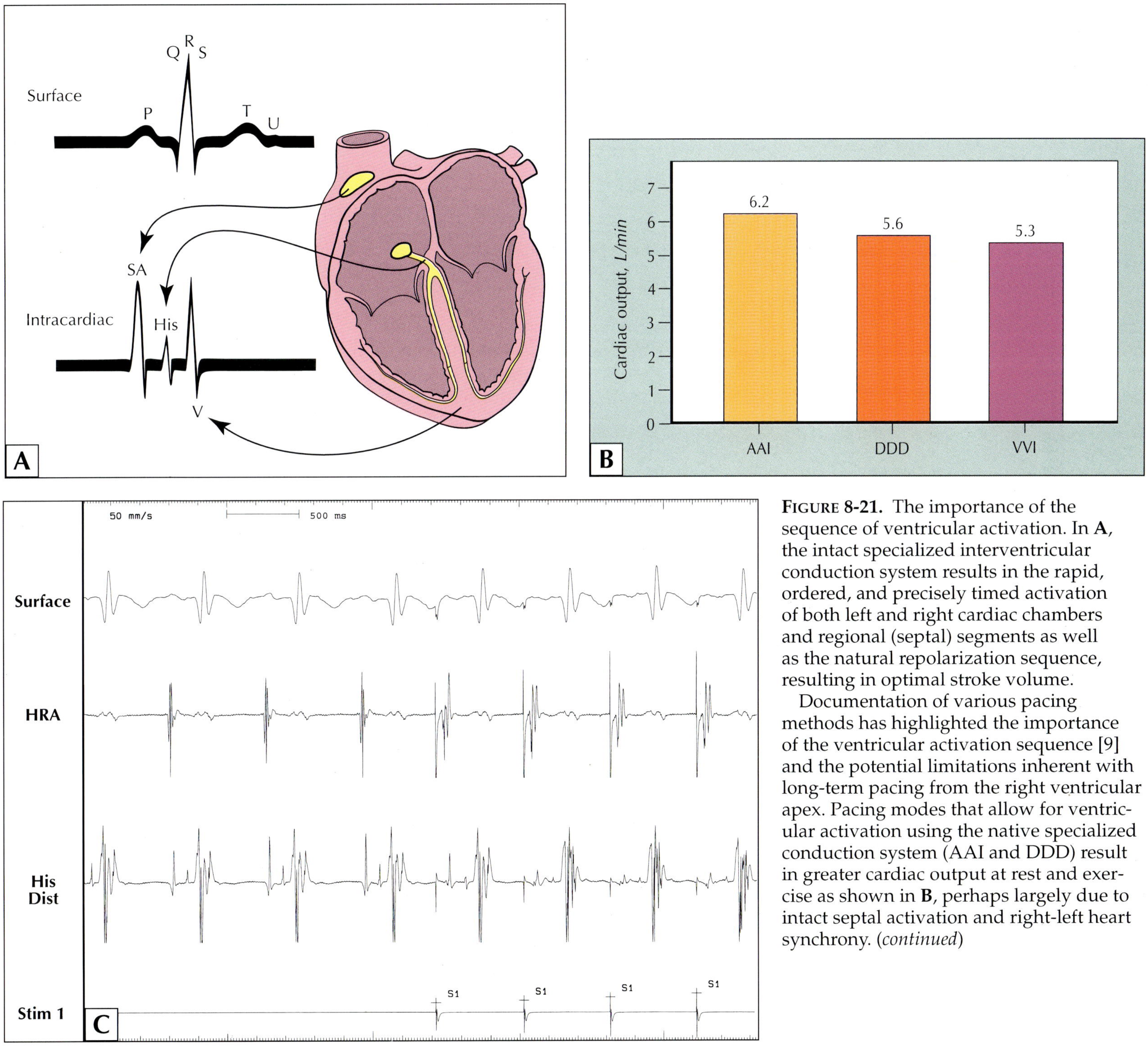

FIGURE 8-21. The importance of the sequence of ventricular activation. In **A**, the intact specialized interventricular conduction system results in the rapid, ordered, and precisely timed activation of both left and right cardiac chambers and regional (septal) segments as well as the natural repolarization sequence, resulting in optimal stroke volume.

Documentation of various pacing methods has highlighted the importance of the ventricular activation sequence [9] and the potential limitations inherent with long-term pacing from the right ventricular apex. Pacing modes that allow for ventricular activation using the native specialized conduction system (AAI and DDD) result in greater cardiac output at rest and exercise as shown in **B**, perhaps largely due to intact septal activation and right-left heart synchrony. (*continued*)

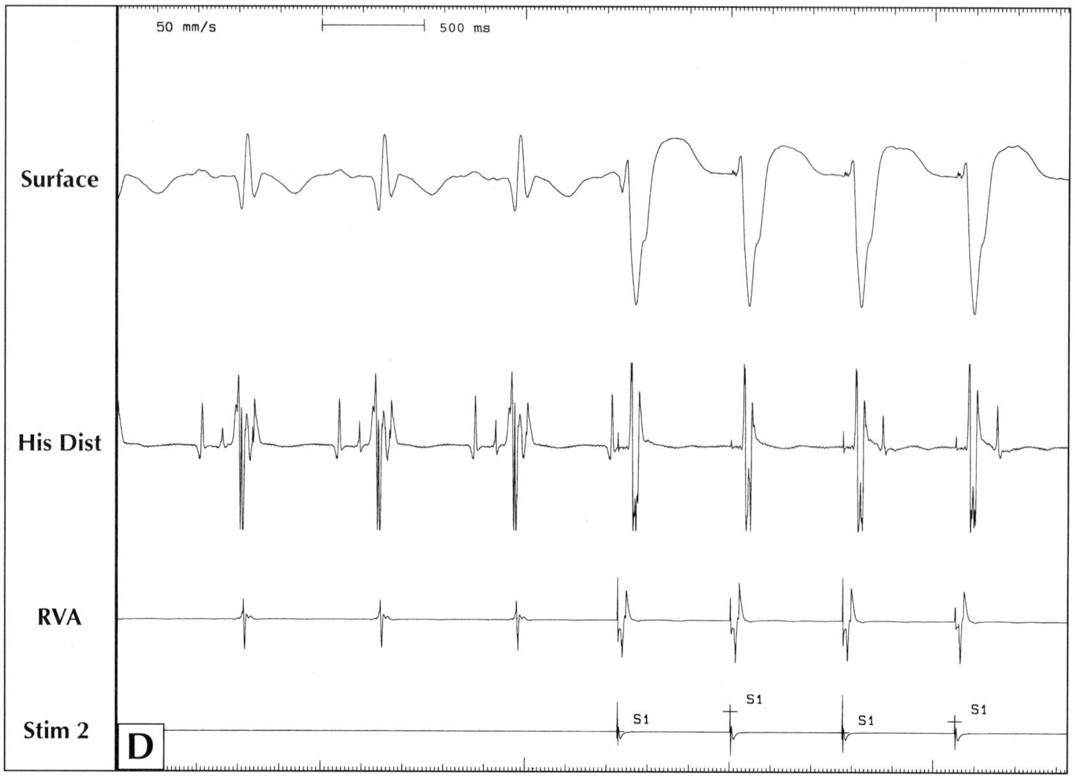

Figure 8-21. *(continued)* **C** and **D** demonstrate the ECG pattern of AAI and VVI pacing, respectively. AAI—atrial pacing, sensing, inhibition; His—His bundle; SA—sinoatrial node; V—ventricular; VVI—ventricular pacing, sensing, inhibition.

Cardiac Pacing and Survival

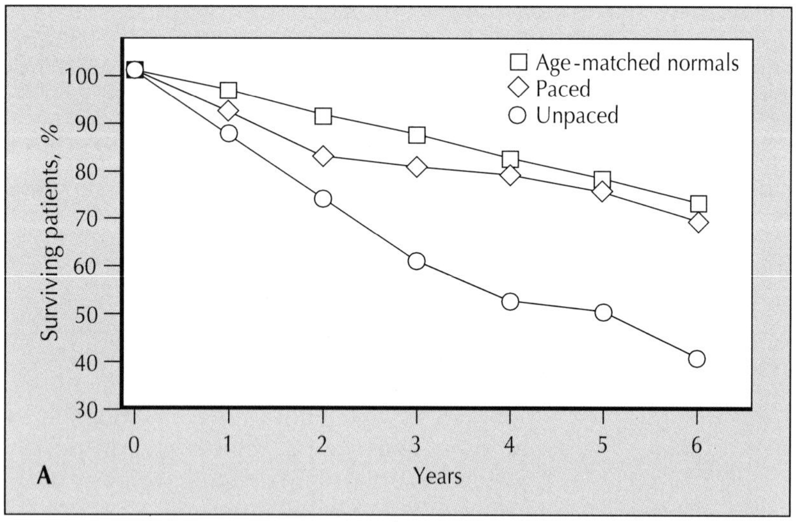

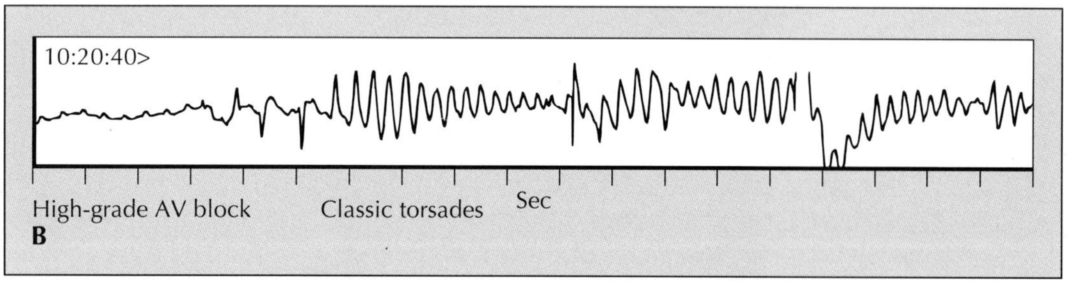

Figure 8-22. Heart block. **A,** Prior to the availability of pacemakers, survival among patients with third-degree heart block was dismal, approaching only 50% at one year and only 10% to 25% survival by five years [10]. Survival among patients with second-degree heart block is about 50% at five years compared with over 75% survival among patients receiving pacemakers [11]. **B,** Pacing prevents catastrophic bradycardia that predisposes patients to serious life-threatening arrhythmias such as torsades or associated trauma from sudden loss of blood pressure.

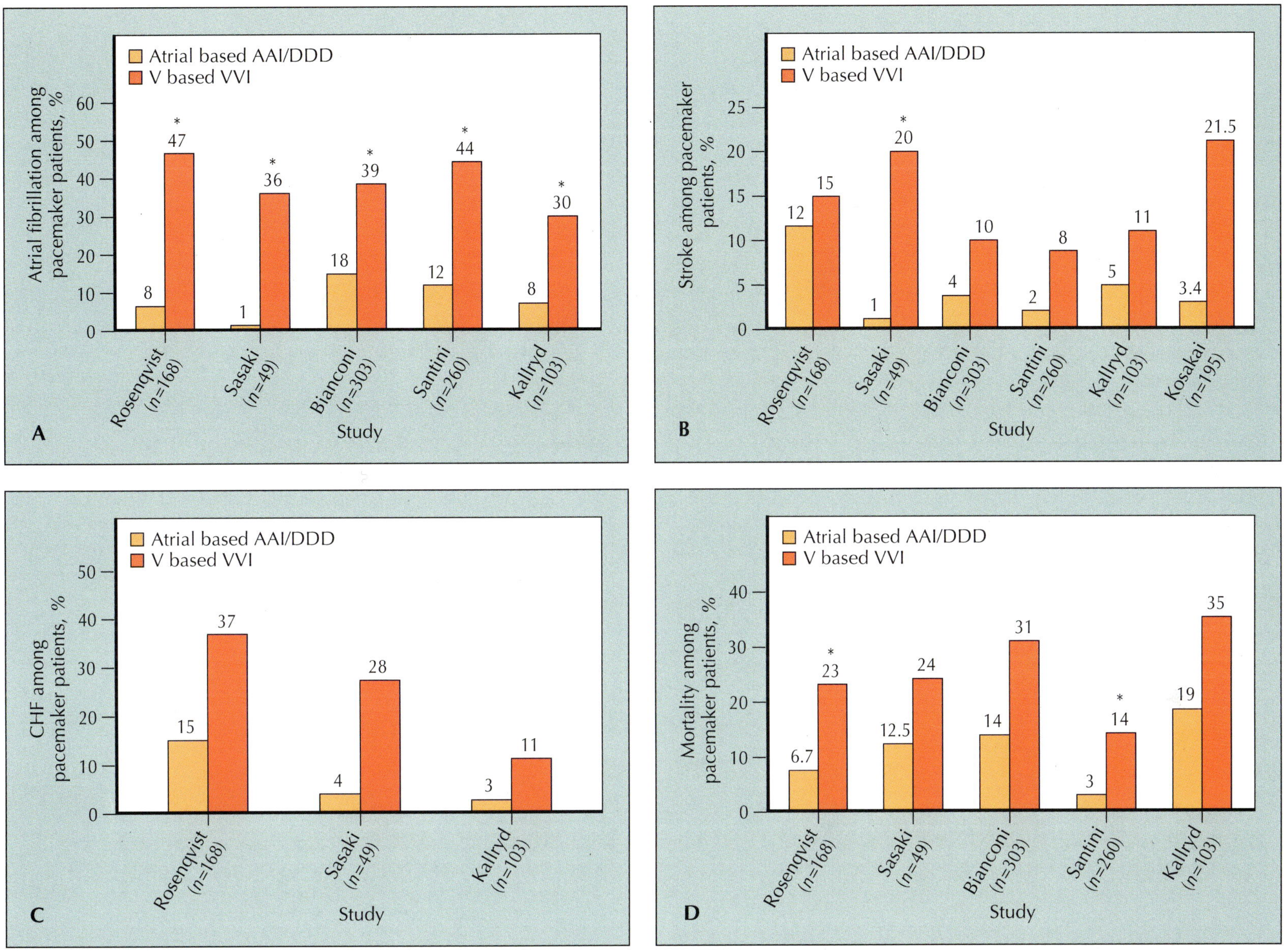

FIGURE 8-23. Sinus node disease. Due to the use of permanent pacemakers for the treatment of sinus node disease, its natural history is poorly understood. There may be a 5% excess mortality rate associated with the (treated) condition, and half of all deaths appear to be due to embolic events. In retrospective comparison studies, atrial or atrioventricular pacing was associated with significantly lower rates of new atrial fibrillation (**A**), stroke (**B**), and congestive heart failure (**C**) when compared with ventricular-based systems. Moreover, atrial or AV sequential pacing mode was associated with lower mortality rates, when compared with the rate associated with single-chamber ventricular pacing (**D**) [12–17]. AAI—atrial-pacing, sensing, inhibition; DDD—dual chamber (atrial and ventricular) pacing, sensing with atrial tracking, and ventricular inhibition; V—ventricular; VVI—ventricular pacing, sensing, inhibition.

Rate-adaptive pacing

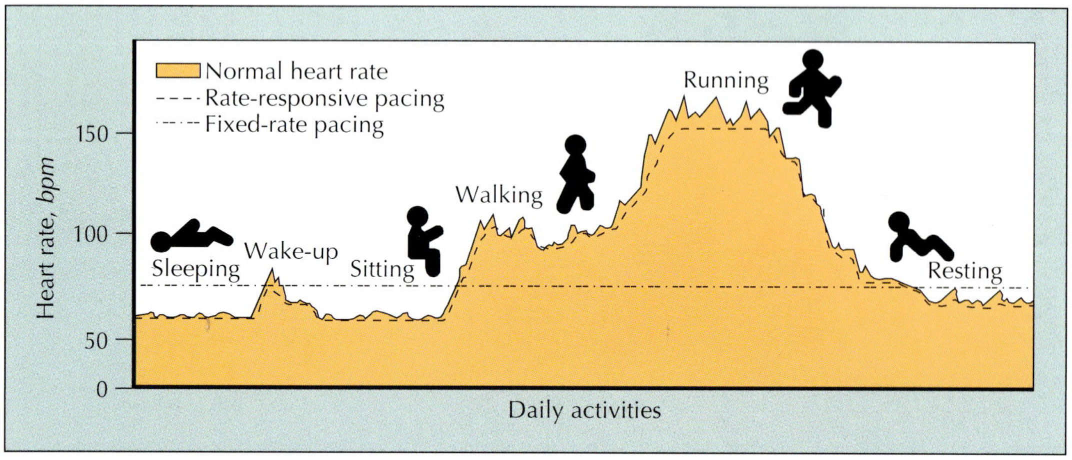

Figure 8-24. Adjusting heart rate to activity. Since the landmark achievement 35 years ago of restoring a stable cardiac rhythm with fixed-rate ventricular pacing (*straight dotted line*), efforts have focused on attempts to faithfully duplicate the rate responsiveness and physiologic characteristics of the native cardiac electrical pacemaking system. In the normal heart, rate (chronotropic) response accounts for a significant amount of the total cardiac reserve output in response to metabolic requirements with exercise (*shaded area*). A significant number, perhaps 50%, of patients receiving pacemakers today show variable amounts of chronotropic incompetence and may potentially benefit from pacing systems that offer chronotropic, rate-adaptive support. In addition, a significant number (estimated at 5% per year) of patients receiving pacing systems initially for heart-block, develop rate-incompetence during follow-up and would benefit from such capability as well. The ideal pacemaker would duplicate the impressive responsiveness of the autonomic and cardiac nervous system, sinus node, and specialized interventricular conduction system to meet the full array of physiologic requirements (dotted line). (*Adapted from* Medtronic, Inc., Minneapolis, MN.)

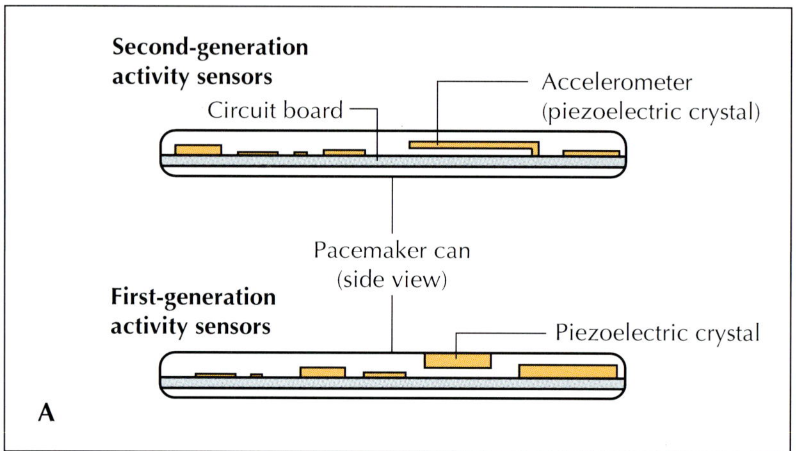

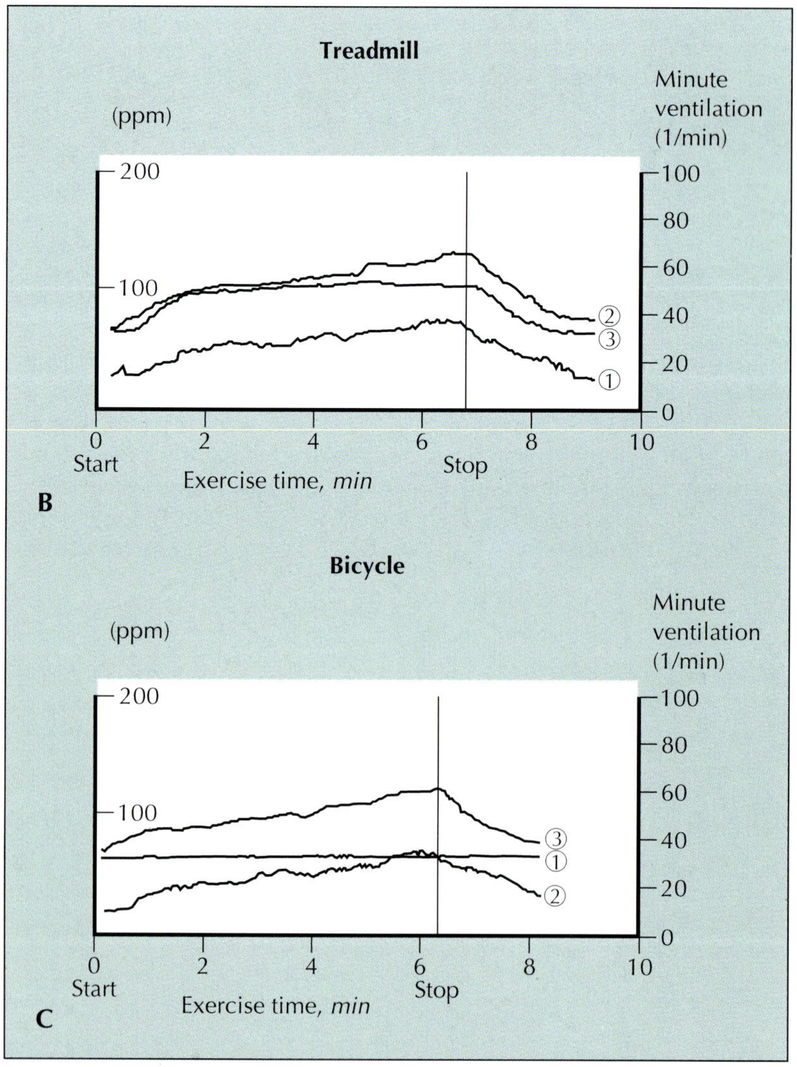

Figure 8-25. Pacemaker sensor systems. Various physiologic sensor systems have been developed to provide heart rate variability in pacemaker systems. Since reports of the initial rate-adaptive system in 1977 [18] several sensors for rate-adaptive systems have evolved. In **A**, direct body activity (motion) sensors mounted within the pacemaker cannister include the use of piezoelectric crystals to detect body activity or acceleration and provide appropriate, programmable sensor-indicated dynamic heart rate variability.

Indirect metabolic sensors, including those that detect respiratory rate or minute ventilation, are presently in use and may provide improved responses to different forms of activity such as that associated with upright (**B**) and bicycle (**C**) exercise. In addition, sensor systems that measure mixed-venous temperature are in clinical use at present. Other sensors, including direct metabolic indicators (central venous pH, mixed-venous O_2 saturation) and nonmetabolic physiologic indices (stim-T interval, QT interval, evoked ventricular potentials, systolic indices and pressure sensors), are in various stages of development. PPM—pulse per minute.

The use of multiple sensor systems is emerging and holds promise for improved, more specific rate adaptation; however, this practice also reflects the limitations inherent with any single sensor system in use at present. ①—first-generation activity sensor; ②—second-generation activity sensor; ③—minute ventilation sensor. Part A *adapted from* Intermedics, Inc. Parts B and C *adapted from* Telectronics, Inc., Englewood, CO.

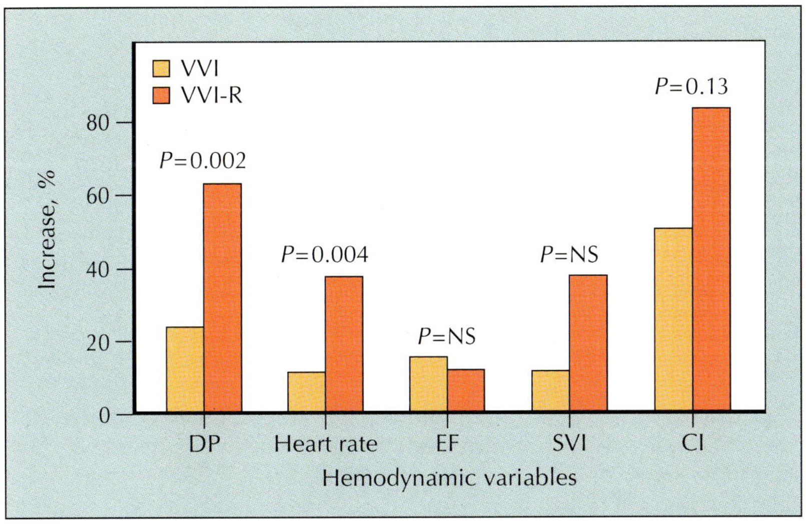

FIGURE 8-26. The benefits of rate-adaptive pacing with exercise. Studies have documented the hemodynamic and symptomatic improvement with single-chamber, rate-adaptive pacing compared with fixed-rate pacing [19]. Using presently available measurement techniques, it has been harder to define measurable differences between single- and dual-chamber rate-adaptive pacing, and this is the subject of ongoing studies. Differences over the long-term remain to be defined. Comparative assessments involving multiple sensor systems, where differences may be subtle, are likely to represent an even greater challenge, given the limitations of present measurement techniques. CI—cardiac index; DP—double products, heart rate × systolic blood pressure; EF—ejection fraction; SVI—stroke volume index; VVI—ventricular pacing, sensing, inhibition; VVI-R— VVI with rate adaptive capability. (*Adapted from* Buckingham and coworkers [19].)

Newer Uses for Cardiac Pacing

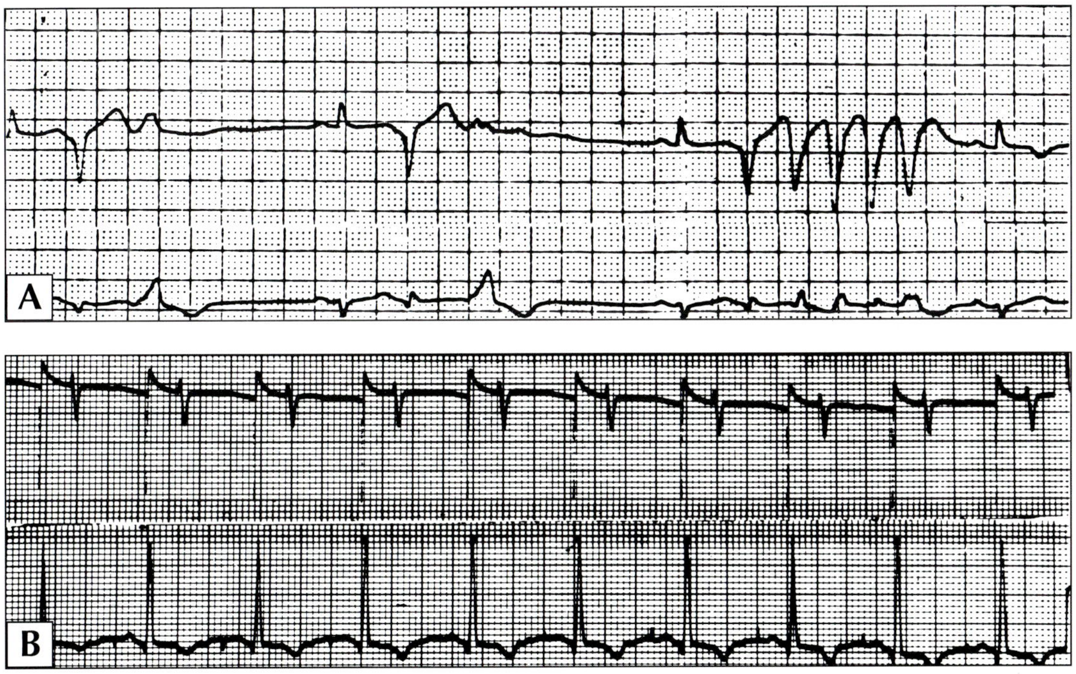

FIGURE 8-27. Disorders of myocardial repolarization. Primary electrical system disease resulting in disordered myocardial repolarization and the potential for malignant arrhythmias (**A**) has emerged as a new indication for cardiac pacing among symptomatic patients [20]. Pacing (**B**) for selected patients with the congenital or acquired long QT syndrome, those with acquired pause-dependent arrhythmias, and patients with the profound (malignant) cardio-inhibitory form of neurally mediated syncope can result in a stable cardiac rhythm and QT interval.

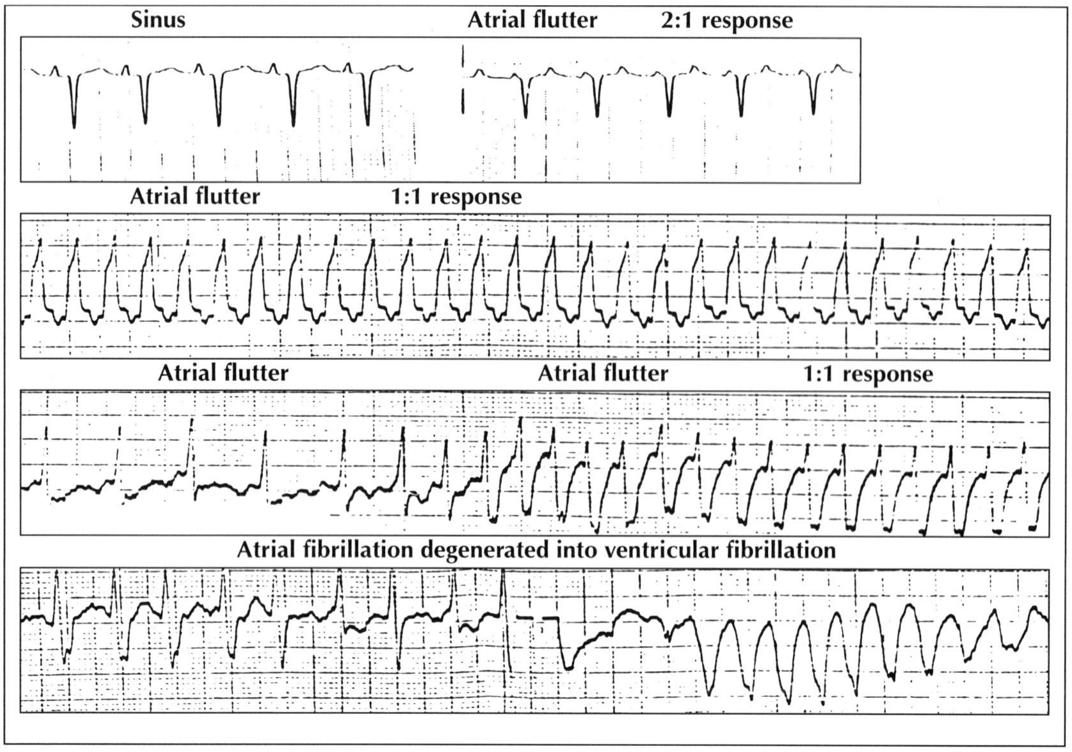

FIGURE 8-28. Refractory atrial arrhythmias. There is increasing experience with patients who suffer limiting symptoms and life-threatening ventricular arrhythmias from atrial fibrillation, flutter, and tachycardia, often in the setting of left ventricular hypertrophy, not responsive or intolerant to medical therapy. Newer nonpharmacologic approaches, including radiofrequency catheter ablation or modification of the atrioventricular junction followed by rate-adaptive pacing have resulted in encouraging results, improvement in symptoms, and possibly improved function [21] in a growing number of patients.

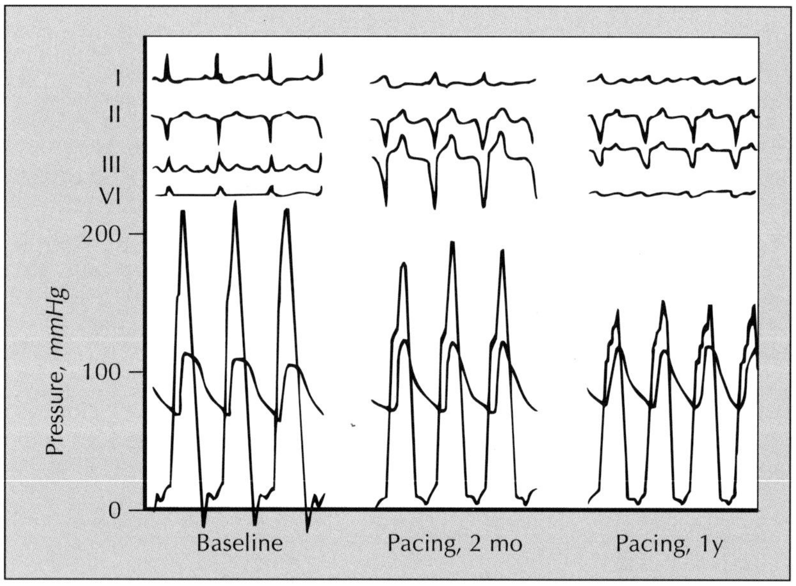

FIGURE 8-29. Hypertrophic obstructive cardiomyopathy. Dual chamber pacing with ventricular control may improve symptoms in a majority of patients with refractory symptoms associated with the dynamic subaortic obstruction. The typical "spike-and-dome" pressure gradient is significantly reduced from that observed during sinus rhythm [22] and may show progressive improvement [23] over time. This approach takes advantage of the hemodynamic effects of pacing from the right ventricular apex and the associated pacing-induced changes due to altered septal activation in the region of the dynamic obstruction at the septum and left ventricular outflow tract.

Historically, patients with symptoms refractory to medical therapy (usually β-blockade or calcium entry blocking drugs such as verapamil) have been candidates for surgery (myectomy) to improve symptoms. Such surgery, however, has been associated with high perioperative morbidity and unpredictable efficacy.

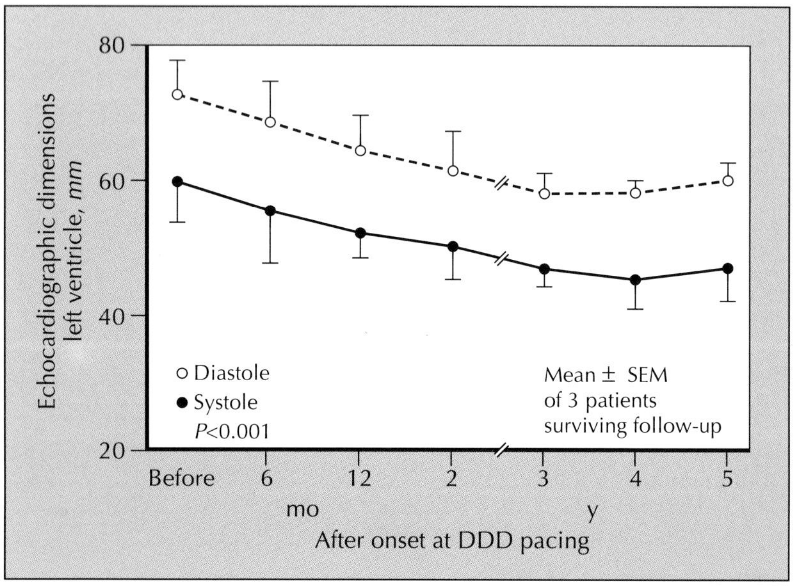

FIGURE 8-30. Idiopathic dilated cardiomyopathy. Patients with advanced cardiomyopathy and symptoms from low-output failure refractory to medical therapy may benefit from dual-chamber pacing therapy [24] to control heart rate and atrioventricular synchrony. In addition to symptomatic improvement, beneficial changes in measured cardiac indices such as echocardiographic internal dimensions may be observed over time. Changes in pacing site, activation sequence, and timing [25,26] may be especially important among these patients.

References

1. Elmquist R, Senning A: Implantable Paemaker for the Heart. In *Medical Electronics: Proceedings of the Second International Conference on Medical Electronics*. Paris, June 1959. Edited by Smyth CN. London: Iliffe & Sons, 1960.
2. Bernstein AD, Camm AJ, Fletcher RD, *et al.*: The NASPE/BPEG generic pacemaker code for antibradyarrhythmia and adaptive-rate pacing and antitachyarrhythmia devices. *PACE* 1987, 10:794.
3. VA National Registry. June 1989–June 1990.
4. Karlof I: Hemodynamic studies at rest and during exercise in patients treated with artificial pacemaker. *Acta Med Scand* 1974, 565(suppl):1–24.
5. Daubert C, Ritter P, Mabo P, *et al.*: Physiologic relationship between AV interval and heart rate in healthy subjects: applications to dual chamber pacing. *PACE* 1986, 9:1032–1039.
6. Benditt DG, Milstein S, Buetikofer J, *et al.*: Sensor-triggered, rate-variable cardiac pacing. *Ann Intern Med* 1987, 107:714–724.
7. Kostis J, Moreyra A, Amendo M, *et al.*: The effect of age on heart rate in subjects free of heart disease. *Circulation* 1982, 65(1):141–145.
8. Bonow RO, Vitale DF, Bacharach SL, *et al.*: Effects of aging on asynchrounous left ventricular regional function and global ventricular filling in normal human subjects. *J Am Coll Cardiol* 1988, 11(1):50–58.
9. Rosenqvist M, Isaz K, Botvinick EH, *et al.*: Relative importance of activation sequence compared to atrioventricular sequence in left ventricular function. *Am J Cardiol* 1991, 67:148–156.
10. Johansson BW: Longevity in complete heart block. *Ann NY Acad Sci* 1969, 167:1031–037.
11. Shaw DB, Kekwick CA, Veal D, *et al.*: Survival in second degree AV block. *Br Heart J* 1990, 53:587–593.
12. Bianconi L, Boccadamo R, Di Florio A, *et al.*: Atrial versus ventricular stimulation in sick sinus syndrome: Effects on morbidity and mortality. *PACE* 1989, 12:1236–242.
13. Kallryd A, Kristensson B-E, Ryden L, *et al.*: Atrial versus ventricular pacing in sinus node disease. Clinical experience. 6th Nordic Synposium on Cardiac Pacing, Arhus, 1990.
14. Rosenqvist M, Brandt J, Schuller H: Long-term pacing in sinus node disease. Effect of stimulation mode on cardiovascular morbidity and mortality. *Am Heart J* 1988, 116:16–22.
15. Santini M, Messina G, Porto MP, *et al.*: Relation of prognosis in sich sinus syndrome to age, conduction defects, and modes of permanent cardiac pacing. *Am J Cardiol* 1990, 65:729–735.
16. Sasaki Y, Shimotori M, Akahane K, *et al.*: Long-term follow-up of patients with sick sinus syndrome: A comparison of clinical aspects among unpaced, ventricular inhibited paced, and physiologically paced groups. *PACE* 1988, 11:1575–1583.
17. Kosakai Y, Ohe T, Kamakura S: Long-term follow-up of incidence of embolism in sich sinus syndrome after pacing. *PACE* 1991, 1,14:680–686.
18. Cammilli L, Adeidi L, Papeschi G: A new pacemaker autoregulating the rate of pacing in relation to metabolic needs. In *Cardiac pacing*. Edited by Watanabe Y. Amsterdam: Excerpta Medica; 1977:4149.
19. Buckingham TA, Woodruff RC, Pennington G, *et al.*: Effect of ventricular function on the exercise hemodynamics of variable rate pacing. *J Am Coll Cardiol* 1988, 11:169–177.
20. Moss AJ, Liu JE, Gottlieb S, *et al.*: Efficacy of permanent pacing in the management of high-risk patients with long QT syndrome. *Circulation* 1991, 84:1524–1529.
21. Kay GN, Bubien RS, Epstein AE, Plumb VJ: Effect of catheter ablation of the atrioventricualr junction on quality of life and exercise tolerance in paroxysmal atrial fibrillation. *Am J Cardiol* 1988, 62:741–744.
22. Fananapazir L, Cannon RO, Tripodi D, Panza JA: Impact of dual-chamber permanent pacing in patients with obstructive hypertrophic cardiomyopathy with symptoms refractory to verapamil and β-adrenergic blocker therapy. *Circulation* 1992, 85:2149–2161.
23. Fananapazir L, Epstein ND, Curiel RV, *et al.*: Long-term results of dual-chamber (DDD) pacing in obstructive hypertrophic cardiomyopathy. *Circulation* 1994, 90:2731–2742.
24. Hochleitner M, Hortnagl H, Ng CK, *et al.*: Usefulness of physiologic dual-chamber pacing in drug-resistant idiopathic dilated cardiomyopathy. *Am J Cardiol* 1990, 66:198–202.
25. Nishimura RA, Hayes DL, Holms DR, Tajik AJ: Mechanisms of hemodynamic improvement by dual-chamber pacing for severe left ventricular dysfunction: an acute doppler and catheterization hemodynammic study. *J Am Coll Cardiol* 1995, 25:281–288.
26. Hochlectness M, Hortnagl H, Fritrich L, Gschnitzer F: Long-term efficacy of physiologic dual-chamber pacing in the treamtent of end-stage idiopathic dilated cardiomyopathy. *Am J Cardiol* 1992, 70:1320–1325.

IMPLANTABLE DEFIBRILLATORS FOR THE MANAGEMENT OF CARDIAC RHYTHM DISORDERS

9

CHAPTER

James L. Cockrell and Andreana Siu

Since the first use in humans in 1980, following the visionary, pioneering efforts of Mirowski and Mower, the novel approach of implantable defibrillator therapy has emerged as the cornerstone of modern antiarrhythmia therapy to treat patients who are at risk for recurrent life-threatening cardiac arrhythmias.

The recent development of smaller, sophisticated implantable devices, capable of advanced diagnostic and therapeutic functions, together with equally impressive advances in implantation techniques, have resulted in the potential for wider application, improved patient outcome and patient acceptance, and reduced associated costs.

The Clinical Problem of Sudden Cardiac Death

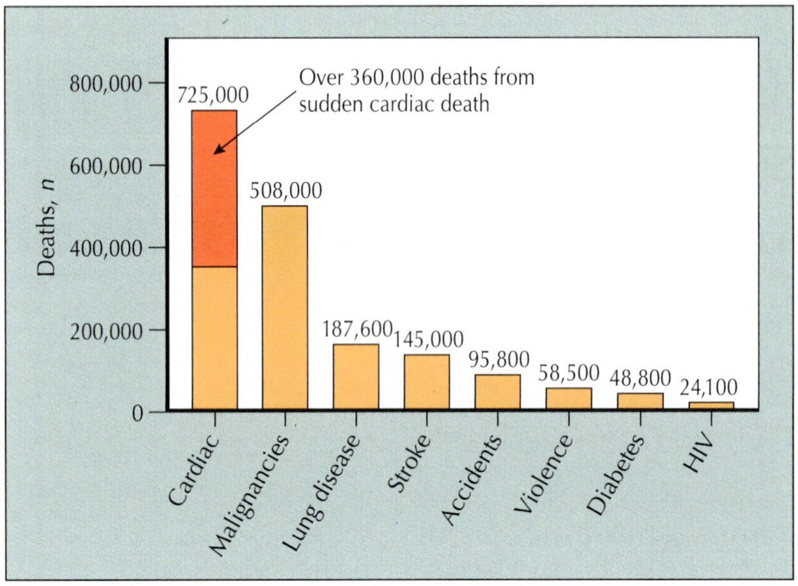

Figure 9-1. Annual deaths in the United States. Sudden cardiac death affects some 360,000 people in North America each year, and the majority of those affected do not survive [1]. Due to public awareness and emergency medical resuscitation efforts, perhaps 10% to 15% are successfully resuscitated and enter the medical system for treatment. (*Adapted from* Statistical Abstract of the United States [1a].)

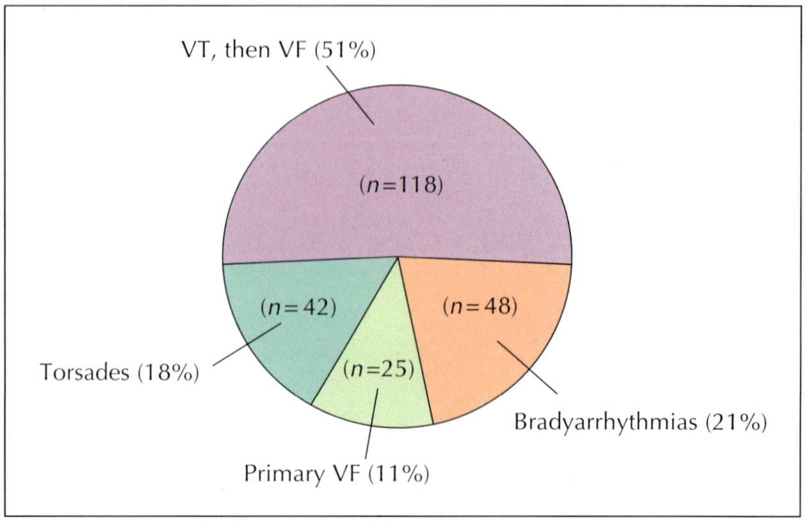

Figure 9-2. Cardiac arrhythmia at the time of sudden death. The cardiac rhythm present at the time of sudden death is usually ventricular tachycardia (VT) or fibrillation (VF) [2] as detected by ambulatory monitoring. The cardiac arrhythmogenic substrate is generally chronic, with various degrees of myocardial fibrosis such as that following myocardial infarction. This predisposes to lethal events following otherwise benign triggering events. (*Adapted from* Bayes and coworkers[2].)

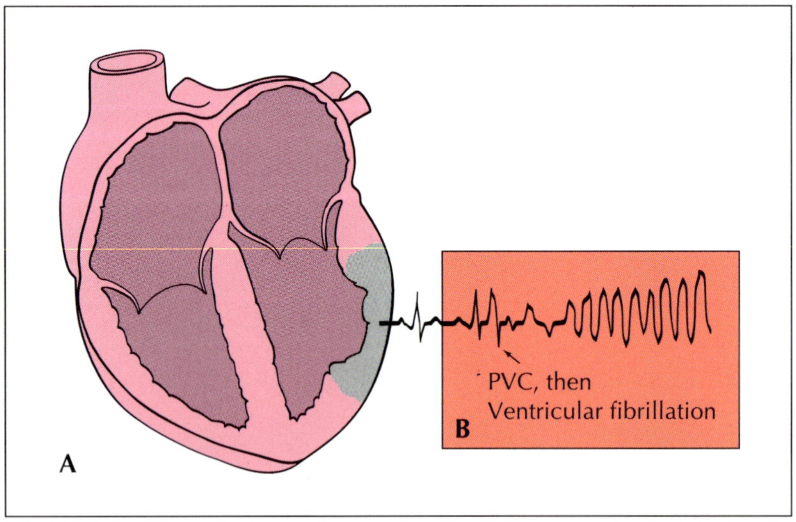

Figure 9-3. Substrate for malignant arrhythmias. **A**, Evidence of healed or recent myocardial infarction (shaded area) [3] and significant coronary artery atherosclerosis [4], even in the absence of a suggestive clinical history [5], have been frequent findings at autopsy following sudden death. **B** shows premature ventricular contraction (PVC), resulting in ventricular fibrillation.

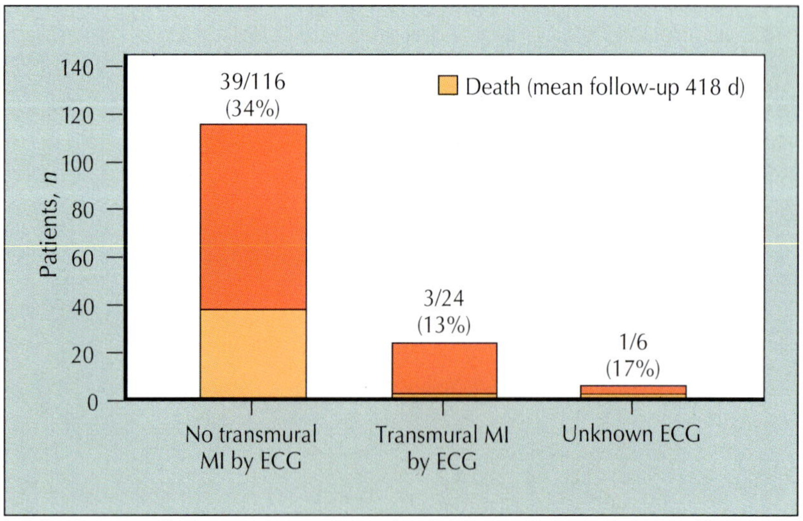

Figure 9-4. Recurrent sudden death after hospital discharge following out-of-hospital ventricular fibrillation. Recurrent sudden death occurs at very high rates, particularly early after the initial event and among patients resuscitated and hospitalized without evidence of new transmural myocardial infarction by ECG [6].

The emergence of implantable cardioverter defibrillator technology is based on the important clinical observation that time to resuscitation is the critical factor for survival. The relatively disappointing results with antiarrhythmic drug treatment to prevent recurrent sudden death has propelled device therapy to the forefront of current therapy. (*Adapted from* Baum and coworkers [6].)

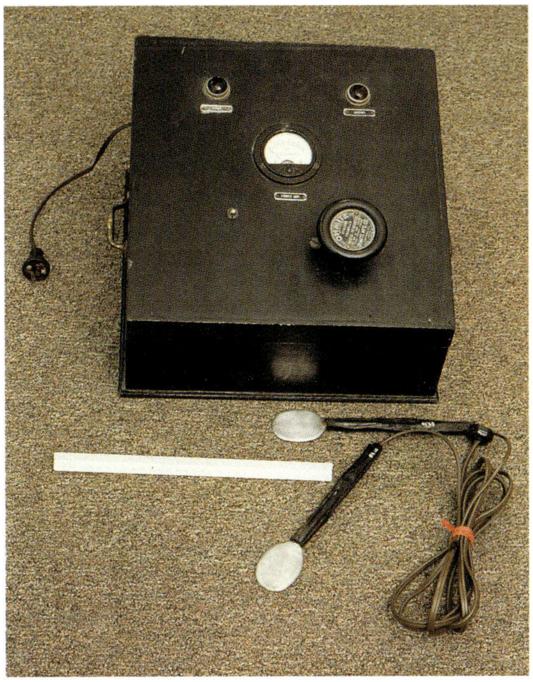

FIGURE 9-5. Early defibrillation in clinical use. The roots of many of the modern concepts of cardiac fibrillation and defibrillation are attributed to the publications of Prevost and Batelli in 1899 and 1900. The vulnerable phase in the cardiac cycle for ventricular fibrillation was described in 1940. The first open chest defibrillation was described in 1947 by Beck, and the first closed-chest in 1957 by Zoll and Linenthal. (*Courtesy of* Medtronics, Inc., Minneapolis, MN; with permission.)

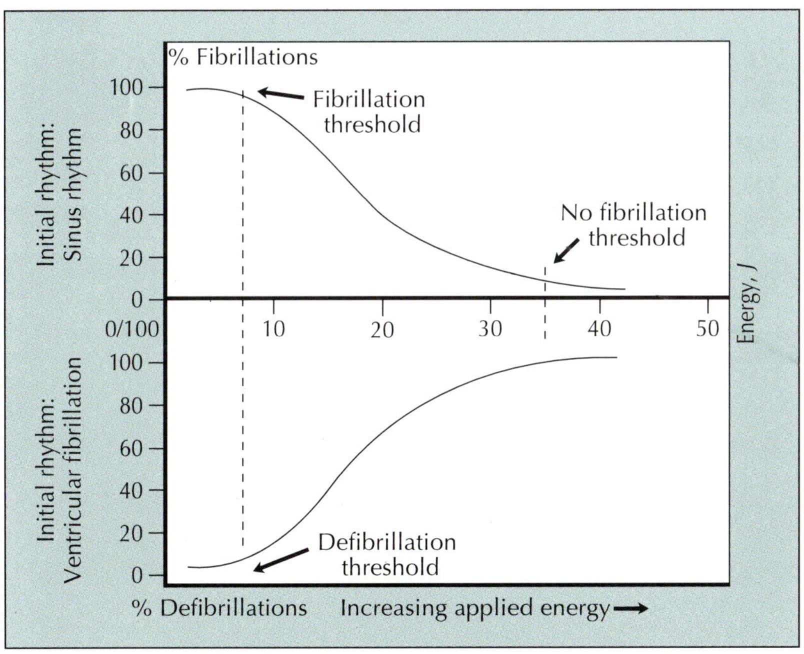

FIGURE 9-6. Cardiac fibrillation and defibrillation are related. Present concepts of the fundamental relation between fibrillation and defibrillation thresholds in the canine model were described in 1965 by Coumel [7]. This set the stage for improvements and wide application of portable external defibrillators and the novel approach for internal defibrillation. Shock energy in the vulnerable period as it relates to cardiac rhythm is shown in this figure. (*Adapted from* Coumel [7].)

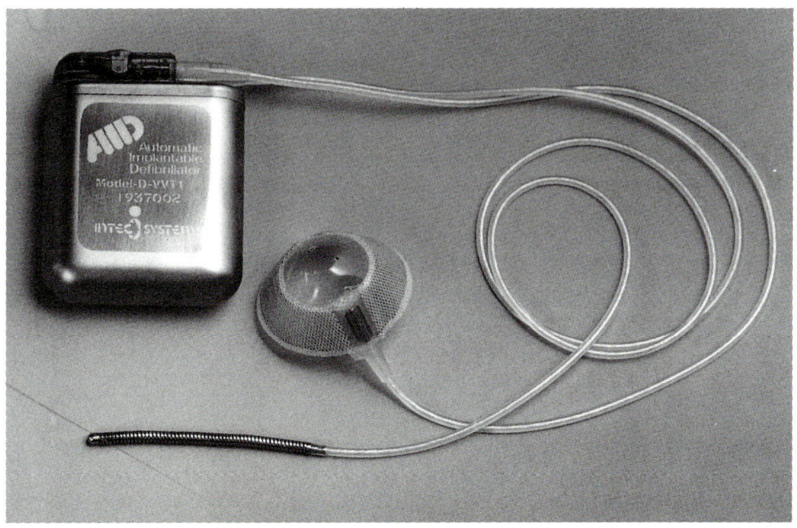

FIGURE 9-7. The first implantable defibrillator. The first implantable defibrillator, described in 1970, was conceived and developed by Mirowski [8] and Mower. In many ways it remains the standard today. It was a single-lead transvenous system that monitored right ventricular pressure and delivered 50 J energy through two electrodes on the same lead. His inspiration led to the first human implant in 1980 at Johns Hopkins Medical Center [9]. (*Courtesy of* Cardiac Pacemakers, Inc., St. Paul, MN; with permission.)

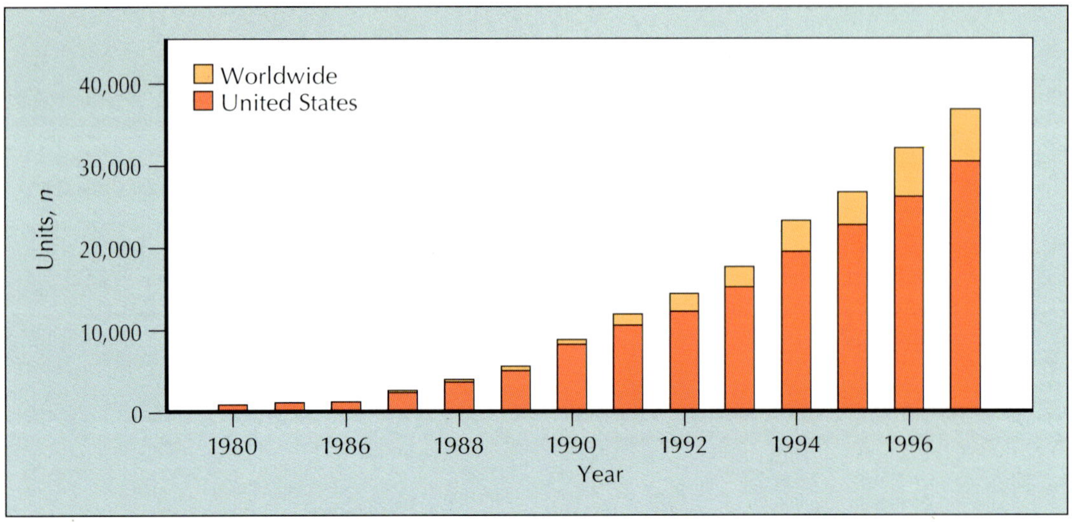

FIGURE 9-8. The growth of defibrillator implantation. To date, four evolutionary generations of devices have been in clinical use, largely to treat patients with a history of ventricular fibrillation or ventricular tachycardia and coronary disease and with reduced left ventricular function. Data shown for 1995 and later are projected figures. (*Data from* Cardiac Pacemakers, Inc., St. Paul, MN.)

PREVENTION OF RECURRENT SUDDEN DEATH

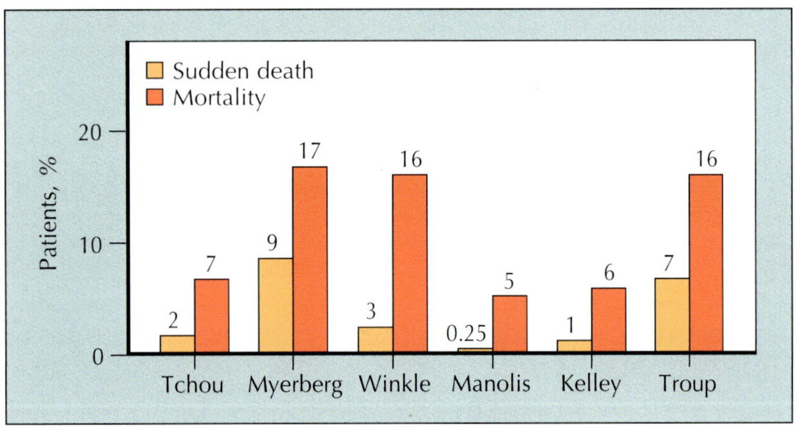

FIGURE 9-9. Improved survival after implantable cardioverter defibrillator therapy. The implantable defibrillator has had a remarkable impact on improving the freedom from recurrent sudden death relative to historical experiences, ranging from 91% at one-year to 96% at five years, in a number of clinical studies [10–18]. Overall survival has been reported to range from 95% [19] at one year to 60% [20] at 3 years. Most deaths are due to congestive heart failure [10,17,19] and a much smaller proportion are due to bradyarrhythmias, electromechanical dissociation, or device failure [20].

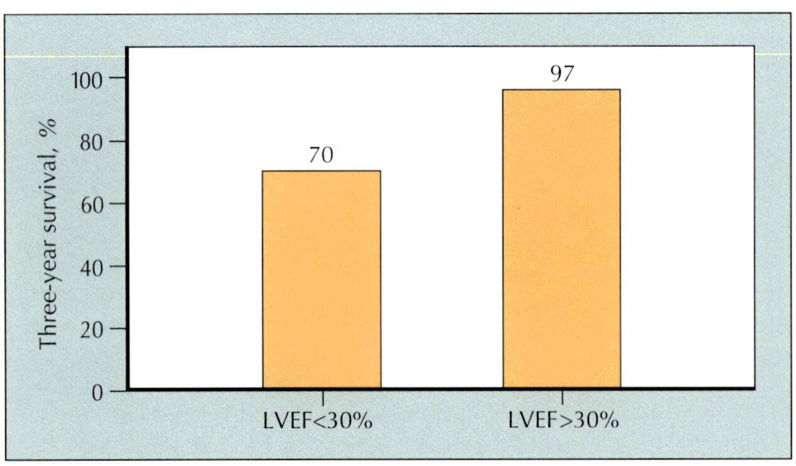

FIGURE 9-10. Effect of severity of cardiac disease on survival. Survival in patients treated with implantable defibrillator therapy is influenced by the type and severity of underlying heart disease [13,17,18,19,21] and functional classification. Three-year survival following implantation was 90% among patients with left ventricular ejection fractions (LVEF) greater than or equal to 30%, and only 70% among patients with an LVEF less than 30% as reported by Kim and coworkers [22]. (*Adapted from* Kim and coworkers [22].)

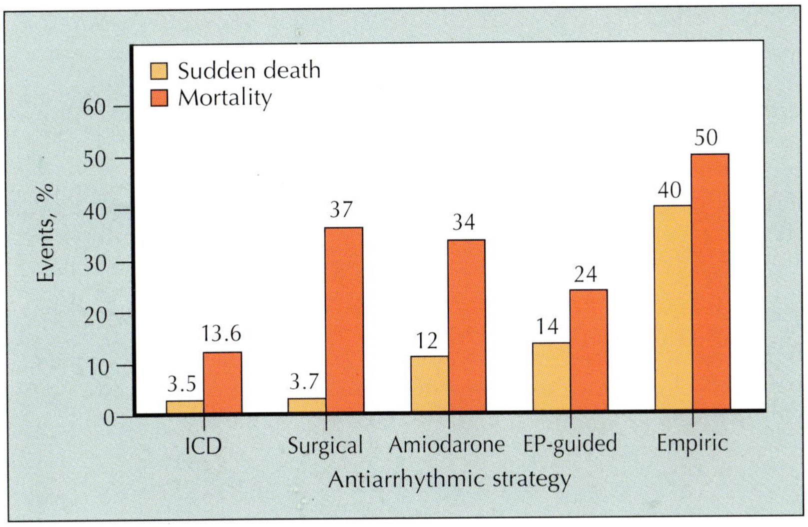

FIGURE 9-11. Two-year results. While the proportion of patients with recurrent sudden death within two years following implantable cardioverter defibrillator (ICD) therapy (3.5%) [13,17,18,23,24] and map-guided arrhythmia surgery (3.7%) [16,25] was similar, the total mortality at two years for ICD (13.6%) and arrhythmia surgery (37%) was quite divergent. The surgical approach was not applicable to all patients with a history of malignant arrhythmias, and it has been associated with higher perioperative mortality rates [26]. Success has been relatively center-specific and less widely available when compared with ICD therapy.

Therapy limited to antiarrhythmic drug treatment, without employing nonpharmacologic options, has been associated with higher two-year cumulative sudden death rates for amiodarone [27] and therapy guided by serial electropharmacologic (EP) testing [28].

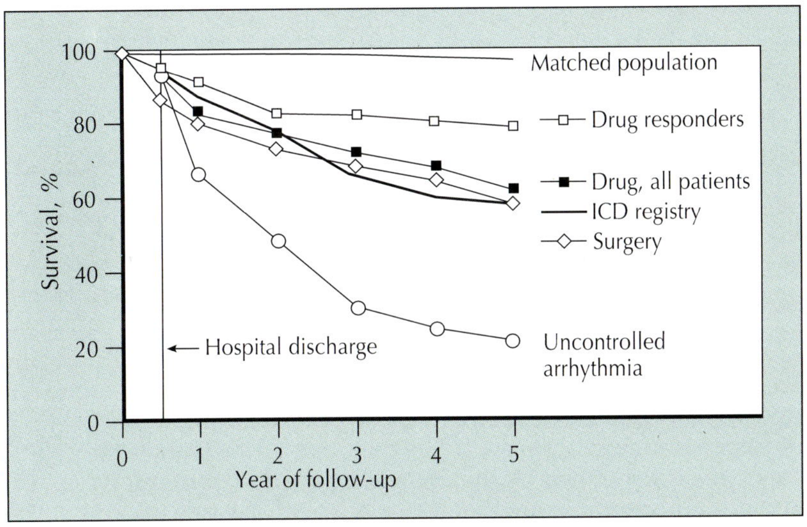

FIGURE 9-12. Five-year results. Survival among patients whose arrhythmias remain uncontrolled has been very poor, approaching only 20% in five years follow-up [29–33]. In contrast, survival among patients whose arrhythmias have remained controlled with specific drug therapy and confirmed by electrophysiologic testing is over 75% [31]. Patients with refractory arrhythmias who have been treated with map-guided surgical therapy [26,34–36] or first- and second-generation implantable cardioverter defibrillator therapy (registry data [38]) for refractory arrhythmias have similar survival at five years, approaching 60%. (*Adapted from* Fisher and coworkers [38a].)

COMPLICATIONS ASSSOCIATED WITH NONTHORACOTOMY ICD THERAPY*

COMPLICATION	INCIDENCE, %
Pace/sense related	0.8
Therapy related	1.2
Pocket related	4.8
Lead related	3.2
Decreased battery voltage	0.5

*757 Patients, Mean Follow-up 11.7 mo

FIGURE 9-13. Long-term complicating factors. Long-term complications, usually requiring specific surgical intervention, include pacing lead under- or over-sensing and loss of capture. Therapy-related complications, particularly increased defibrillation requirements in the setting of additional antiarrhythmic drug therapy [39], are observed. Pocket-related complications, including pulse generator migration (reported in 0.7% to 1.2% of recipients [39]), infection due to *Staphylococcus epidermidis*, skin erosion, seroma, and hematoma, are all largely related to the size of the pulse generator. Lead-related complications, including dislodgement, fracture, and perforation, have declined relative to that (5% to 8% [20,41] of patients) reported with earlier experience. (*Adapted from* Medtronic, Inc., Report No. UC9302830aEN, 1994.)

Components of a Defibrillator

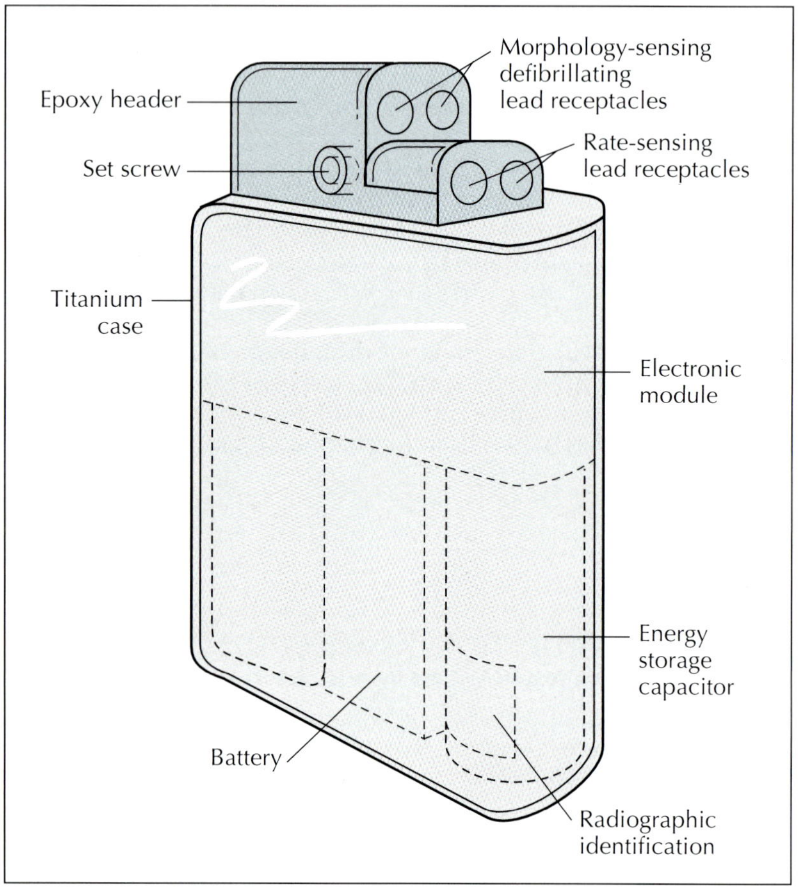

Figure 9-14. Pulse generator battery. Most of the pulse generator size results from the battery and capacitor(s) necessary for high energy shock delivery. While most implantable pacemakers employ lithium-iodine polyvinyl-pyridine batteries, these cells cannot provide the current required for rapid charging of the high-voltage capacitors in implantable defibrillators.

The first defibrillators in clinical use contained a lithium-vanadium pentoxide cell that was capable of rapidly charging the high-voltage capacitor but exhibited a life-span of only 1 to 2 years and lacked a reliable indicator of battery reserve. The newer lithium-silver-vanadium oxide cell, in use at present, appears to have a 3- to 5-year life-span and a relatively reliable correlation between battery voltage and battery reserve. (*Adapted from* Medtronic, Inc., Minneapolis, MN.)

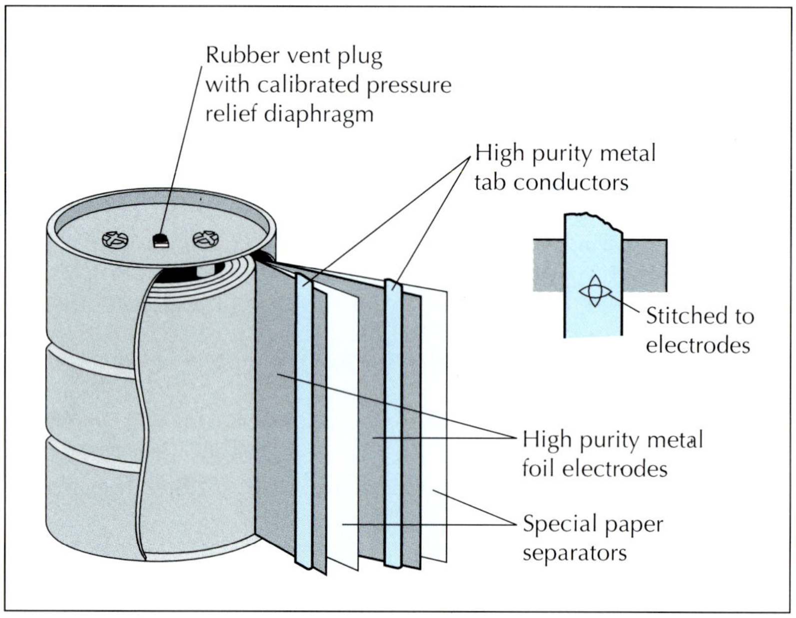

Figure 9-15. Capacitor. The aluminum-based electrolytic capacitor, similar to those used in photoflash applications, is the industry standard at present. The dielectric of such an electrolytic capacitor is generated by the voltage-dependent formation of a layer of aluminum oxide that forms between the two capacitor plates when DC voltage is applied to the plates and the electrolyte ammonium borate at the time of manufacture. This thin (a few angstroms thick) aluminum oxide layer breaks down over time in the absence of applied voltage through a process termed "deformation," which results in charge dissipation (as leakage current) through defects in the disintegrating aluminum oxide layer. Periodic manual or automatic "reformation" is required to keep these electrolytic capacitors functional. (*Adapted from* Medtronic, Inc., Minneapolis, MN.)

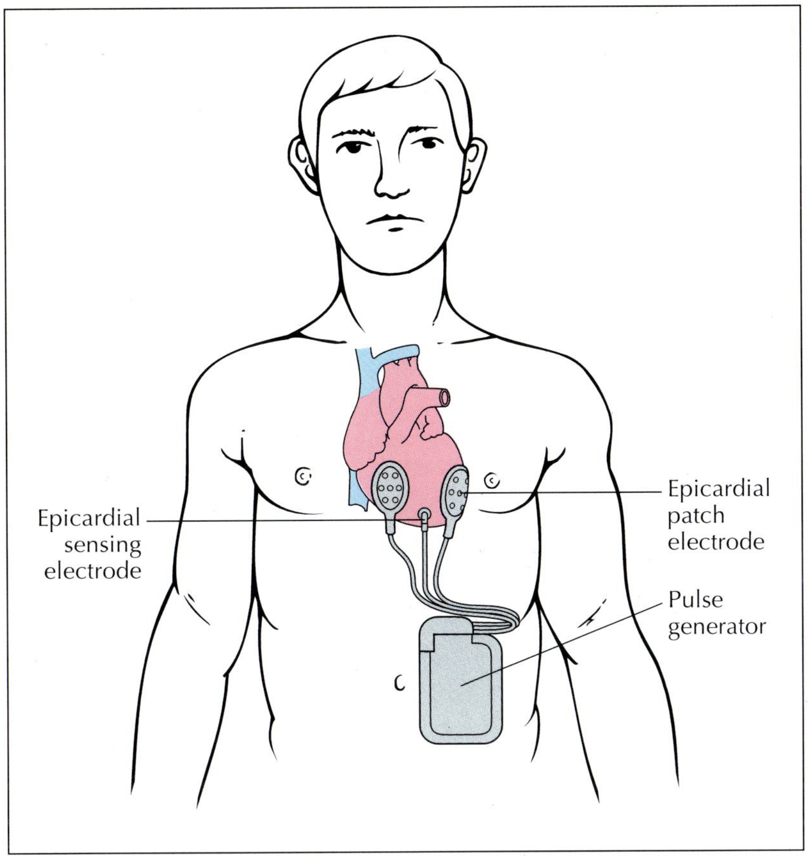

Figure 9-16. Thoracotomy lead system. While the initial concept of the implantable cardioverter defibrillator was that of an entirely transvenous system, early results from human and animal studies suggested that one or more of the defibrillating electrodes could be placed on the surface of the heart or pericardium to reduce energy requirements. This required a thoracotomy from the lateral median sternotomy or subxyphoid surgical approach. (*Adapted from* Cardiac Pacemakers, Inc., St. Paul, MN.)

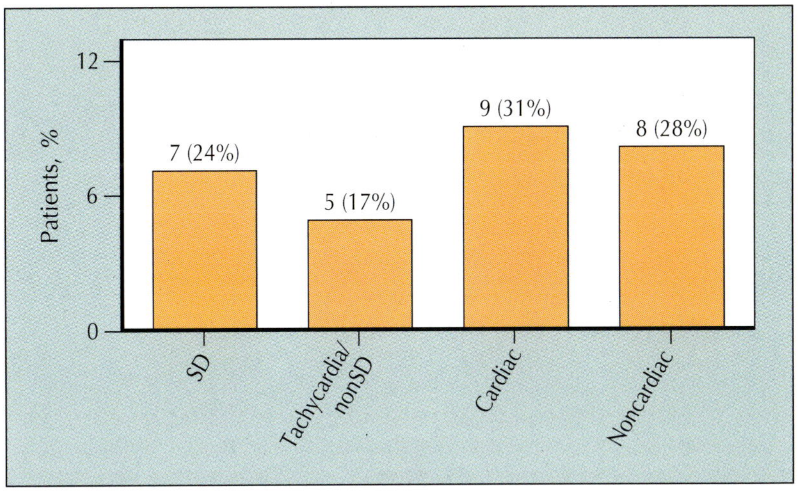

Figure 9-17. Operative risks associated with thoracotomy implantation. The 30-day operative mortality was substantial among those patients with advanced heart disease receiving defibrillator therapy using the thoracotomy approach. While nearly half of the deaths remained arrhythmia-related, the majority were non–arrhythmia-related. Graph shows distribution of deaths in 29 patients of 939 consecutive patients receiving implantable cardioverter defibrillators. SD—sudden death. (*Adapted from* Mosteller [41].)

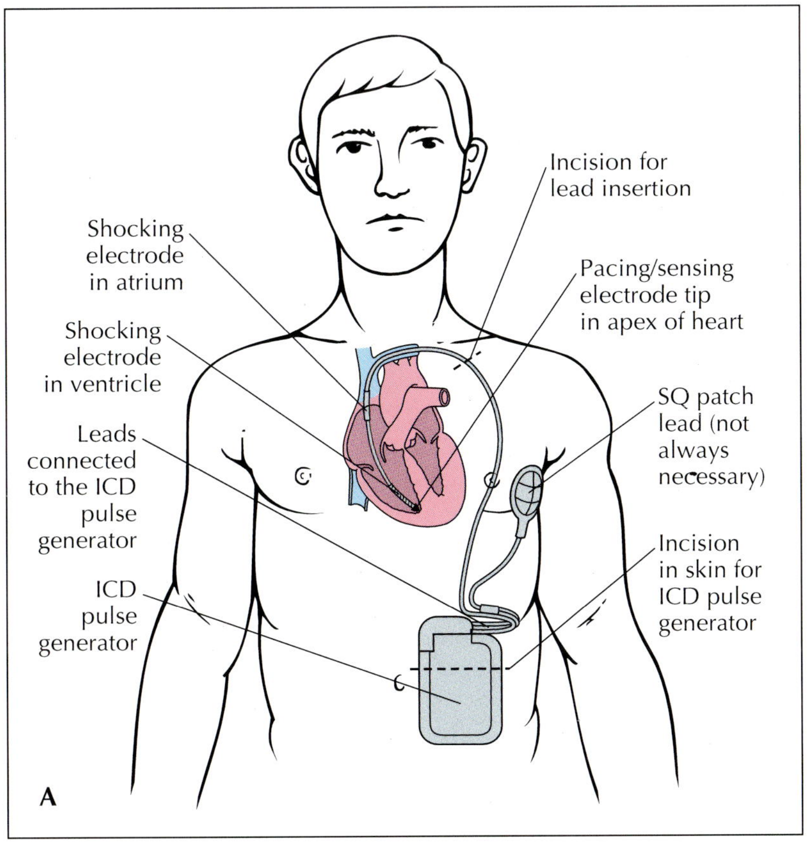

Figure 9-18. Nonthoracotomy lead system. Perhaps the single most significant advance in implantable defibrillator technology to date has been the development of transvenous lead systems that do not require thoracotomy for implantation. **A**, Nonthoracotomy system and incision sites for implantation. (*continued*)

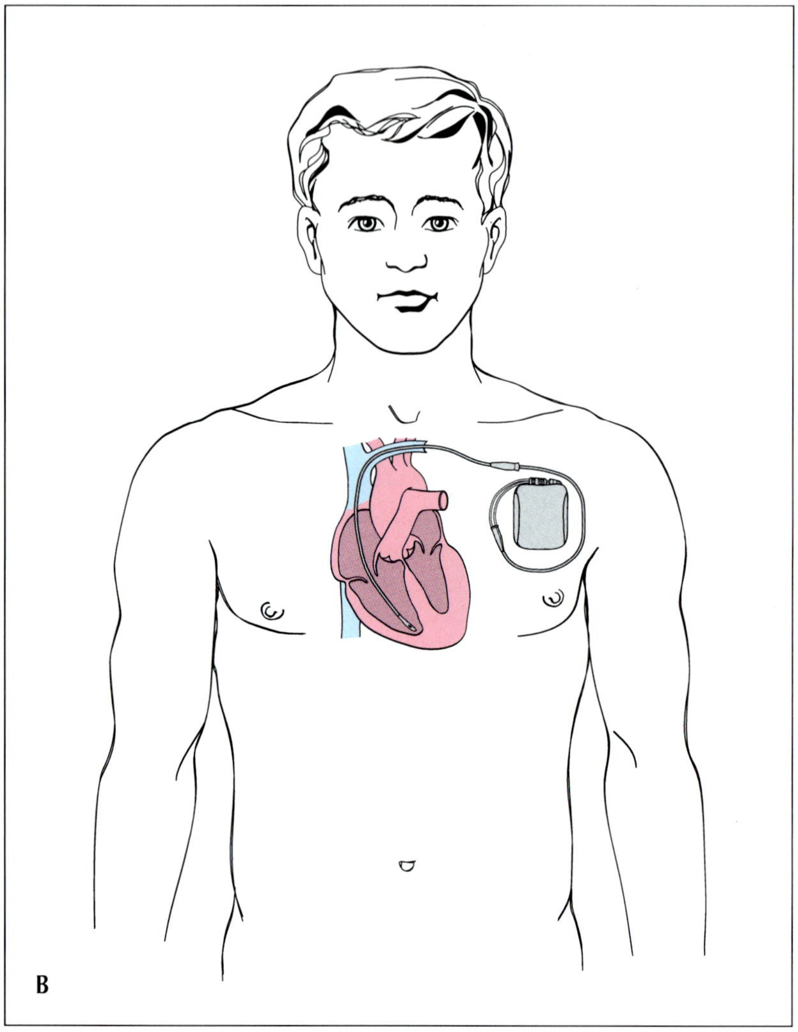

FIGURE 9-18. (*continued*) **B**, Pectoral implantation single-lead technology. (A *Adapted from* Cardiac Pacemakers, Inc, St. Paul, MN; B *adapted from* Medtronic, Inc., Minneapolis, MN.) ICD—implantable cardioverter defibrillator; SQ—subcutaneous.

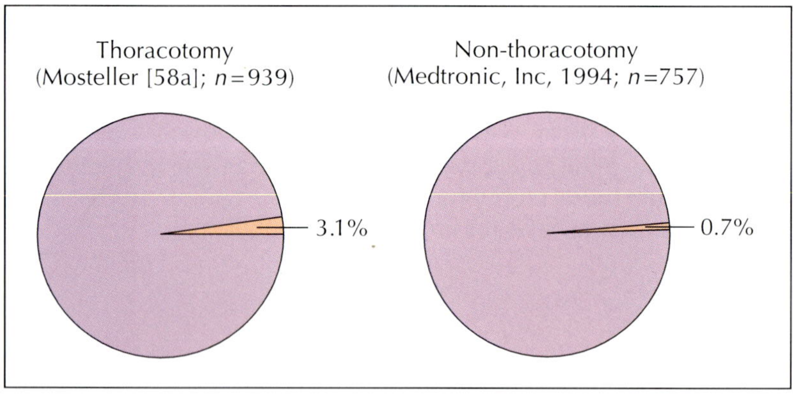

FIGURE 9-19. Operative risks associated with nonthoracotomy implantation. Early experience has shown that the nonthoracotomy approach dramatically lowers the 30-day perioperative mortality rate, approaching 1%, and may have the potential to lower the associated cost, largely through shorter hospitalizations. (*Data from* Mosteller [41] and Medtronic, Inc., Minneapolis, MN.)

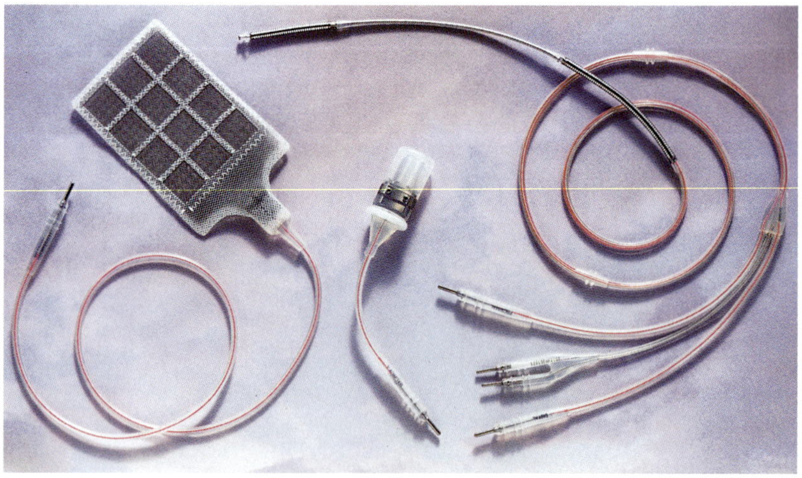

FIGURE 9-20. Nonthoracotomy leads. Impressive advances in engineering design technology have made possible the nonthoracotomy approach. The lead system shown here, the results of decades of engineering technology, is a tripolar, tined endocardial system for both sensing and pacing as well as high-energy (shock) delivery. It has a patch electrode and "Y" connector for lateral subcutaneous/submuscular patch or array implantation if necessary in some patients. The lead system is then tunneled subcutaneously to the pulse generator implantation site. (*Courtesy of* Cardiac Pacemakers, Inc., St. Paul, MN; with permission.)

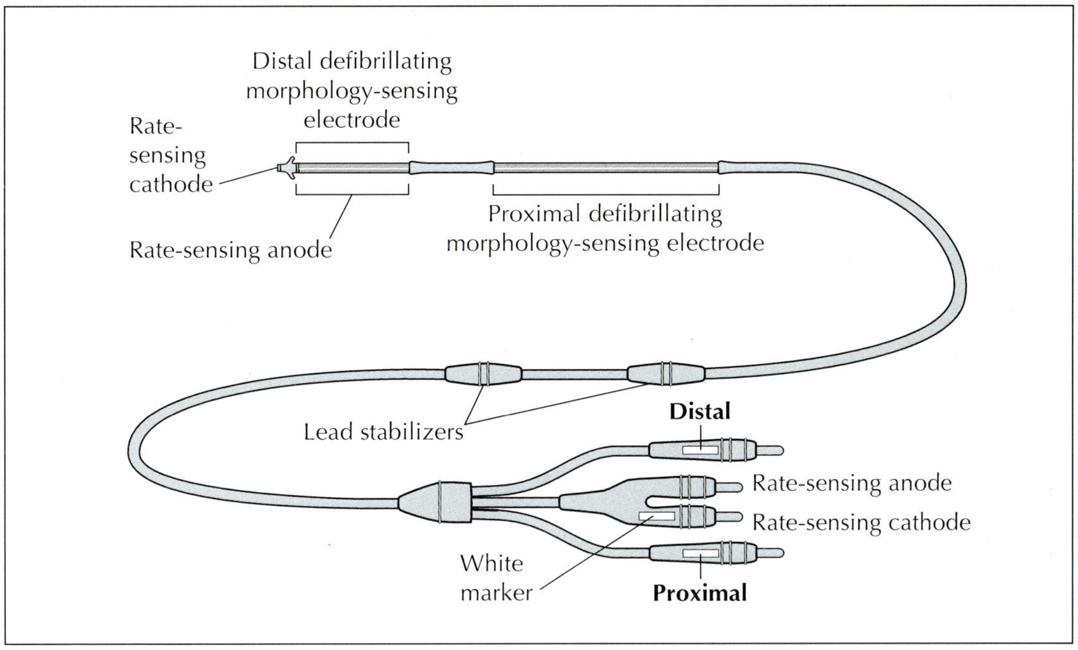

Figure 9-21. Tripolar intregrated bipolar endocardial lead. The porous tip electrode serves as the cathode for intracardiac rate sensing and pacing. The spring electrodes offer large surface areas for improved defibrillation and cardioversion. (*Adapted from* Cardiac Pacemakers, Inc., St. Paul, MN.)

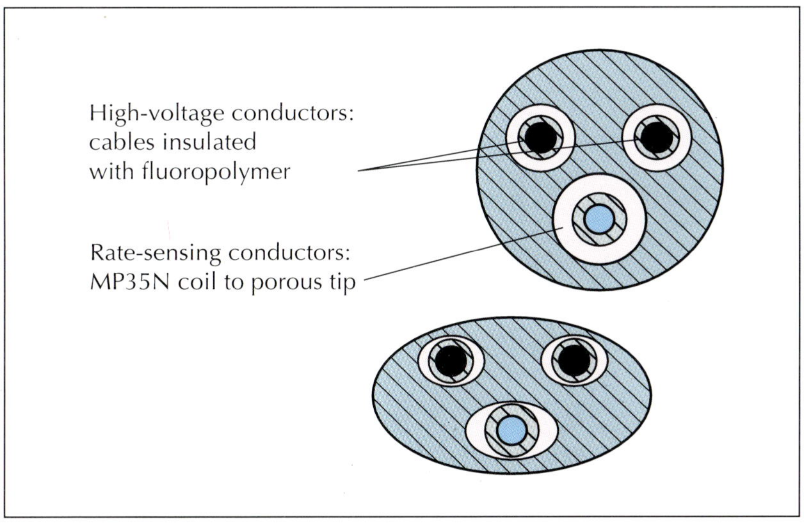

Figure 9-22. Tripolar lumen design. The lead body contains one conductor for rate sensing and two conductors for morphology sensing/defibrillation. The conductors are insulated in separate lumens within the silicone rubber lead body that is resistant to crush- and stress-related damage such as may occur as the lead crosses the region of the clavicle and first rib. (PTFE—polytetrafluoroethylene) (*Adapted from* Cardiac Pacemakers, Inc., St. Paul, MN.)

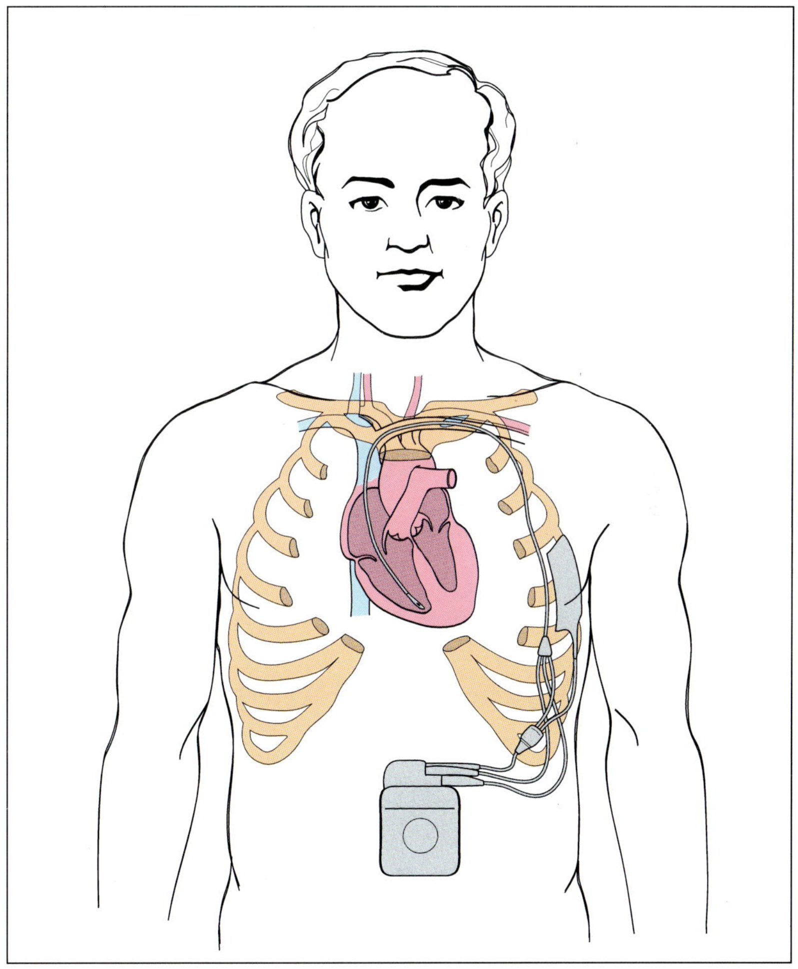

Figure 9-23. Nonthoracotomy system in place. The majority of configurations use a right ventricular lead for sensing and either the right ventricular lead alone or additional leads, including a submuscular patch or array (necessary in less than 5% of patients at present), or a superior vena cava/coronary sinus lead system for defibrillation. (*Adapted from* Cardiac Pacemakers, Inc., St. Paul, MN.)

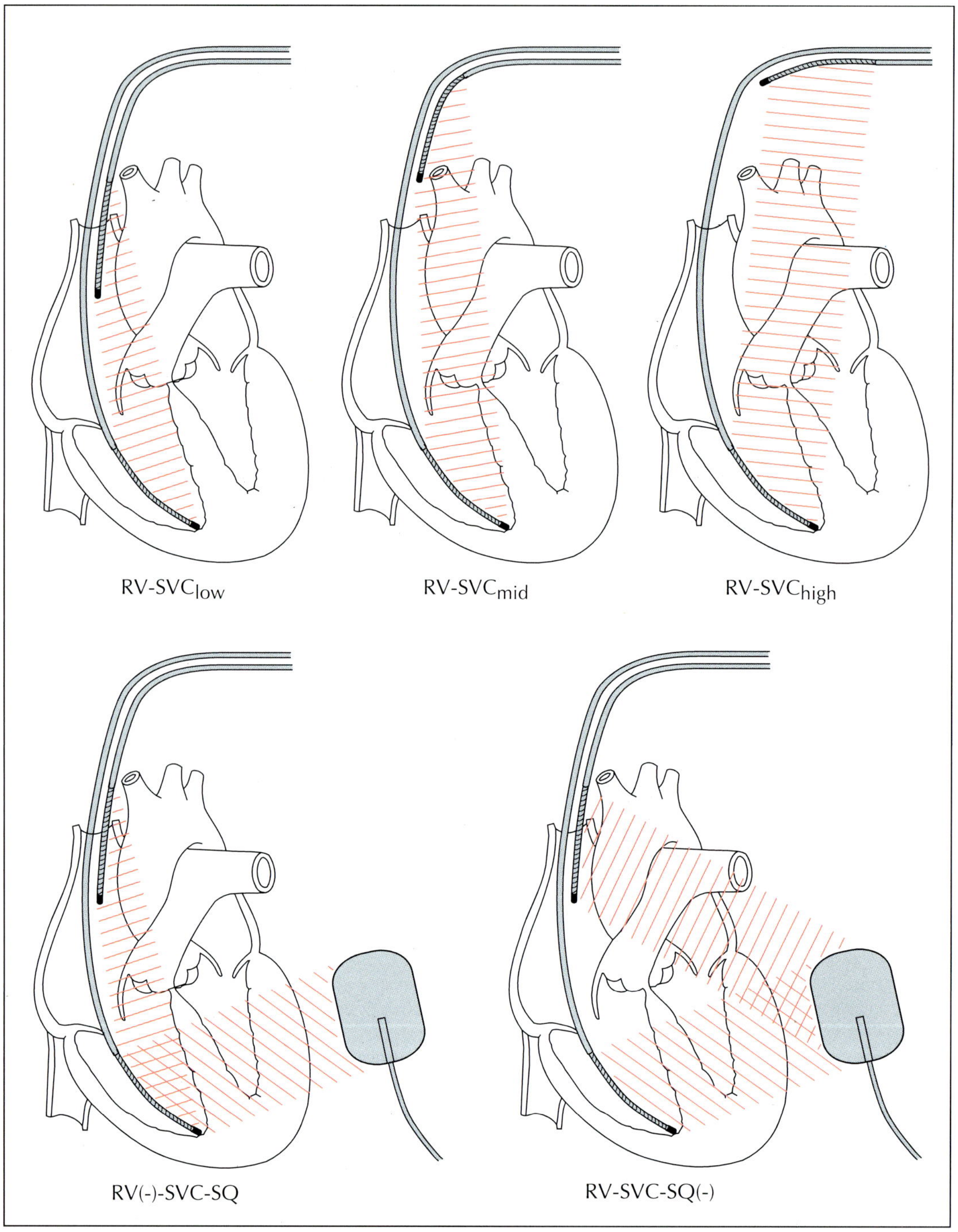

FIGURE 9-24. Lead polarity configuration. The high-energy delivery lead system employs a cathodal electrode or electrodes designated (-) together with an anodal electrode(s) designated (+) for defibrillation or cardioversion. RV—right ventricular; SQ—subcutaneous patch electrode; SVC—superior vena cava. (*Adapted from* Cardiac Pacemakers, Inc., St. Paul, MN.)

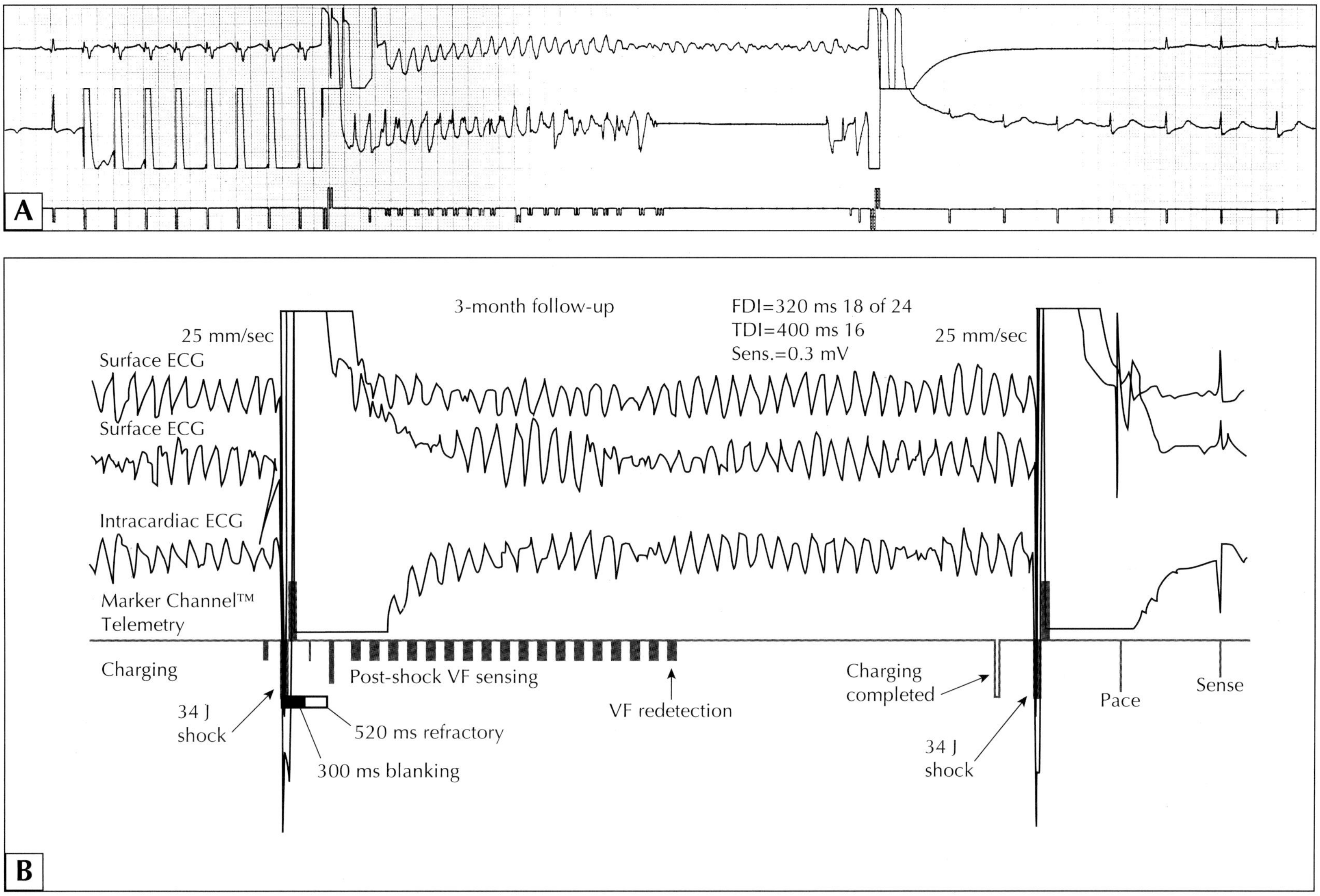

FIGURE 9-25. Rapid response to malignant arrhythmias. The implantable defibrillator serves as an integrated testing and therapeutic system for patients with life-threatening arrhythmias. During defibrillator system testing, after a series of paced beats, a critically timed low-energy pulse during the cardiac vulnerable period at the peak of the "T" wave results in ventricular fibrillation. The arrhythmia is then detected (**A**) or redetected if initial therapy fails (**B**) by way of an amplifier with continuous sensing and logic circuit designed to detect the arrhythmia on the basis of specific programmable detection criteria. Once detection criteria are satisfied, the power source charges the capacitor, and the charge is then delivered through the load (lead system and heart) to defibrillate, thereby restoring a normal cardiac rhythm. ATP—antitachycardia pacing; FDI—fibrillation detection interval; VF—ventricular fibrillation; TDI—tachycardia detection interval. (*Adapted from* Medtronic, Inc., Minneapolis, MN.)

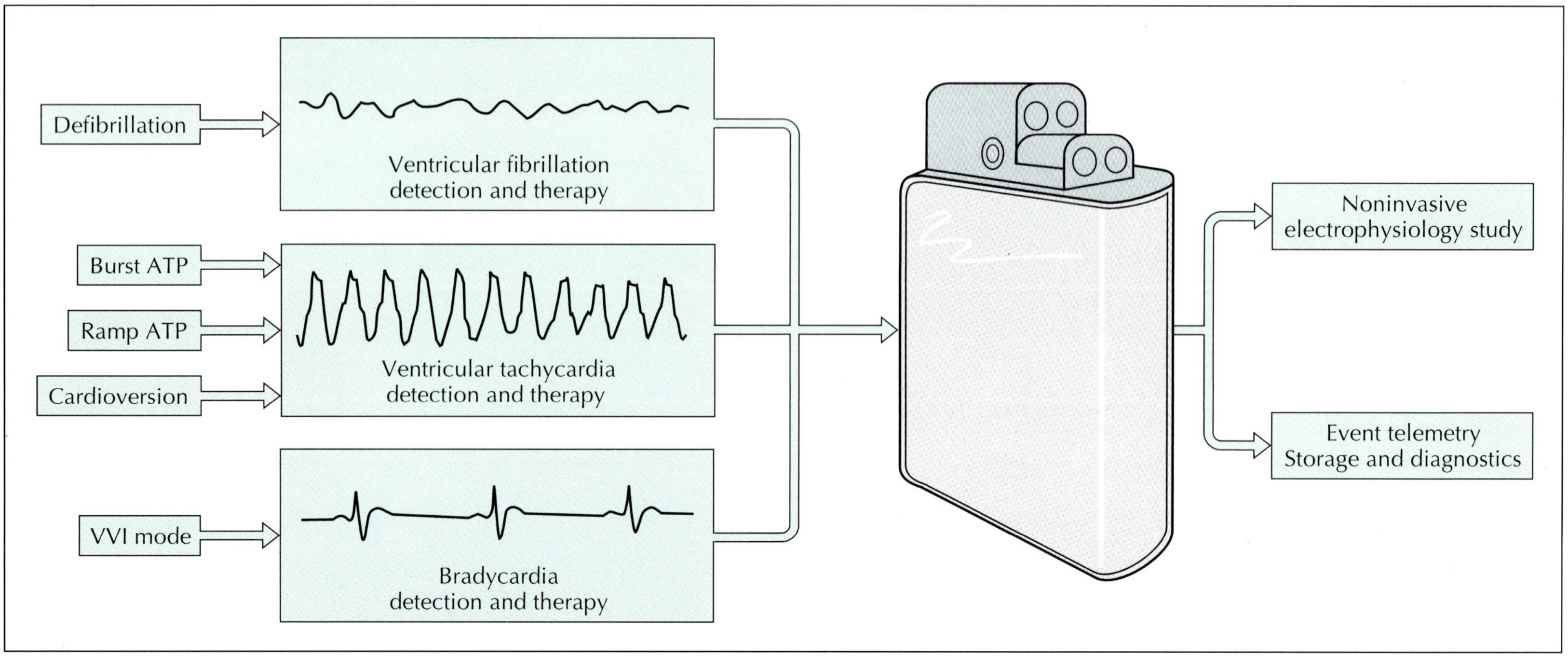

FIGURE 9-26. Tiered-therapy defibrillators. In addition to defibrillation, the implantable defibrillator has the capacity for several "tiered" functions including bradycardia pacing, antitachycardia pacing, and cardioversion. Therapy may be specifically programmed for individual patient needs and may include one or more "heart rate zones" based on both electrophysiologic testing and device-based testing after implantation. ATP—antitachycardia pacing; VVI—ventricular pacing, sensing, inhibiting. (*Adapted from* Medtronic, Inc., Minneapolis, MN.)

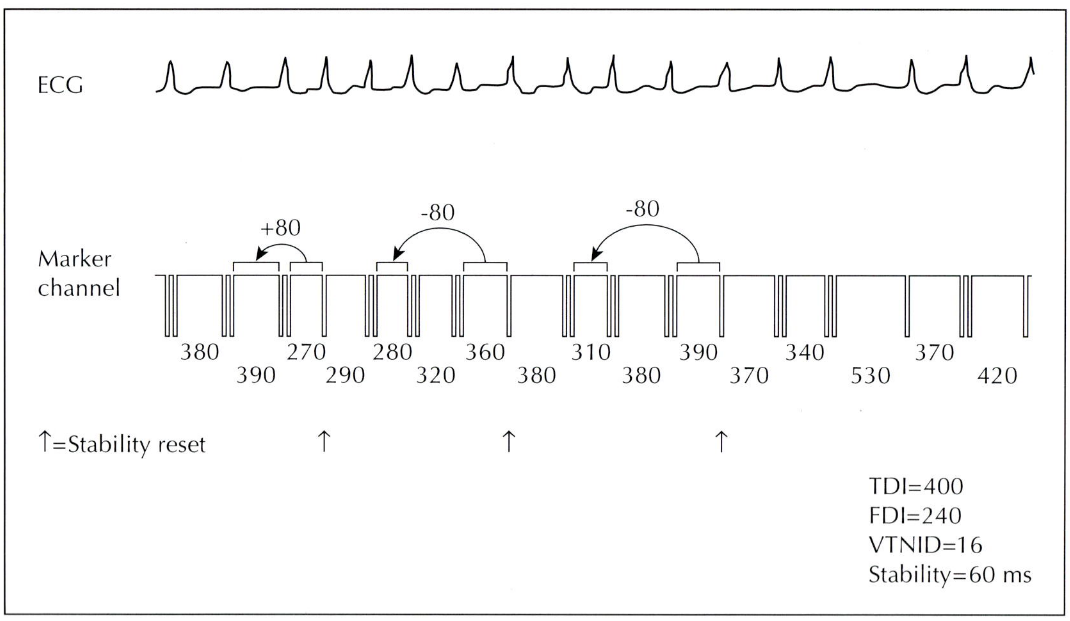

FIGURE 9-27. Enhanced tachycardia recognition. Atrial fibrillation with a rapid ventricular response may result in inappropriate device therapy based on rate criteria alone. Engineering advances such as programmable rate stability criteria that result in device rejection or resetting offer improved therapeutic specificity. Additional detection criteria, including QRS morphology, sudden onset, and arrhythmia duration are used as well. Future devices may employ atrial sensing functions to improve recognition accuracy. FDI—fibrillation detection interval; TDI—tachycardiac detection interval; VTNID—ventricular tachycardia number of intervals to detect. (*Adapted from* Medtronic, Inc., Minneapolis, MN.)

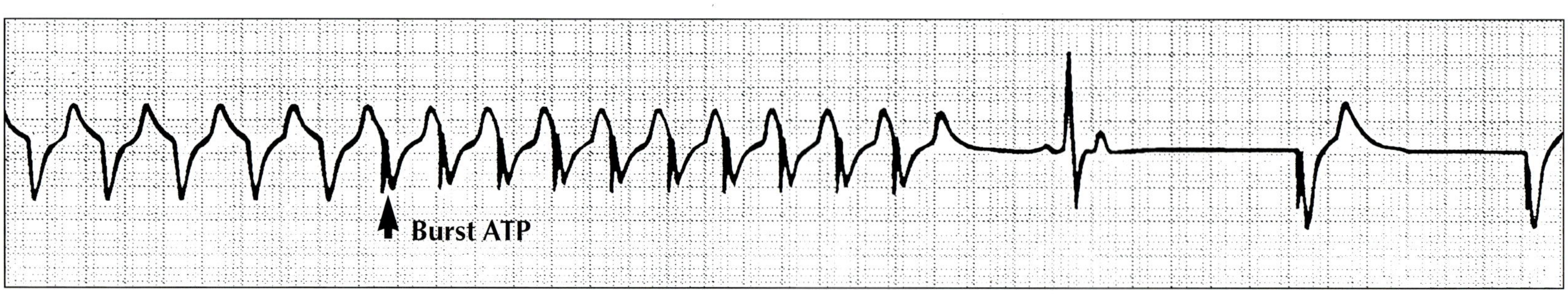

FIGURE 9-28. Antitachycardia pacing. A programmable number (burst) of low-energy pacing pulses at a percentage (adaptive rate) of the sensed tachycardia rate may be used to interrupt with block in two directions to terminate reentrant tachycardia. Basic cycle length= 300 ms; delay= 352 ms; tachycardia cycle length= 400 ms. ATP—antitachycardia pacing.

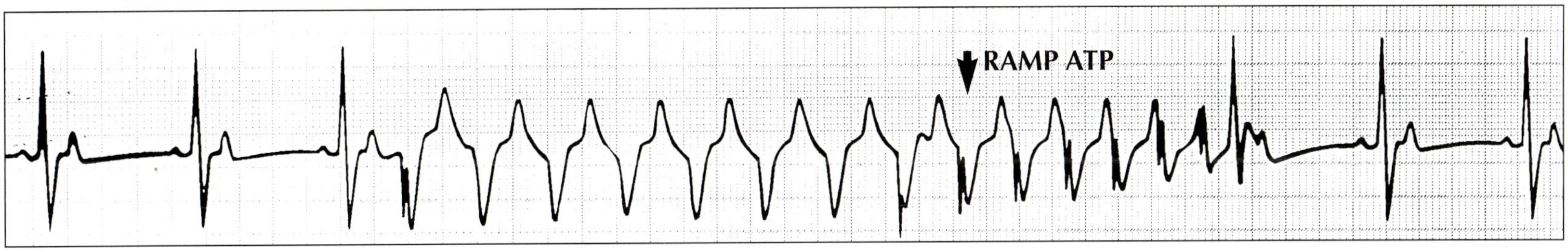

FIGURE 9-29. Antitachycardia pacing. Effective antitachycardia pacing burst patterns include those with between-burst decrement (SCAN) with or without an additional within-burst decrement (RAMP) pattern. In a randomized, controlled trial reported by Newman and colleagues [42], laboratory administration of adaptive SCAN or RAMP antitachycardia pacing patterns had a similar efficacy of 85% and 90% successful conversion among 29 patients with 65 inducible ventricular tachycardias. Acceleration due to antitachycardia pacing was observed in 7 (5 SCAN, 2 RAMP) of 65 (11%) tachycardias. Failure to convert tachycardia was associated with a shorter tachycardia cycle length. Basic cycle length=240–340 ms; delay= 36 ms. ATP—antitachycardia pacing.

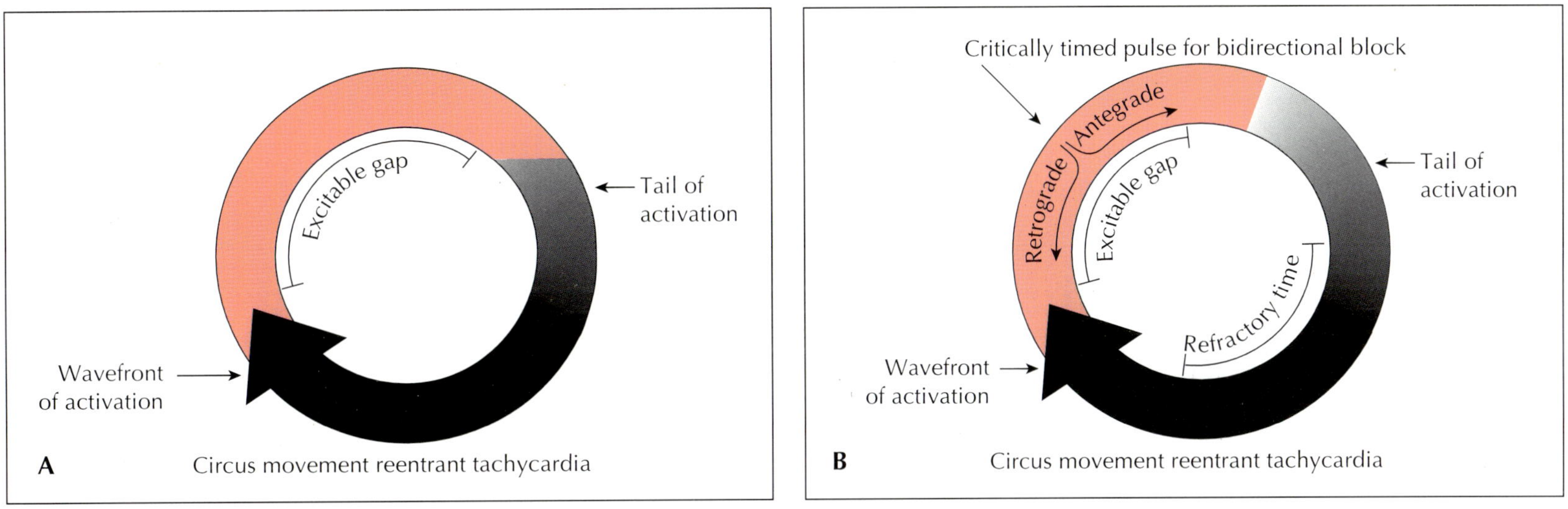

FIGURE 9-30. Reentrant tachycardia (**A**) may be terminated with critically timed stimulation resulting in twin propagated wavefronts (**B**) of depolarization in both antegrade and retrograde directions along the excitable reentrant pathway, resulting in bidirectional block to terminate the reentrant arrhythmia.

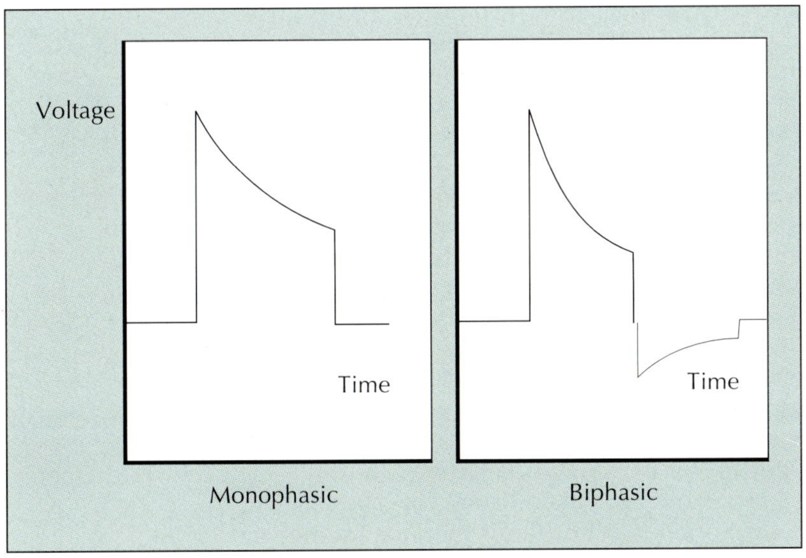

FIGURE 9-31. Defibrillator output waveform. Present devices employ a truncated output waveform from capacitor discharge through the predominantly resistive load, represented by the electrode system and heart. Truncated pulses were developed in order to avoid the potential adverse consequences of refibrillation or failure to defibrillate [43,44] that could result from the low voltage "tail" near the end of untruncated capacitor discharges.

Research has been directed at reducing the amount of energy required for cardiac defibrillation. This research has shown that altering the path [45] of the defibrillating current, the output waveform [46–48], or the separation of sequential pulses [49] results in lower energy requirements.

Clinical Uses of Defibrillator Therapy

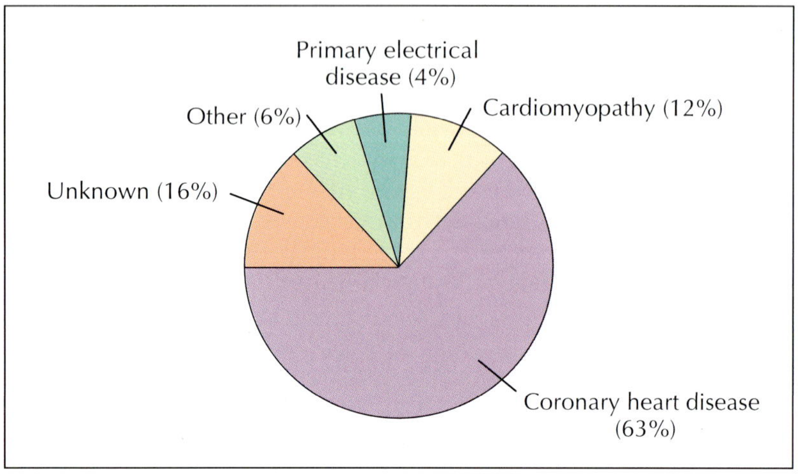

Figure 9-32. Primary cardiac disease. While the majority of patients treated with implantable defibrillator therapy have a history of coronary heart disease and depressed left ventricular function, other patient groups have included those with hypertrophic heart disease or idiopathic dilated cardiomyopathy, patients awaiting heart transplantation, and patients without demonstrable structural heart disease but with a history of malignant arrhythmias. (*Adapted from* Cardiac Pacemakers, Inc., St. Paul, MN.)

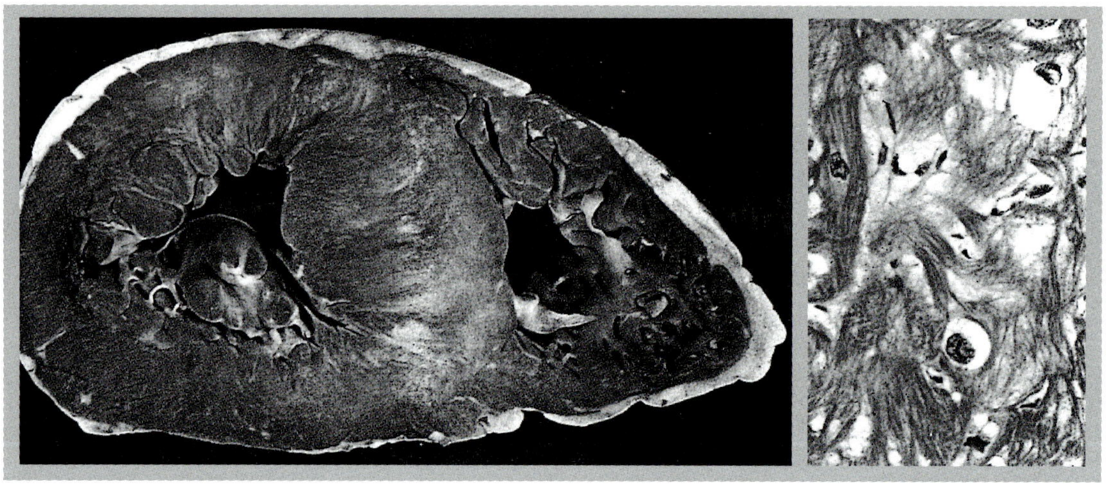

Figure 9-33. Hypertrophic cardiomyopathy. The annual incidence of sudden cardiac death among patients with familial hypertrophic cardiomyopathy has been found to be 2% to 4% of adults, and perhaps 4% to 6% of children, and this generally represents about half of all deaths [50]. A history of cardiac arrest or syncope and inducible sustained ventricular arrhythmias at electrophysiologic study have been found to be independently predictive [51] of subsequent cardiac events. A family history of sudden death, young age, and ventricular ectopy associated with symptoms of impaired consciousness may identify patients at additional risk.

Perhaps up to two thirds of patients with a history of documented ventricular tachycardia or ventricular fibrillation have inducible malignant ventricular arrhythmias with electrophysiologic testing [52,53], and perhaps 40% of those patients without such a history of documented malignant ventricular arrhythmias have inducible arrhythmias as well, depending on the stimulation protocol used at the time of study. While controversy exists over the efficacy of drug therapy [54], it is clear that pharmacologic therapy has not had a great impact on the prevention of recurrent sudden death [55,56] and may be harmful. Myectomy [57,58] and more recently ventricular-control atrioventricular sequential pacing therapy [59] among patients with obstructive hypertrophic cardiomyopathy may improve symptoms, but these modalities at present have an unknown impact on survival. These factors have led to the emergence of implantable cardioverter defibrillator therapy among these patients. (*Adapted from* Hurst [59a].)

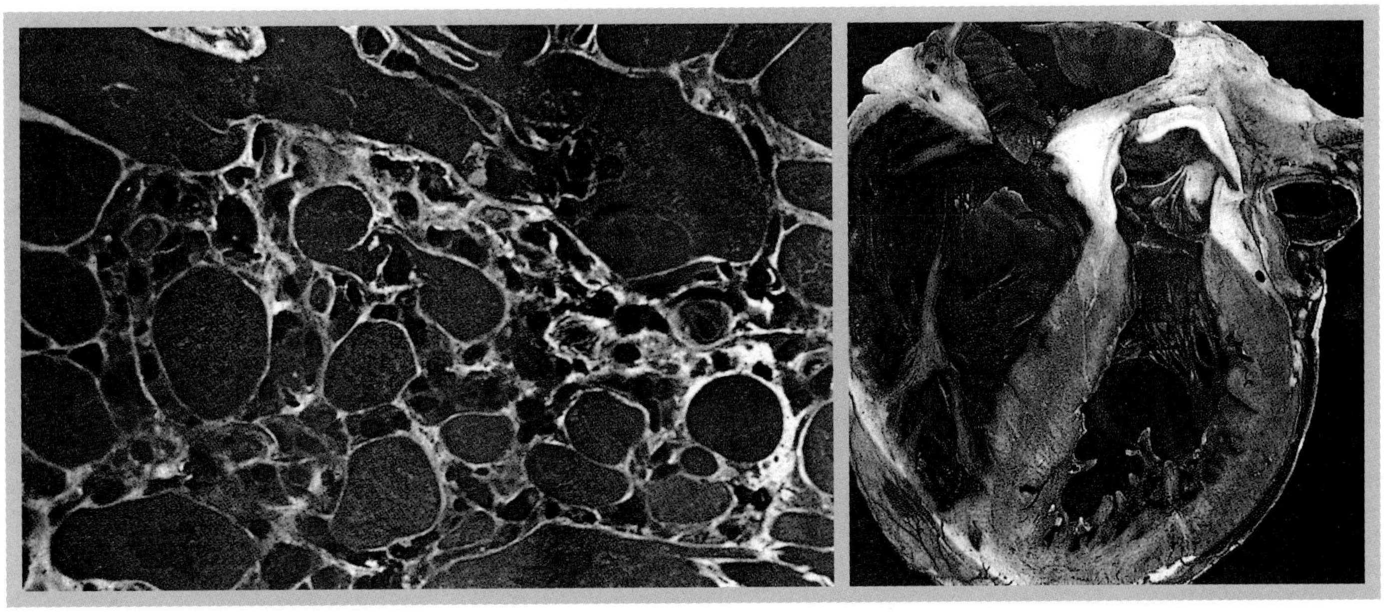

Figure 9-34. Dilated cardiomyopathy. The evaluation and treatment of malignant arrhythmias for patients with dilated cardiomyopathy remain a clinical enigma. Perhaps up to 40% of asymptomatic patients undergoing electrophysiologic testing have inducible malignant ventricular arrhythmias in the laboratory. However, the results of such testing may not be predictive of subsequent malignant clinical events [60,61]. Inducible ventricular tachycardia or ventricular fibrillation may be present in 50% to 65% [62] of patients with a clinical history of malignant ventricular arrhythmias, but a minority of these patients (perhaps up to 30%) are found to be suppressible with drug therapy. Despite suppression, a significant proportion of these patients, perhaps 11%, have recurrent sudden death within the first year of therapy. This dilemma has led to the emergence of implantable cardioverter defibrillator therapy for patients with a history of aborted sudden death and medically refractory malignant arrhythmias at electrophysiologic testing or for patients with a similar history of malignant ventricular arrhythmias but without inducible arrhythmias with laboratory testing. (*Adapted from* Hurst [59a].)

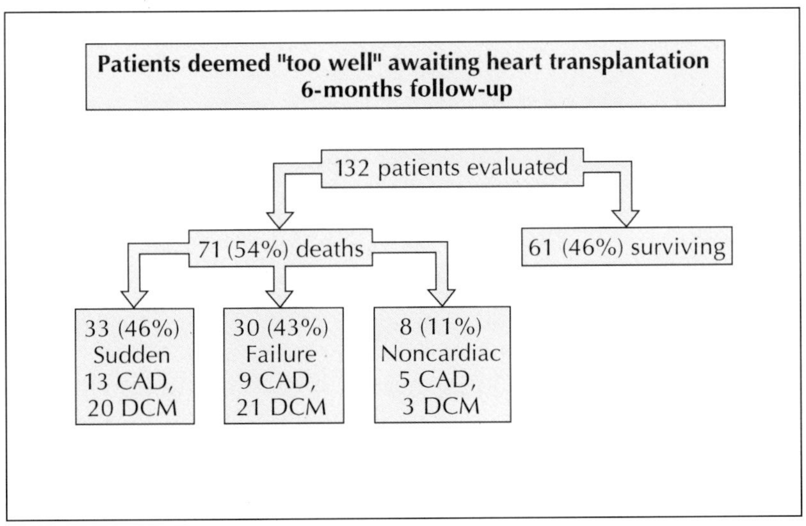

Figure 9-35. Implantable cardioverter defibrillator therapy (ICD) as a bridge to heart transplantation. Survival while awaiting heart transplant is poor. As reported by Haverich and colleagues [63], 71 of 132 patients (54%) deemed "too well" for transplant died during a mean follow-up of 5.6 months, and 33 of these 71 patients (46%) died suddenly. In contrast, 30 of 38 patients (78.4%) with limited heart failure referred primarily for intractable arrhythmias that were treated with ICD therapy while awaiting transplantation survived at a mean follow-up of 19 months. Perioperative mortality was 2.6%, and 31 of 37 patients (84%) experienced ICD discharges in the follow-up period. From their retrospective analysis, there were no preoperative factors that identified patients who may have been at particularly high risk for sudden death while awaiting transplantation. The authors concluded that while bridge ICD therapy may be warranted in some patients, prospective studies are needed to clarify the role of such therapy. CAD—coronary artery disease; DCM—dilated cardiomyopathy.

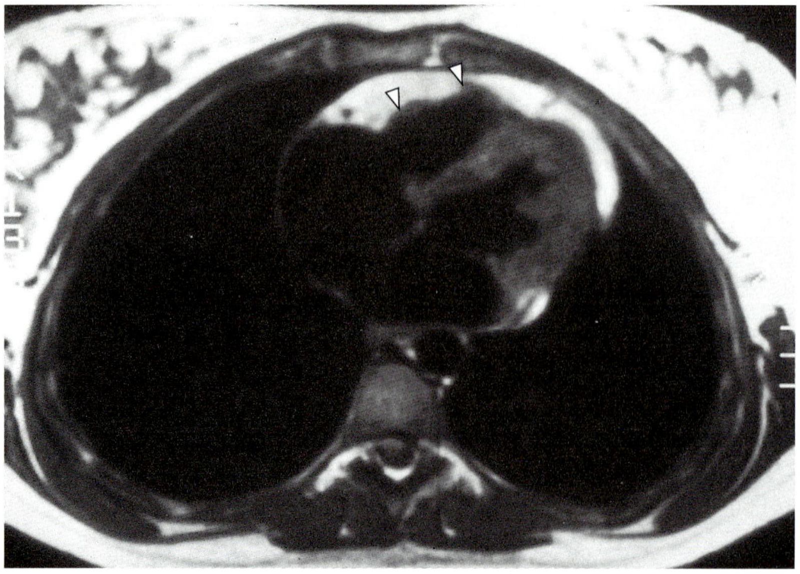

Figure 9-36. Malignant ventricular arrhythmias without structural heart disease. While most patients who develop malignant arrhythmias have underlying structural heart disease, it is well understood that a minority of those patients have no identifiable abnormality other than the cardiac arrhythmia. In one large series [64], 15% of 516 patients undergoing electrophysiologic testing for a history of symptomatic ventricular arrhythmias fell into this category. Specialized imaging techniques may identify minimal "fatty change" in the region of the right ventricular outflow tract in some patients (*arrowheads*).

Among these patients, a history of cardiac arrest seems to identify a group of patients at particularly high risk of recurrent life-threatening events. While electrophysiologic testing among these patients may reveal inducible sustained ventricular arrhythmias in perhaps 50%, the rate of recurrent sudden death is remarkably high [65,66]. These patients may be candidates for implantable cardioverter defibrillator therapy.

Socioeconomic Issues Associated with Defibrillator Therapy

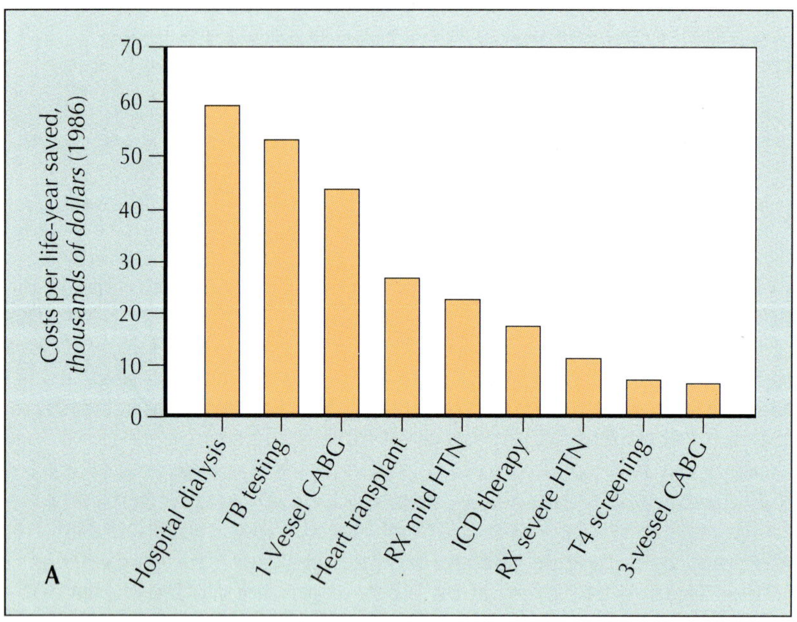

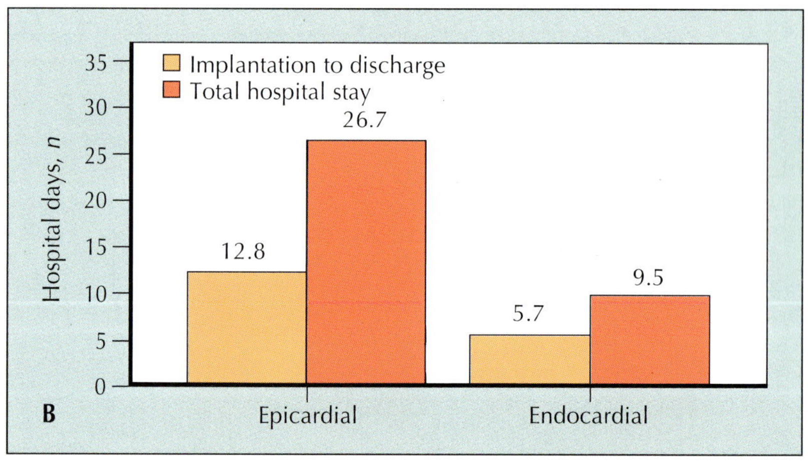

Figure 9-37. The cost of defibrillator therapy. The success of implantable cardioverter defibrillator (ICD) therapy together with substantial return to productive life and employment among patients treated may help offset the substantial price of implantation and for replacement of the pulse generator, which is necessary periodically. The estimated cost per year of life saved with first- and second-generation device therapy was reported at $17,000 indexed to 1986 [67] and another at $29,200 indexed to 1989 [68]. Despite such costs, ICD therapy may compare favorably with other life-saving medical interventions, including antiarrhythmic drug therapy, antihypertensive therapy, coronary artery bypass surgery (CABG), and kidney dialysis (**A**).

The costs associated with more recent tiered therapy nonthoracotomy defibrillator therapy may be significantly lower not only due to improved device longevity but also to greatly simplified implantation techniques and significantly shortened hospital stay (**B**). HTN—hypertension; RX—medication; TB—tuberculosis. (A *Adapted from* Kuppermann and coworkers [67]; B *adapted from* Baxter and coworkers [69].)

References

1. Greene LH, *et al.*: Sudden arrhythmic cardiac death mechanisms, resuscitation and classification: the Seattle perspective. *Am J Cardiol* 1990, 65:4b.

1a. Statistical Abstract of the United States, 1990; The National Data Book (Bureau of the Census), 1992.

2. Bayes de Luna AJ, Soldevila JG, Prat XV: Do silent myocardial ischemia and ventricular arrhythmias interact to result in sudden death? *Clin Cardiol* 1992, 10:449–459.
3. Myerberg RJ, Castellanos A: Cardiac Arrest and Sudden Cardiac Death. In: *Heart Disease: A Textbook of Cardiovascular Medicine*, 3rd ed. Edited by Braunwald E. Philadelphia: WB Saunders; 1988:742–747.
4. Kuller L, Cooper M, Perper J: Epidemiology of sudden death. *Ann Intern Med* 1972, 129:714–719.
5. Newman WP, 3d, Strong JP, Johnson WD, *et al.*: Community pathology of atherosclerosis and coronary heart disease in New Orleans. Morphologic findings in young black and white men. *Lab Invest* 1981, 44:496–501.
6. Baum RS, Alvarez H, Cobb LA: Survival after resuscitation from out-of-hospital ventricular fibrillation. *Circulation* 1974, 50:1231–1235.
7. Coumel P: Etude experimentale des effets cardizques des courants electriques. (Thesis) Paris, 1965.
8. Mirowski M: Standby automatic defibrillator. An approach to prevention of sudden coronary death. *Arch Intern Med* 1970, 126:158–161.
9. Mirowski M, Reid RP, Mower MM, *et al.*: Termination of malignant ventricular arrhythmias with an implanted automatic defibrillator in human being. *N Engl J Med* 1980, 303:322–324.
10. Winkle RA, Mead RH, Ruder MA, *et al.*: Long-term outcome with the automatic implantable cardioverter defibrillator. *J Am Coll Cardiol* 1988, 13:1353–1361.
11. Veltri EP, Mower MM, Mirowski M, *et al.*: Follow-up of patients with ventricular tachyarrhythmias treated with the automatic implantable cardioverter-defibrillator: Programmed electrical stimulation results do not predict clinical outcome. *J Electrophysiol* 1989, 3:467–476.
12. Forgoros RN, Elson JJ, Bonnet CA, *et al.*: Efficacy of the automatic implantable cardioverter defibrillator in prolonging survival in patients with severe underlying cardiac disease. *J Am Coll Cardiol* 1990, 16:381–386.
13. Kelley PA, Cannom DS, Garon H, *et al.*: The automatic implantable cardioverter defibrillator: Efficacy, complications, and survival in patients with malignant ventricular arrhythmias. *J Am Coll Cardiol* 1988, 11:1278–1286.
14. Olinger GN, Chapman PD, Troup PJ, *et al.*: Stratified application of the automatic implantable cardioverter defibrillator. *J Thorac Cardiovasc Surg* 1988, 96:141–149.
15. Manolis AS, Tan-deguzman W, Lee MA, *et al.*: Clinical experience in seventy-seven patients with the automatic implantable cardioverter-defibrillator. *Am Heart J* 1989, 118:445–450.
16. Hargrove WC, Josephson ME, Marchlinski FE, *et al.*: Surgical decisions in the management of sudden cardiac death and malignant ventricular arrhythmias. Subendocardial resection, the automatic internal defibrillation, or both. *J Thorac Cardiovasc Surg* 1989, 97:923–928.
17. Tchou PJ, Kadri N, Anderson J, *et al.*: Automatic implantable cardioverter defibrillators and survival of patients with left ventricular dysfunction and malignant ventricular arrhythmias. *Ann Intern Med* 1988, 109:529–534.
18. Myerberg RJ, Luceri RM, Thurer R, *et al.*: Time to first shock and clinical outcome in patients receiving an automatic cardioverter defibrillator. *J Am Coll Cardiol* 1989, 14:508–514.
19. Luceri RM, Habal SM, Castallanos A, *et al.*: Mechanism of death in patients with the automatic implantable cardioverter defibrillator. *PACE* 1988, 11:2015–2022.
20. Marchlinski FE, Flores BT, Buxton AE, *et al.*: The automatic implantable cardioverter defibrillator: Efficacy, complication and device failures. *Ann Intern Med* 1986, 104:481–488.
21. Forgoros RN, Elson JJ, Bonnet CA, *et al.*: Efficacy of the automatic implantable cardioverter defibrillator in prolonging survival in patients with severe underlying cardiac disease. *J Am Coll Cardiol* 1990, 16:381–386.
22. Kim SG, Fisher JD, Chung WC, *et al.*: Left ventricular function on outcome with implantable defibrillators. *Circulation* 1992, 85:1304–1310.
23. Winkle RA, *et al.*: Long-term outcome with the automatic implantable cardioverter defibrillator. *J Am Coll Cardiol* 1989, 13:1353–1361.
24. Manolis AS, *et al.*: Clinical experience in seventy-seven patients with the automatic implantable cardioverter defibrillator. *Am Heart J* 1989, 118:445–450.
25. Hargrove WC, Miller JM: Risk stratification and management of patients with recurrent ventricular tachycardia and other malignant ventricular arrhythmias. *Circulation* 1989, 79(Suppl 1):178–181.
26. Borggrefe M, Podczeck A, Ostermeyer J, *et al.*: Long-term results of electrophysiologically guided antitachycardia surgery in ventricular tachyarrhythmias: A collaborative report in 665 patients. In *Nonpharmacological Therapy of Tachyarrhythmias*. Edited by G Breithardt, M Borggrefe, DP Zipes. Mount Kisco, NY: Futura Publishing; 1987:109–132.
27. Herre JM, Sauve MJ, Malone P, *et al.*: Long-term results of amiodarone therapy in patients with recurrent sustained ventricular tachycardia or ventricular fibrillation. *J Am Coll Cardiol* 1989, 13:442–449.
28. Wilber DJ, *et al.*: Out-of-hospital cardiac arrest. Use of electrophysiologic testing in the prediction of long-term outcome. *N Engl J Med* 1988, 318:19–24.
29. Swerdlow CD, Winkle RA, Mason JW: Determinants of survival in patients with ventricular tachyarrhythmias. *N Engl J Med* 1983, 24:1436–1442.
30. Roy D, Waxman HL, Kienzle MG, *et al.*: Clinical characteristics and long-term follow-up in 119 survivors of cardiac arrest: relation to inducibility at electrophysiologic testing. *Am J Cardiol* 1983, 52:969–974.
31. Waller TJ, Kay HR, Spielman SR, *et al.*: Reduction in sudden death and total mortality by antiarrhythmic therapy elevated by electrophysiologic drug testing: Criteria of efficacy in patients with sustained ventricular tachyarrhythmia. *J Am Coll Cardiol* 1987, 10:83–89.
32. Howowitz LN: Sudden arrhythmic death: Prediction and prevention. In *Cardiac Arrhythmias: Recent Progress in Investigation and Management*. Edited by T Iwa, G Fontaine. New York: Elsevier Science Publishers; 1988:165–170.
33. Wilbur DJ, Garan H, Finkelstein D, *et al.*: Out-of-hospital cardiac arrest. Use of electrophysiologic testing in the prediction of long-term outcome. *N Engl J Med* 1988, 318:19–24.
34. Ostermeyer J, Kirklin JK, Borggrefe M, *et al.*: Ten years of electrophysiologically guided direct operations for malignant ischemic ventricular tachycardia: results. *Thorac Cardiovasc Surgeon* 1989, 37:20–27.
35. McGiffin DC, Kirklin JK, Plumb EH, *et al.*: Relief of life-threatening ventricular tachycardia and survival after direct operations. *Circulation* 1987, 76:93–103.

36. Miller JM, Kienzle MG, Harken AH, *et al.*: Subendocardial resection for ventricular tachycardia: Predictors for surgical success. *Circulation* 1984, 70:624–631.

37. Song SL and the Nine-Center Study Group: The Bilitch Report: Performance of implantable cardiac rhythm management devices. *PACE* 1993, 16:129–131.

38. Jung W, Manz M, Luderitz B: Effects of antiarrhythmic drugs on defibrillation threshold in patients with the implantable cardioverter defibrillator. *PACE* 1992, 15:645–648.

38a. Fisher JD, Broadman RF, Kim SG, *et al.*: VT/VF: 60/60 protection. *PACE* 1990; 13:218–227.

39. Watkins L, Mirowski M, Mower MM, *et al.*: Implantation of the automatic defibrillator: The subxiphoid approach. *Ann Thorac Surg* 1982, 34:515–520.

40. Mirowski M, Reid PR, Winkle RA, *et al.*: Mortality in patients with implanted automatic defibrillators. *Ann Intern Med* 1983, 98:585–588.

41. Mosteller RD, Lehmann MH, Thomas AC, Jackson K: Operative mortality with implantation of the automatic cardioverter-defibrilatior. *Am J Cardiol* 1991, 68(13):1340–1345.

42. Newman D, Dorian P, Hardy J: Randomized controlled comparison of antitachycardia pacing algorithms for termination of ventricular tachycardia. *J Am Coll Cardiol* 1993, 21:1413–1418.

43. Schuder JC, Stoeckle H, Keskar PY, *et al.*: Transthoracic ventricular defibrillation in the dog with unidirectional rectangular double pulses. *Cardiovasc Res* 1970, 4:497–501.

44. Geddes LA, Tacker WA: Engineering and physiological considerations of direct capacitor-discharge ventricular defibrillation. *Med Biol Eng* 1971, 9:185–199.

45. Hauser RG, Mower MM, Mitchell M, Nisam S: Current Stats of the Ventak PRx pulse generator and Endotak nonthoracotomy lead system. *PACE* 1992, 15(part III):671–677.

46. Jones SL, Jones RE: Improved defibrillator waveform safety factor with biphasic waveforms. *Am J Physiol* 1983, 245:H60–H65.

47. Dixon EG, Tang AS, Wolf PD, *et al.*: Improved defibrillation thresholds with large contour epicardial electrodes in biphasic waveforms. *Circulation* 1987, 76:1176–1184.

48. Winkle RA, MEad RH, Ruder MA *et al*: Improved low-energy defibrillaion in man with the use of a biphasic truncated exponential waveform. *Am Heart J* 1989, 117:122–127.

49. Cooper RAS, Wallenius St, Smith WM, *et al.*: Effect of phase separation on biphasic waveform defibrillation. *PACE* 1993, 16:471.

50. McKenna WJ: Sudden death in hypertrophic cardiomyopathy: Identification of the "high risk" patient. In *Cardiac Arrhythmias: Where To Go From Here?* Edited by P Brugada, HJ Wellens. Mount Kisco, NY: Futura Publishing; 1987:353–365.

51. Fananapazir L, Chang AC, Epstein SE, *et al.*: Prognostic determinants in hypertrophic cardiomyopathy. Prospective evaluation of a therapeutic strategy based on clinical, holter, hemodynamic, and electrophysiological findings. *Circulation* 1992, 86:730–740.

52. Fananapazir L, Tracy CM, Leon MB, *et al.*: Electrophysiologic abnormalities in patients with hypertrophic cardiomyopathy: A consecutive analysis in 155 patients. *Circulation* 1989, 80:1259–1268.

53. Kuck KH, Kunze KP, Schluter M, *et al.*: Programmed electrical stimulation in hypertrophic cardiomyopathy. Results in patients with and without cardiac arrest or syncope. *Eur Heart J* 1988, 9:177–185.

54. McKenna WJ, Oakley CM, Krikler DM, *et al.*: Improved survival with amiodarone in patients with hypertrophic cardiomyopathy and ventricular tachycardia. *Br Heart J* 1985, 53:412–416.

55. Fananapazir L, Leon MB, Bonow RO, *et al.*: Sudden death during empiric amiodarone therapy in symptomatic hypertrophic cardiomyopathy. *Am J Cardiol* 1991, 67:169–174.

56. Fananapazir L, Epstein SE: Value of electrophysiologic studies in hypertrophic cardiomyopathy treated with amiodarone. *Am J Cardiol* 1991, 67:175–182.

57. Borggrefe M, Kuhn H, Koniger HH, *et al.*: Arrhythmias in hypertrophic obstructive and nonobstructive cardiomyopathy. *Eur Heart J* 1983, 4(Suppl F):245–251.

58. Borggrefe M, Martinezz-Rubio A, Block M, *et al.*: Hypertrophic cardiomyopathy: Electrophysiologic findings and management of survivors of cardiac arrest. *Eur Heart J* 1989, 10(Suppl):316.

59. Fananapazir L, Cannon III RO, Tripodi D, Panza JA: Impact of dual-chamber permanent pacing in patients with obstructive hypertrophic cardiomyopathy with symptoms refractory to verampamil and β-adrenergic blocker therapy. *Circulation* 1992, 85:2149–2161.

59a. Hurst W: Atlas of the Heart. New York: Gower Medical Publishing, 1988.

60. Stevenson WG, Stevenson LW, Weiss J, *et al.*: Inducible ventricular arrhythmias and sudden death during vasodilator therapy of severe heart failure. *Am Heart J* 1988, 116:1447.

61. Meinertz T, Treese N, Kasper W, *et al.*: Determinants of prognosis in idiopathic dilated cardiomyopathy as determined by programmed electrical stimulation. *Am J Cardiol* 1985, 56:337–341.

62. Borggrefe X: Clinical value of programmed ventricular stimulation in dilative cardiomyopathy: Acute and long-term results. (in preparation) *PACE* 1992, 15:616–626.

63. Haverich A, Troster J, Wahlers T, *et al.*: The automatic implantable cardioverter defibrillator (AICD) as a bridge to heart transplantation. *PACE* 1992, 15(III):701–707.

64. Zipes DP: Specific arrhythmias: Diagnosis and treatment. In *Heart Disease*. Edited by E Braunwald. Philadelphia: WB Saunders; 1984:683–743.

65. Wever E, Hauer R, Oomen A, *et al.*: Unfavorable outcome in patients with primary electrical disease who survived unexpected cardiac arrest [abstract]. *Eur Heart J* 1991, 12(Suppl):86.

66. Poole JE, Mathisen T, Kudenchuk PJ, *et al.*: Long-term outcome in patients who survive out of hospital ventricular fibrillation and undergo electrophysiologic studies: evaluation by electrophysiologic subgroups. *J Am Coll Cardiol* 1990, 16:657–665.

67. Kupperman M, Luce BR, McGovern B, *et al.*: An analysis of the cost effectiveness of the implantable defibrillator. *Circulation* 1990, 81:91–100.

68. Larsen GC, Manolis AS, Sonnenberg FA, *et al.*: Cost-effectiveness of the implantable cardioverter-defibrillator: Effect of improved battery life and comparison with amiodarone therapy. *J Am Coll Cardiol* 1992, 19:1323–1334.

69. Baxter JM, Beachamp DV, Goldberg HR, *et al.*: Nonthoracotomy vs thoracotomy implantable cardioverter defibrillator lead system implantation: comparison of cost and length of stay. *PACE* 1992, 15(part II):539.

Surgical Treatment of Cardiac Arrhythmias

10

CHAPTER

Gerard M. Guiraudon

Most cardiac arrhythmias are associated with a reentrant mechanism. Arrhythmias are currently classified according to the site of origin, that is, atrial tachycardias, atrioventricular nodal tachycardias, His bundle tachycardias, ventricular tachycardias, and atrioventricular reentrant tachycardias (which requires the presence of an accessory atrioventricular connection) [1]. The arrhythmogenic anatomic substrate is either the anatomic site of the mechanism or a specific segment of the reentrant mechanism that is necessary for the perpetuation of the tachycardia [2].

Cardiac arrhythmias may be associated with cardiac pathology, the pathologic lesions being either discrete or diffuse, quiescent or progressive. The lesions are either primary or secondary to the tachycardia (tachycardias induce cardiomyopathy). Electrophysiologic testing is paramount. It identifies the mechanism and localizes the anatomic substrate. Electrophysiologic testing is performed preoperatively, intraoperatively (cardiac mapping), and postoperatively [3].

Surgery for cardiac arrhythmias is intended to neutralize the arrhythmogenic anatomic substrate, using the concept of either exclusion [4] or ablation [5]. The exclusion of the anatomic substrate confines the abnormal impulses within the encircled area and prevents them from activating the rest of the heart. The ablation of the anatomic substrate uses either actual surgical removal or *in situ* modification by freezing (cryoablation), heating (laser energy), or chemical destruction (alcohol). If electrophysiologic testing fails or is not feasible, a comprehensive preoperative surgical plan is initiated, with the surgical technique guided by intraoperative mapping as well. The surgical techniques involve exclusion or ablation of the arrhythmogenic anatomic substrate and ancillary procedures such as thoracotomy, cardiopulmonary bypass, myocardial preservation, and aortic cross-clamping. Each of these is associated with inherent risks and these are responsible for most of the surgical risk (morbidity and mortality) [6]. Consequently, surgical therapy is only indicated after thorough consideration of other electrophysiologic nonpharmacologic interventions: catheter ablation techniques, antitachycardia devices, or implantable cardioverter defibrillator (ICD).

Historically, surgery for cardiac arrhythmias was the first electrophysiologic nonpharmacologic intervention, and it provided documentation that cardiac arrhythmias could be "cured" by addressing the anatomical substrate. Currently, the role of surgery is confined to failures or complications of catheter technique and is the primary intervention only in rare and selected patients with atrial fibrillation or ventricular arrhythmias. Surgery for ventricular tachycardias, albeit associated with low risk and high efficacy in selected patients, is infrequently used in current practice. ICD implantation by itself or combined with coronary artery bypass graft [7] is the preferred technique. Surgery for atrial fibrillation is still in a developing and creative period in which clinicians are striving to identify the rationales associated with "minimal surgery."

Wolff-Parkinson-White Syndrome

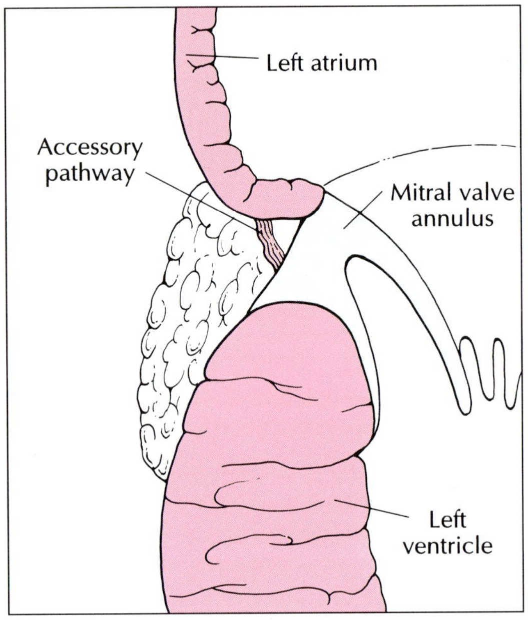

Figure 10-1. The Wolff-Parkinson-White syndrome is associated with an accessory atrioventricular connection distinct from the normal atrioventricular node–His bundle system. This accessory connection is made of normal working myocardium that bridges the atrioventricular attachment. In this figure, the cross section of the left coronary sulcus shows the left atrium, the mitral valve annulus, the left ventricle, and the accessory pathway with para-annular attachment onto the left atrium.

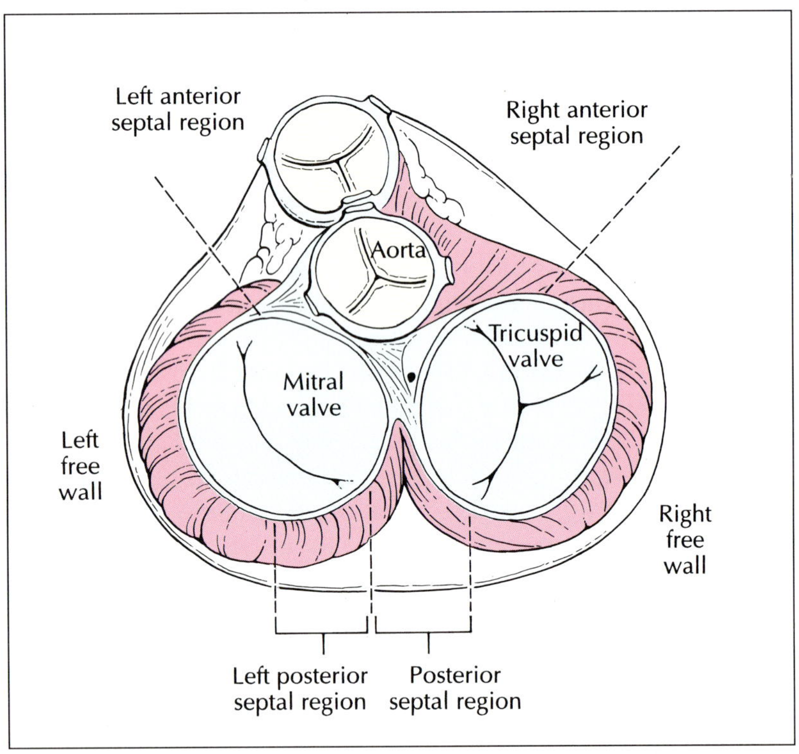

Figure 10-2. The atrioventricular (AV) attachment is a complex structure in its medial segment ("septum") because of the presence of the aortic root and its appended membranous structures harboring the AV node–His bundle. Laterally, the AV attachment is part of the coronary sulcus, which is divided into four regions: left free wall, posterior septal, right free wall, and anterior septal regions. Shown in the figure are the base of the heart with the coronary sulcus and its various regions and the medial segment (septal) of the AV attachment with the aortic root and its appended membranous structures. The *solid black circle* indicates the location of the His bundle within the membranous septum.

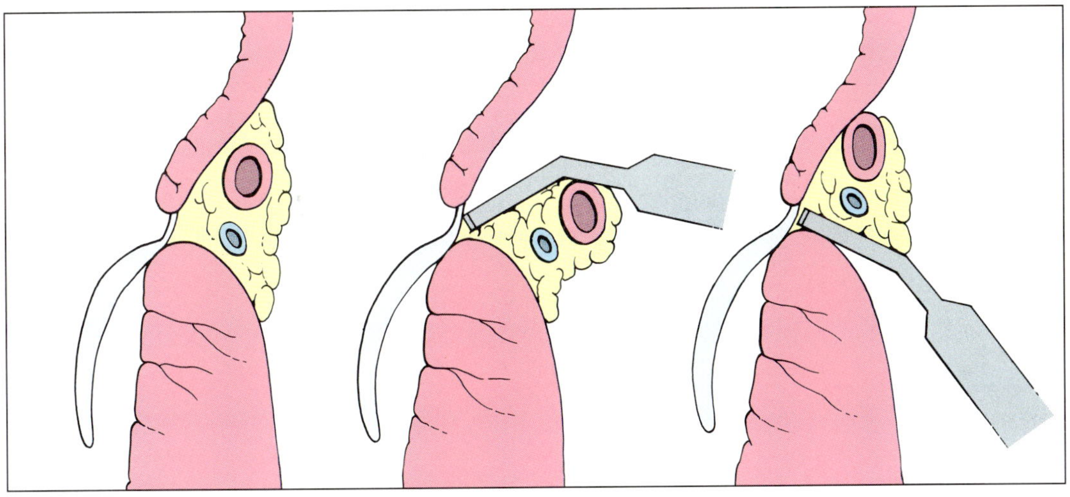

FIGURE 10-3. The rationale for surgical treatment of the Wolff-Parkinson-White syndrome is the ablation of the accessory AV connection. Two approaches have been described: the endocardial and the epicardial. The epicardial approach combines the exposure and cryoablation of the segment of interest on the AV attachment. This figure depicts the epicardial dissection in the left free wall region. Cardiopulmonary bypass is not required in most cases. We reported 502 patients, whose accessory AV connections were ablated using epicardial dissection [8,9]. There was no mortality. The accessory AV connection was ablated in more than 99% of patients.

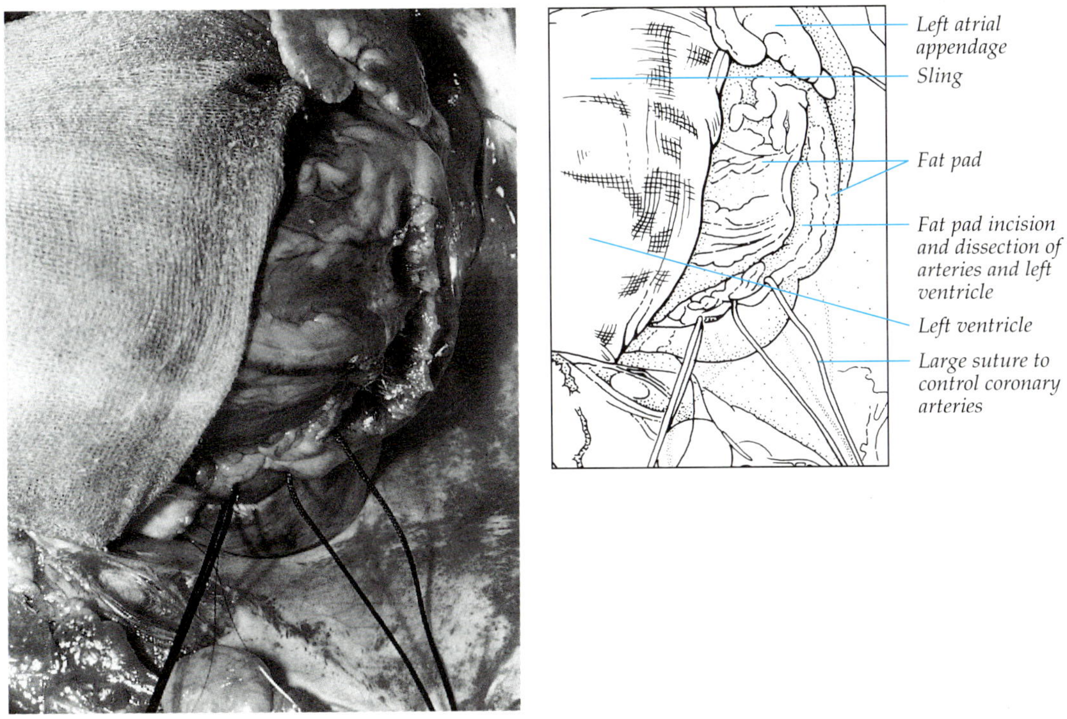

FIGURE 10-4. Left free wall dissection. The exposure uses a sling that provides adequate approach without the need for cardiopulmonary bypass. Large sutures identify dissected coronary arteries.

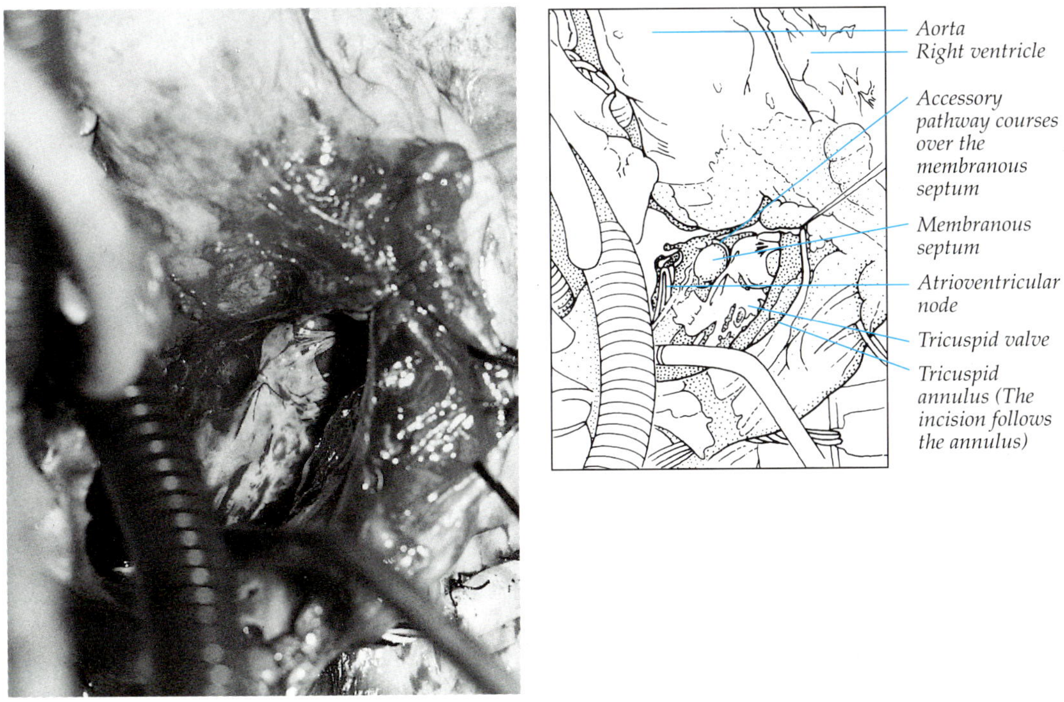

FIGURE 10-5. Operative view of an anterior septal dissection combined with exposure and dissection of the atrial membranous septum under normothermic cardiopulmonary bypass for pathways situated near the AV node–His bundle.

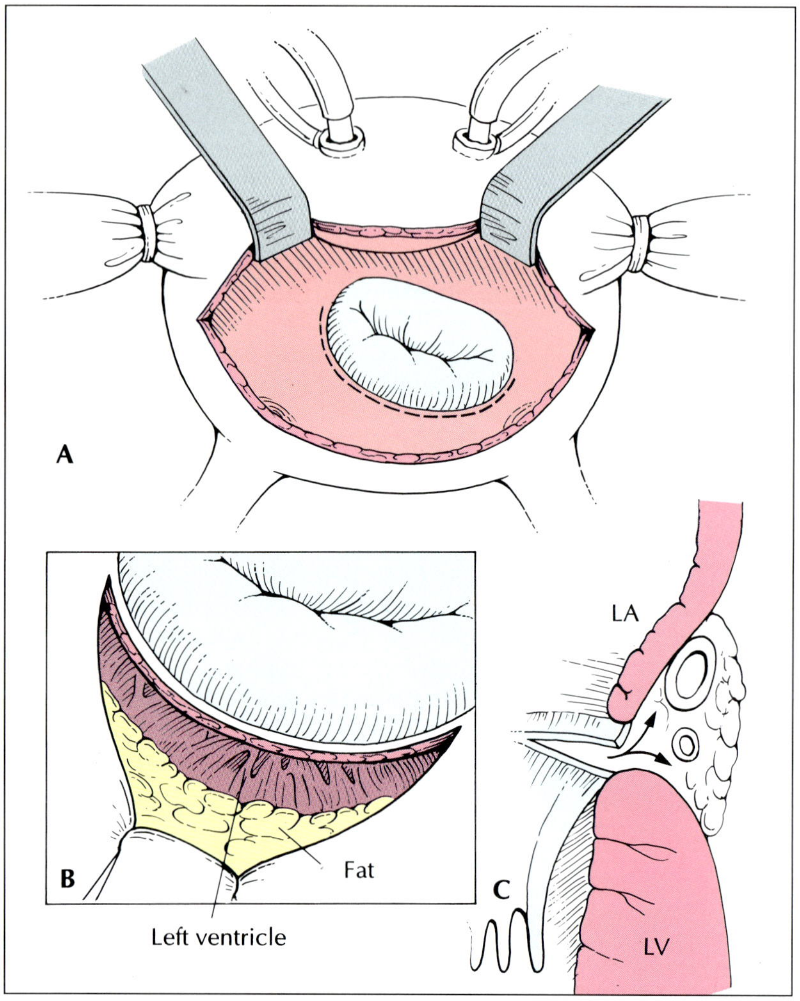

Figure 10-6. The endocardial approach using a left ventricular free wall location of the accessory AV connection. **A,** The mitral valve annulus is exposed using a conventional exposure via the interatrial sulcus. The *dotted line* indicates the site of the para-annular incision of the left atrial wall to enter the AV sulcus. **B,** The blunt dissection of the left ventricular wall within the AV sulcus. **C,** The atrial wall dissected free for better results. The endocardial approach yields results similar to the epicardial approach [10].

AV Nodal Tachycardias

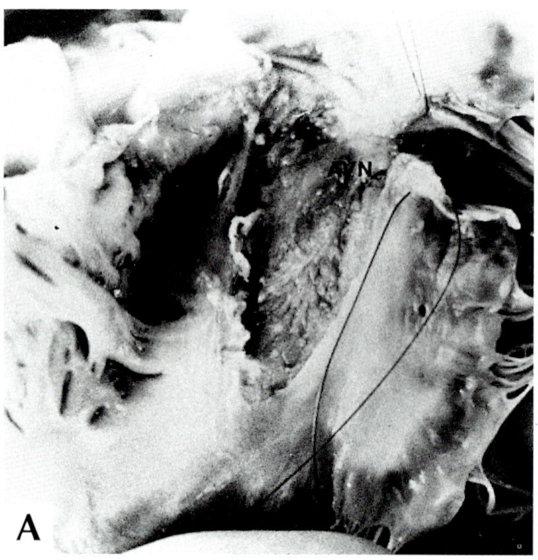

Figure 10-7. The reentrant mechanism associated with atrioventricular (AV) nodal reentrant tachycardia was initially described to be within the compact node (nodal tissue within the central fibrous body), until surgical therapy suggested that the reentrant mechanism involved the intermediate node, which is made up of atrial bundles connecting the atria tissue and the compact node, as limbs of the reentry loop. This concept implies the presence of a large AV nodal area, the limits of which go far beyond the actual node described by pathologists. **A,** A macroscopic dissection of the greater AV node of a human heart specimen. The compact AV node (*AVN*) is exposed after resection of the membranous septum. The atrial myocardial fibers that connect to the AV node include those of the intermediate node, which is in direct continuity with the atrial myocardium without discrete limits (atrial inputs). (*continued*)

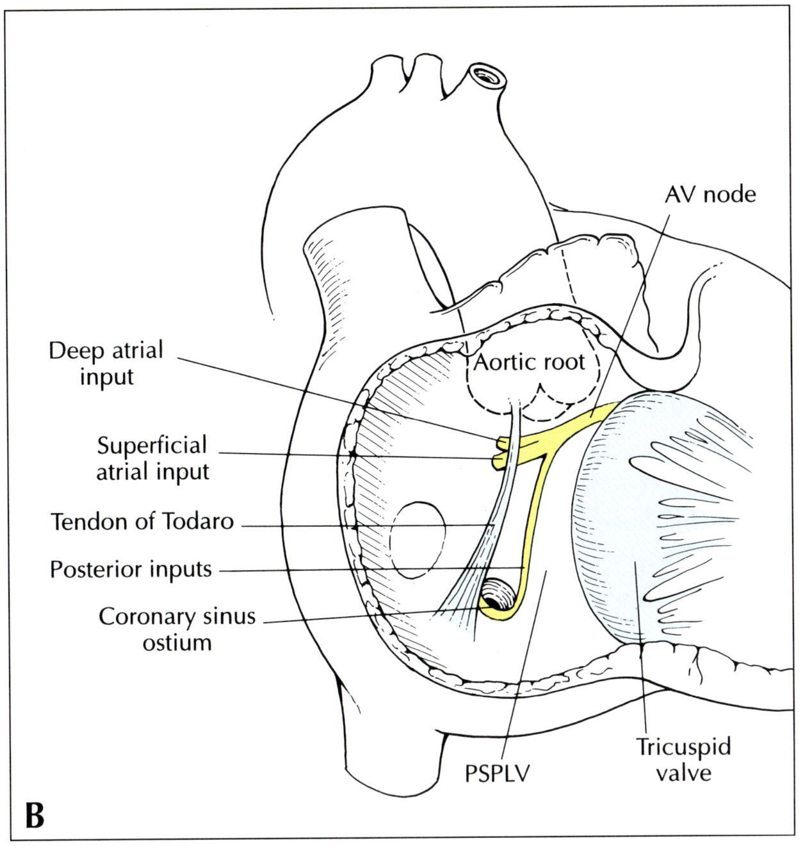

Figure 10-7. (*continued*) **B,** A schematic depiction of the greater AV node. The atrial output materializes AV nodal routes with specific electrophysiologic characteristics: posterior inputs have slow conduction velocity, while the superficial (anterior) inputs have fast conduction velocity. Surgical dissection [11] or cryoablation [12] could ablate or modify the atrial inputs and interrupt the tachycardias. Selective radiofrequency catheter ablation of the slow (posterior) or fast (superficial) inputs also interrupts the AV nodal tachycardias with very high success and minimal morbidity [13,14]. PSPLV—posterior superior process of the left ventricle.

Atrial Fibrillation

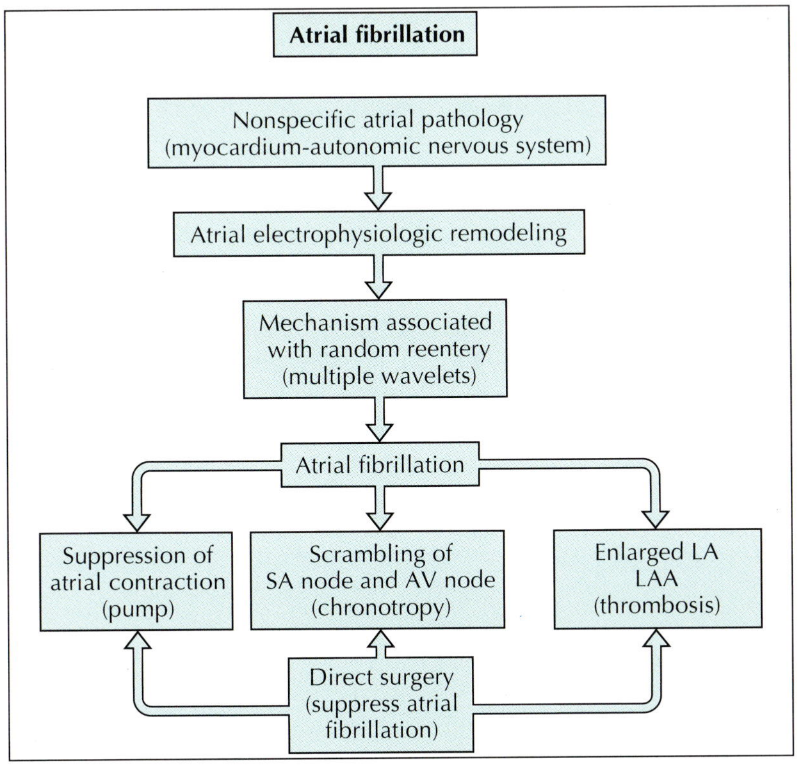

Figure 10-8. Flow chart for surgical treatment of atrial fibrillation. Atrial electrophysiologic remodeling is defined as the electrophysiologic changes in conduction velocity and refractoriness induced by atrial fibrillation itself that produce a new milieu that favors perpetuation of atrial fibrillation. AV—atrioventricular; LA—left atrium; LAA—left atrial appendage; SA—sinoatrial.

ATRIAL FIBRILLATION SURGICAL OPTIONS

Atrial Fibrillation Mechanism Requires Critical Surface Area, which can be altered by

- Exclusion/reduction (reduces area)
- Channelling (alters geometry = one-way channels)
- Fragmentation traps reentrant wavelets

Figure 10-9. Atrial fibrillation surgical options. Exclusion, channeling, and fragmentation are three techniques that have been successful in eliminating atrial fibrillation.

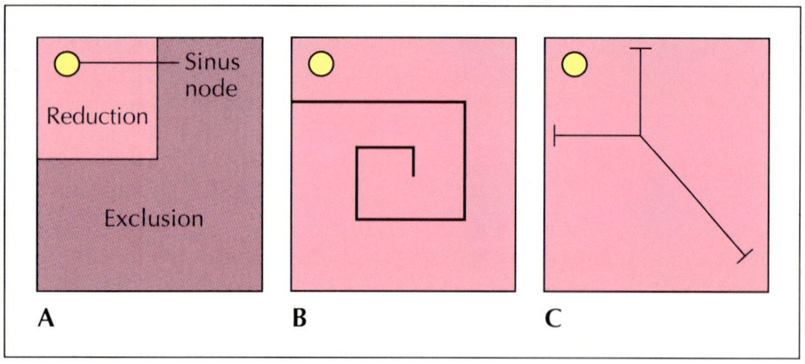

FIGURE 10-10. Rationales for the surgical techniques used for atrial fibrillation. **A,** In reduction/exclusion the clear small square is excluded from the rest of the fibrillation atrial tissue. Because its surface is less than the critical surface area required to support the arrhythmia, it does not fibrillate. **B,** In channeling, the atrial tissue is made unidirectional by adequate incision (spiral). This narrow band becomes a one-way channel and prevents reentry. **C,** In fragmentation, incisions construct quasi-isolated segments of atrial tissue in which the impulses are trapped. Consequently, the reentry mechanism is disabled. The *square* represents the entire surface area of the atrial tissue; the *circle* represents the sinoatrial node.

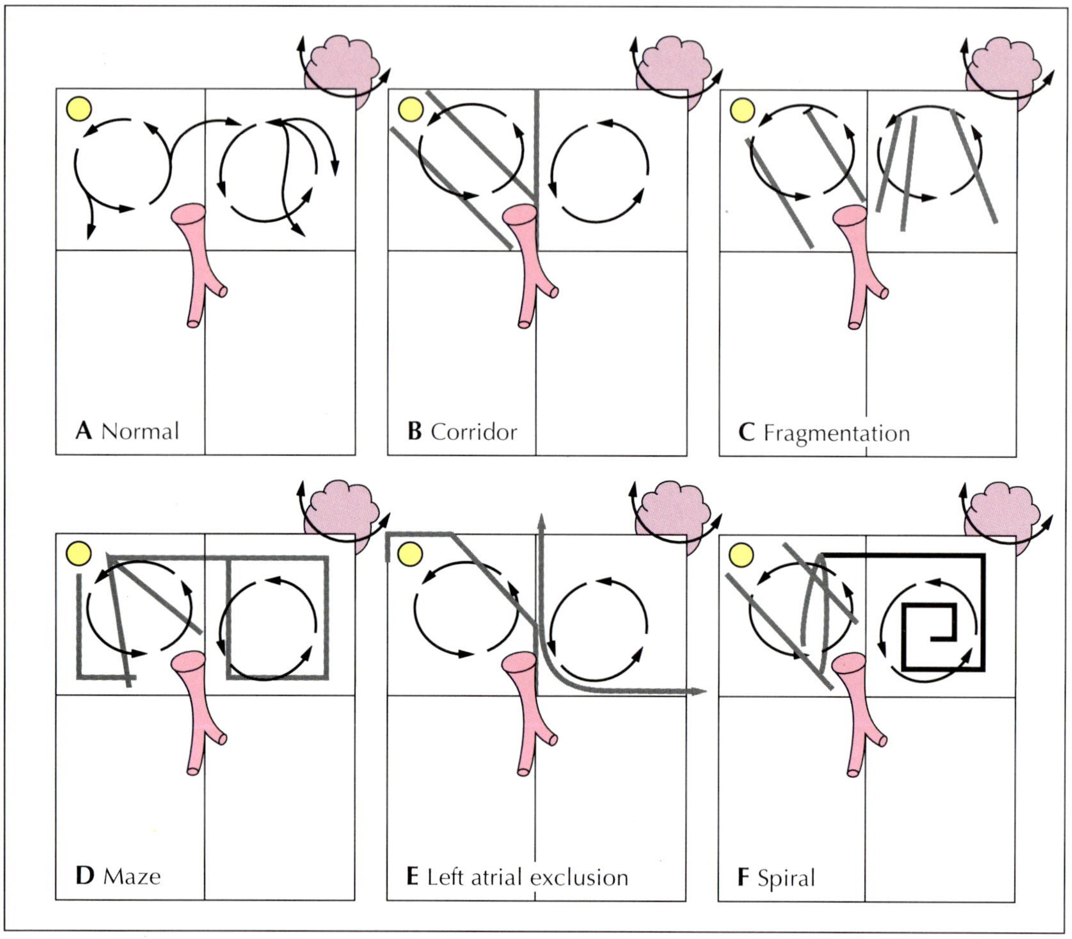

FIGURE 10-11. Surgical techniques for atrial fibrillation. The heart is depicted by four squares, with the sinoatrial (SA) node shown as a circle and the atrioventricular (AV) node within the shaded area. **A,** Normal heart. **B,** Corridor operation [15,16,17] using exclusion/reduction rationale. A strip of atrial tissue (reduction) harboring the SA node and the AV node is separated (exclusion) from the rest of the atrial tissue to restore and preserve chronotropic function. **C,** Compartment operation [18]. The three atrial segments (fragmentation) that are isolated in the corridor operation are left connected by tiny atrial bridges. **D,** The Maze operation [19,20], so called because of multiple complex incisions and the use of the three approaches: exclusion/reduction, fragmentation, and channelling.
It combines subtotal exclusion of the left atrium with multiple right and left atrial incisions. These incisions have evolved over time, the inventor having recently described Maze III. **E,** Left atrial exclusion [21]. This technique excludes the left atrial free wall in patients with mitral valve disease, because the left atrium is thought to house the fibrillating mechanism.
F, The spiral operation is essentially based on the rationale of channelling. The left atrium is entirely channelled by a spiraling incision. The right atrium is incised extensively. *All techniques include the amputation of the left atrial appendage.*

Surgical techniques have various end points (restoring sinus rhythm, right or left atrial contraction, and thrombus prevention). The Maze, the spiral, and the compartment operations aim at the three end points. Surgical results may be altered by myocardial pathology associated with loss of contraction and sinus node dysfunction.

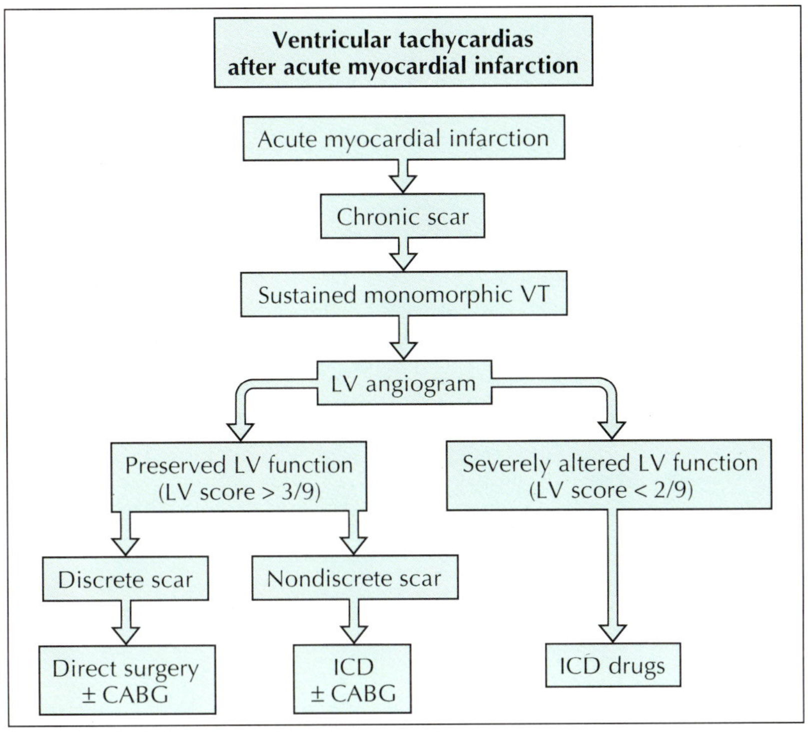

FIGURE 10-12. Development of ventricular tachycardia following myocardial infarction. The left ventricle (LV) score uses the same method as described in the Coronary Artery Surgery Study (CASS) (normal score 9/9) [22]. No electrophysiologic intervention, that is, drugs, direct surgery, coronary artery bypass graft (CABG), or implantable cardioverter defibrillator (ICD), in isolation or in combination, is associated with a better documented outcome in terms of survival. VT—ventricular tachycardia.

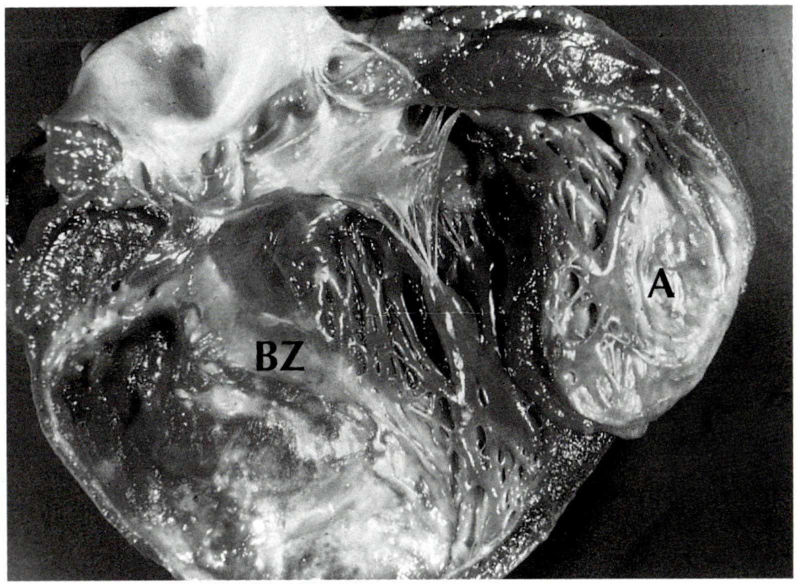

FIGURE 10-13. Typical pathology of a left ventricular aneurysm. The left ventricle is half opened. The border zone (BZ) covered by the whitish endocardial fibrosis circumscribes the central fibrotic segment of the aneurysm (A). The endocardial fibrosis is a reliable marker of the subendocardial ischemia.

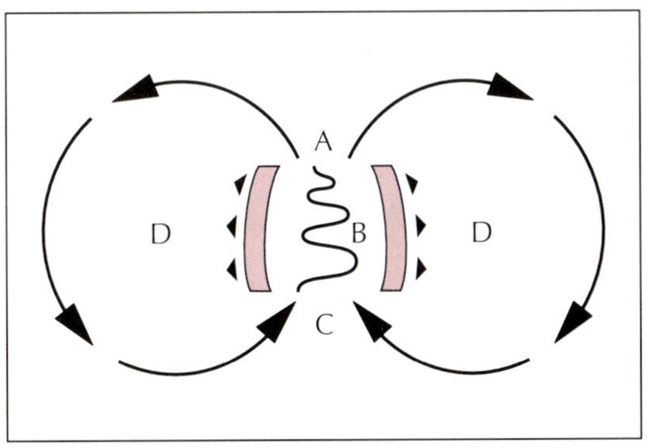

FIGURE 10-14. Schematic depiction of the reentrant circuit using figure-of-eight concept. There is a pathway of slow conduction (*B*) walled by an area of block. The activation front enters the slow conduction path in C and exits in *A*. The rest of the circuit is open and activation involves the remaining myocardium (QRS activation) and surrounding scar tissue. The anatomic arrhythmogenic substrate involves the slow conduction pathway and its input and output, as well as adjacent scar. D—segment of the scar not involved in the mechanism.

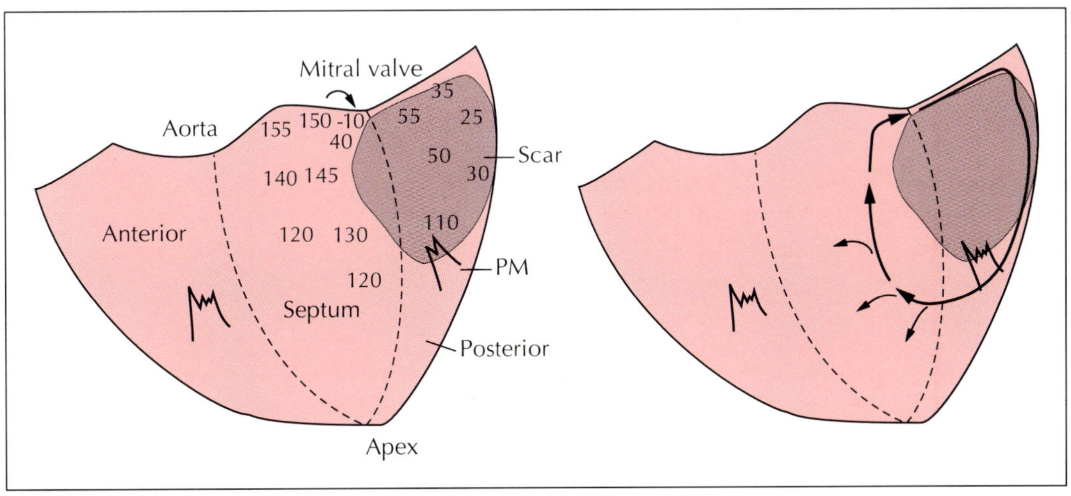

FIGURE 10-15. Endocardial mapping of a posterior scar (*shaded area*). The activation circulates around the scar (*arrows*). The area of slow conduction (arrhythmogenic substrate) is located between the mitral annulus and the scar. The numbers shown refer to activation time in ms—time zero at the onset of QRS. PM—posterior papillary muscle.

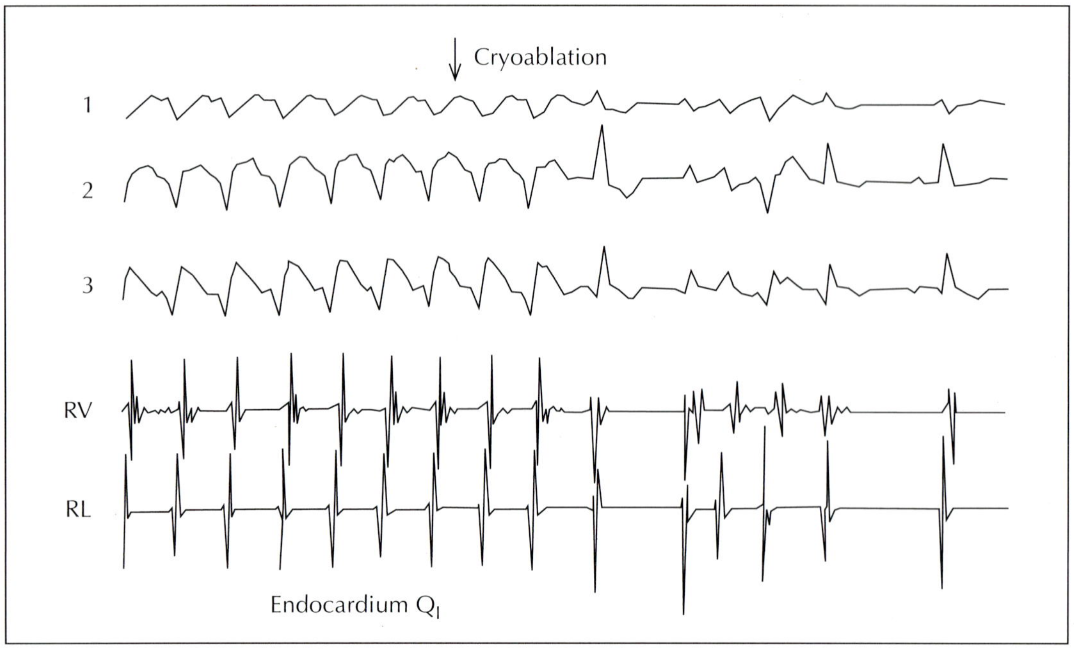

FIGURE 10-16. Cryoablation of the narrow slow pathway interrupts the tachycardia, as seen in this electrocardiographic tracing. RL—roving electrode; RV—right ventricular reference electrode.

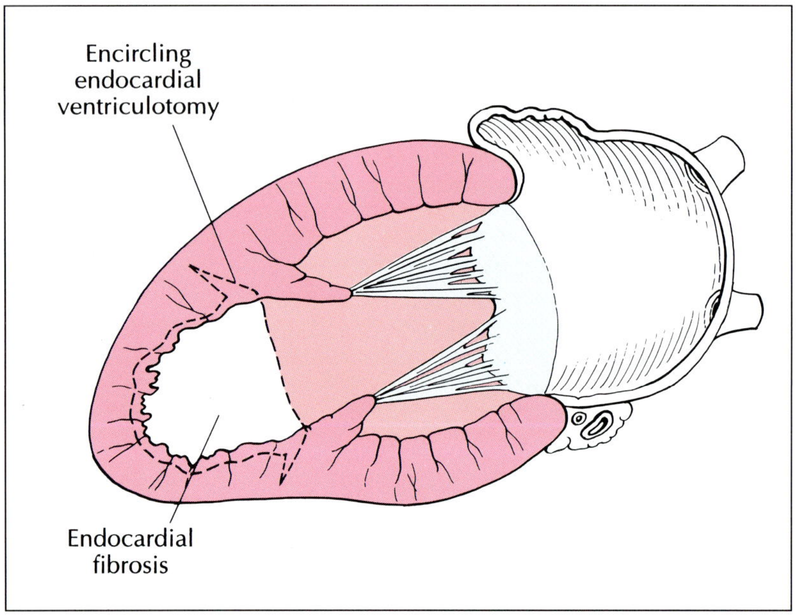

FIGURE 10-17. Encircling endocardial ventriculotomy. Based on the concept of "exclusion," an encircling ventriculotomy, which follows the limits of endocardial fibrosis, circumscribes the potentially arrhythmogenic border zone [4].

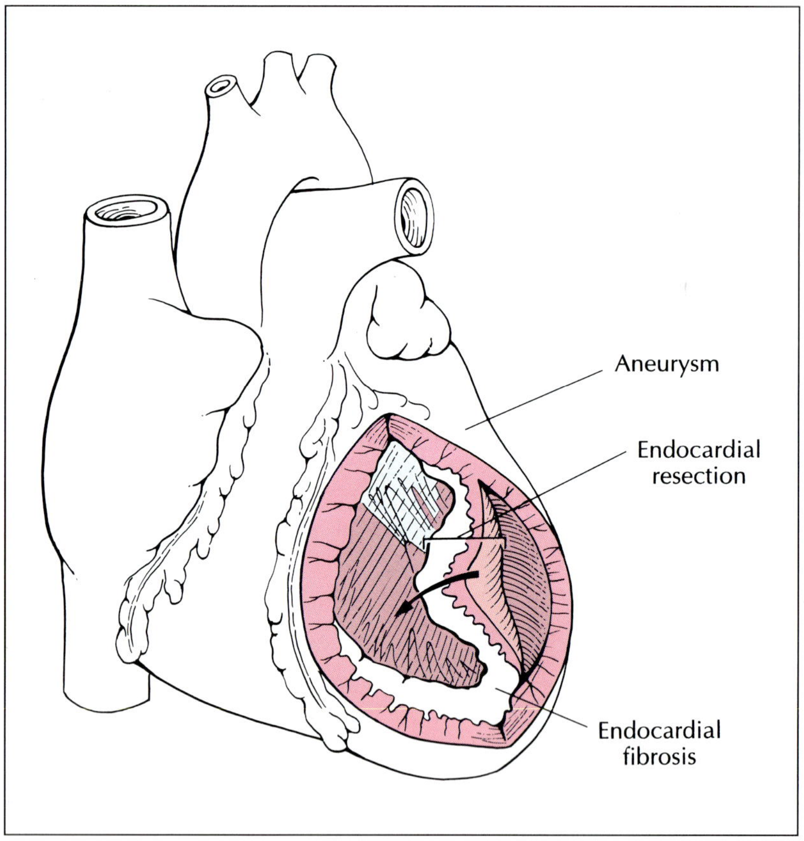

FIGURE 10-18. Endocardial resection (Pennsylvania peel). A segment of endocardial fibrosis and subjacent endocardial myocardium, identified by endocardial mapping as arrhythmogenic, is resected [5,23] or peeled away.

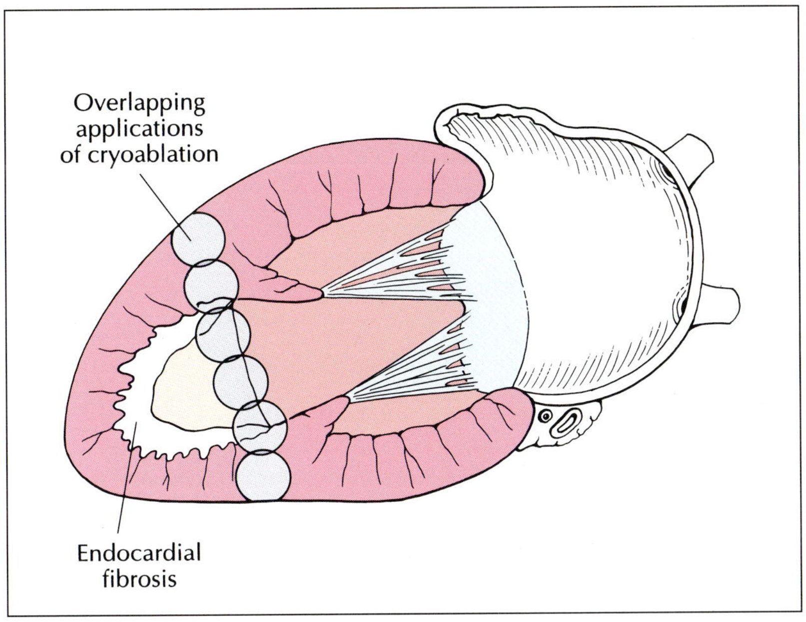

FIGURE 10-19. Encircling endocardial cryoablation. The entire border zone is cryoablated using overlapping applications of a large cryoprobe.

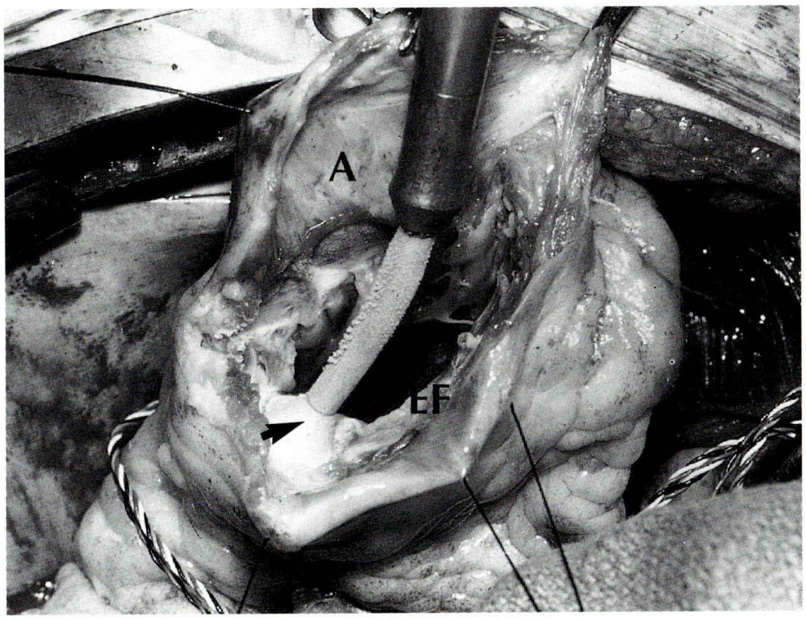

FIGURE 10-20. Operative view of cryoablation of ventricular tachycardia. The aneurysm (A) is opened. The cryoprobe (*arrow*) is applied to the border zone over the endocardial fibrosis (EF).

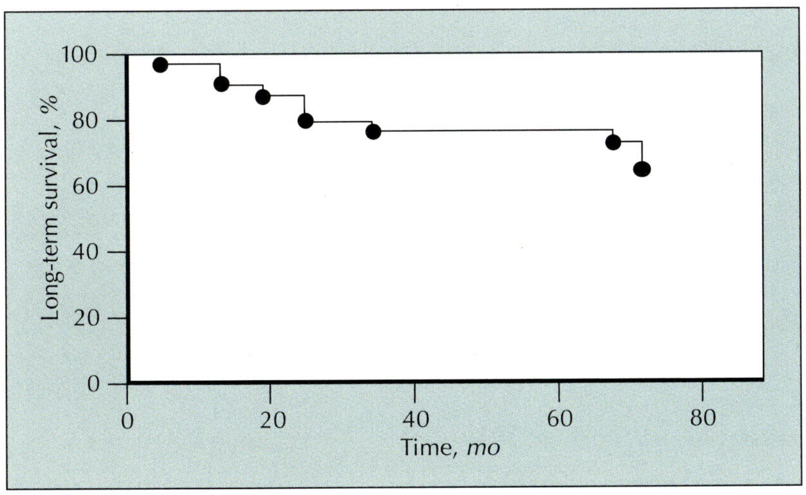

FIGURE 10-21. Long-term results of surgical ablation of ventricular tachycardia [24]. The five-year actuarial survival is over 70%. Most patients died of heart failure or associated noncardiac diseases.

Right Ventricular Free Wall Disconnection for Arrhythmogenic Right Ventricular Dysplasia

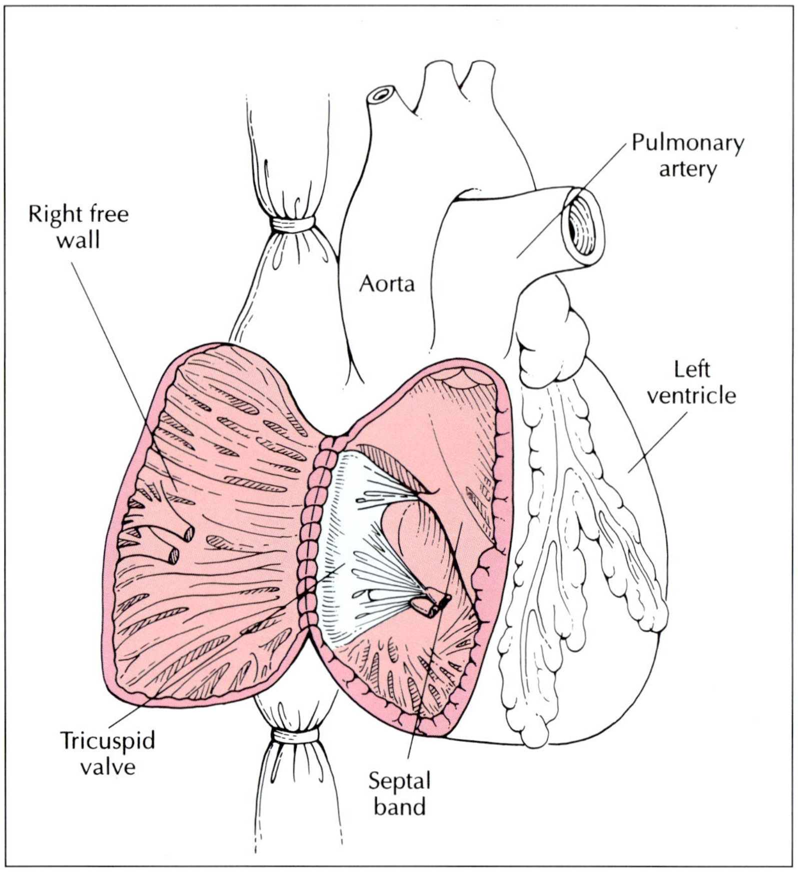

Figure 10-22. The entire arrhythmogenic right ventricular free wall is disconnected. This extensive surgical procedure is still used in rare selected cases [25].

References

1. Guiraudon GM, Klein GJ, Yee R: Surgery for cardiac tachyarrhythmias. *Highlights* 1990, 6:2–10.
2. Guiraudon GM, Klein GJ, Sharma AD, *et al.*: Use of old and new anatomic, electrophysiologic, and technical knowledge to develop operative approaches to tachycardias. In *Cardiac Arrhythmias: Where To Go From Here?* Edited by Brugada P, Wellens HJJ. Mount Kisco, NY: Futura Publishing Company, Inc.; 1987:639.
3. Gallagher JJ, Kasell J, Sealy WC, *et al.*: Epicardial mapping in the Wolff-Parkinson-White syndrome. *Circulation* 1978, 57:854.
4. Guiraudon G, Fontaine G, Frank R, *et al.*: Encircling endocardial ventriculotomy: A new surgical treatment for life-threatening ventricular tachycardias resistant to medical treatment following myocardial infarction. *Ann Thorac Surg* 1978, 26:438–444.
5. Josephson ME, Harken AH, Horowitz LN: Endocardial excision: a new surgical technique for the treatment of recurrent ventricular tachycardia. *Circulation* 1979, 60:1430–1439.
6. Kirklin JK: Prospects for understanding and eliminating the deleterious effects of cardiopulmonary bypass. *Ann Thorac Surg* 1991, 51:529–531.
7. Guiraudon GM: Surgical therapy for cardiac arrhythmias (overview). *Coron Artery Dis* 1992, 3:171–174.
8. Guiraudon GM, Klein GJ, Sharma AD, *et al.*: Closed-heart technique for Wolff-Parkinson-White syndrome: further experience and potential limitations. *Ann Thorac Surg* 1986, 42:651.
9. Guiraudon GM, Klein GJ, Sharma AD, *et al.*: Surgery for the Wolff-Parkinson-White syndrome—the epicardial approach. *Semin Thorac Cardiovasc Surg* 1989, 1:21–33.
10. Cox JL, Gallagher JJ, Cain ME: Experience with 118 consecutive patients undergoing operation for the Wolff-Parkinson-White syndrome. *J Thorac Cardiovasc Surg* 1985, 90:490.
11. Guiraudon GM, Klein GJ, Sharma AD, *et al.*: Skeletonization of the atrioventricular node surgical alternative for AV nodal reentrant tachycardia. Experience with 32 patients. *Ann Thorac Surg* 1990, 49:565.
12. Cox JL, Holman WL, Cain ME, *et al.*: Cryosurgical treatment of atrioventricular node reentrant tachycardia. *Circulation* 1987, 76:1329.
13. Jackman W, Beckman K, McClelland J, *et al.*: Treatment of supraventricular tachycardia due to atrioventricular nodal reentry by radiofrequency catheter ablation of slow-pathway conduction. *N Engl J Med* 1992, 327:313–318.
14. Wathen M, Natale A, Wolfe K, *et al.*: An anatomically guided approach to atrioventricular node slow pathway ablation. *Am J Cardiol* 1992, 70:886–889.
15. Guiraudon GM, Campbell CS, Jones DL, *et al.*: Combined sinoatrial node atrioventricular isolation: a surgical alternative to His bundle ablation in patients with atrial fibrillation [abstract]. *Circulation* 1985, 72:III–220.

16. Leitch JW, Guiraudon GM, Klein GJ, *et al.*: Surgical management of symptomatic atrial fibrillation. In *Atrial Fibrillation: Mechanism and Management*. Edited by Falk RH, Podrid PJ. New York: Raven Press; 1992:375–387.
17. van Hemel NM, Defauw JJAMT, Kingma JH, *et al.*: Longterm results of the "corridor" operation for atrial fibrillation. *Br Heart J* 1994, 71:170–176.
18. Shyu K-G, Cheng J-J, Chen J-J, *et al.*: Recovery of atrial function after atrial compartment operation for chronic atrial fibrillation in mitral valve disease. *J Am Coll Cardiol* 1994, 24:392–398.
19. Cox JL, Schuessler RB, D'Agostino HJ, Jr, *et al.*: The surgical treatment of atrial fibrillation. III. Development of a definite surgical procedure. *J Thorac Cardiovasc Surg* 1991, 101:569–583.
20. Cox JL, Boineau JP, Schuessler HB, *et al.*: Successful surgical treatment of atrial fibrillation. *JAMA* 1991, 266:1976–1980.
21. Graffigna A, Pagani F, Minzioni G, *et al.*: Left atrial isolation associated with mitral valve operations. *Ann Thorac Surg* 1992, 54:1093–1098.
22. van Hemel NM, Kingma JH, Defauw JAM, *et al.*: Left ventricular segmental wall motion score as a criterion for selecting patients for direct surgery in the treatment of postinfarction ventricular tachycardia. *Eur Heart J* 1989, 10:304–315.
23. Hargrove WC, III, Josephson ME, Harken AH, *et al.*: Endocardial resection for ventricular tachycardia in 353 patients [abstract]. *J Am Coll Cardiol* 1994, 1A:480A.
24. Guiraudon GM, Klein GJ, Yee R, *et al.*: Encircling endocardial cryoblation for ventricular tachycardia after myocardial infarction—experience with thirty-three patients. *Am Heart J* 1994, 128:982–989.
25. Guiraudon GM, Klein GJ, Gulamhusein SS: Total disconnection of the right ventricular free wall: surgical treatment of right ventricular tachycardia associated with right ventricular dysplasia. *Circulation* 1983, 67:463–470.

Catheter Ablation

11

CHAPTER

Harlan R. Grogin

There have been tremendous advances in our understanding of the mechanisms of arrhythmias over the past twenty years and in our ability to offer curative therapy for these arrhythmias. Surgical therapy for arrhythmias was pioneered by Sealy, Cox, and Guiraudon and their colleagues. Catheter techniques for the destruction of the atrioventricular (AV) junction were introduced in 1982 by Gonzalez and Scheinman for patients with drug refractory atrial arrhythmias. Since then, refinements in energy sources, advances in catheter technology, and innovations in ablative techniques have virtually replaced the need for surgical intervention in patients with both supraventricular and ventricular arrhythmias. This chapter provides a review of the approaches for catheter ablation in patients with Wolff-Parkinson-White syndrome, AV node reentry, atrial fibrillation, atrial flutter, and atrial tachycardia. Catheter ablation for management of ventricular arrhythmias is discussed in Chapter 6.

Carefully performed electrophysiologic studies are the key elements in directing nonpharmacologic treatment. Precise localization of abnormal foci or pathways is achieved by endocardial mapping. Radiofrequency energy is currently the energy source of choice for ablative purposes, because it does not carry the potential risks of barotrauma and it eliminates the need for general anesthesia. Other methods of ablation, *ie*, chemicals, laser, cryoablation, and microwave, are not discussed in this chapter because they are investigative technologies.

Overview of Catheter Ablation

OVERVIEW OF CATHETER ABLATION

TYPE OF ARRHYTHMIA	SUCCESS RATE FOR CATHETER ABLATION (%)	ACCESS
WPW	85–95 (Right-sided) 95+ (Left-sided)	Transseptal or retrograde aortic approach for left-sided accessory pathways. Femoral right internal jugular or right subclavian for right-sided pathways.
AV node reentry	95+	Femoral
Atrial fibrillation: AV Junction	95+	Femoral
Atrial flutter	80–90 for "typical atrial flutter"; 50–60 for "atypical atrial flutter"	Femoral
Atrial tachycardia	70–80	Femoral for right-sided atrial tachycardia; transseptal for left-sided atrial tachycardia

Figure 11-1. Summary of catheter ablation outcomes. In a number of large series [1,2], catheter ablation was used for treatment of the Wolff-Parkinson-White (WPW) syndrome. Approaches for left-sided accessory pathways have been highly successful. Transseptal approaches are highly useful in patients with aortic valve replacements, disease of the aortic arch, or congenital heart disease (associated with atrial septal defect). Patients with right-sided accessory pathways and Ebstein's anomaly may benefit from coronary artery mapping [1]. With atrioventricular (AV) node modification, the preferred approach is ablation of the slow AV nodal pathway rather than the fast pathway. With slow pathway modification, there is a less than 1% risk of requiring a permanent pacemaker [3]. Complete AV junction ablation requires the placement of a permanent pacemaker and anticoagulation for chronic atrial fibrillation. The His bundle may need to be ablated from the left ventricular septum if necessary. AV modification is a means of altering AV node conduction without causing complete AV node block, thus making a permanent pacemaker unnecessary [4]. There is now investigation into reproducing the surgical Maze procedure with catheter techniques for cure of atrial fibrillation. Up to one third of patients may have a recurrence of their atrial flutter after an ablation and require a second ablation. A subset of patients may have recurrent (more stable) atrial fibrillation but not atrial flutter. The complications of an invasive procedure include bleeding, infection, emboli, and blood clots. The risk of tamponade (from catheter perforation), stroke, or death is less than 1%.

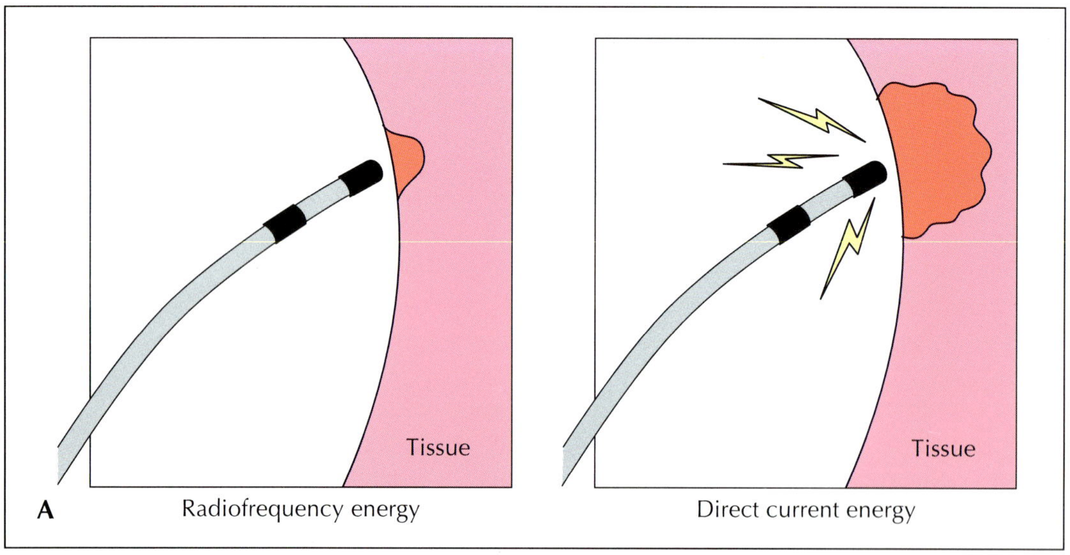

Figure 11-2. Radiofrequency versus direct current energies (**A** and **B**). The first catheter ablations were performed with direct current (DC) energy, which delivered high energy (1–2 KV) for 5 to 6 ms between the catheter tip and an electrode patch on the patient's back. This discharge resulted in internal generation of light, heat, and pressure, and tissue destruction was proportional to the energy used. It was characterized by inhomogeneous areas of myocytolysis and contraction bands. Later, short duration nonarcing DC current was applied, which was associated with less barotrauma. (*continued*)

B. RADIOFREQUENCY VERSUS DIRECT CURRENT ENERGIES

FACTOR BEING COMPARED	RADIOFREQUENCY	DIRECT CURRENT
Lesion	Controllable size, uniform	Large but nonuniform
Energy	5–60 W	2000–3000 V
Sedation	Mild	General anesthesia
Potential complications	Coagulum formation	Barotrauma, arcing, tamponade, sudden death

FIGURE 11-2. (*continued*) Radiofrequency energy, 5–60 W at a frequency of 500–750 kHz, produces smaller but more homogeneous lesions. This results in less arrhythmogenesis and eliminates the requirement of general anesthesia. Other forms of ablation include introducing chemical agents (alcohol) into selective coronary arteries supplying the region of the arrhythmic focus, *eg*, the atrioventricular (AV) nodal artery for atrioventricular nodal reentry tachycardia. Research continues on the development of new energy sources such as microwave antenna or cryoenergy.

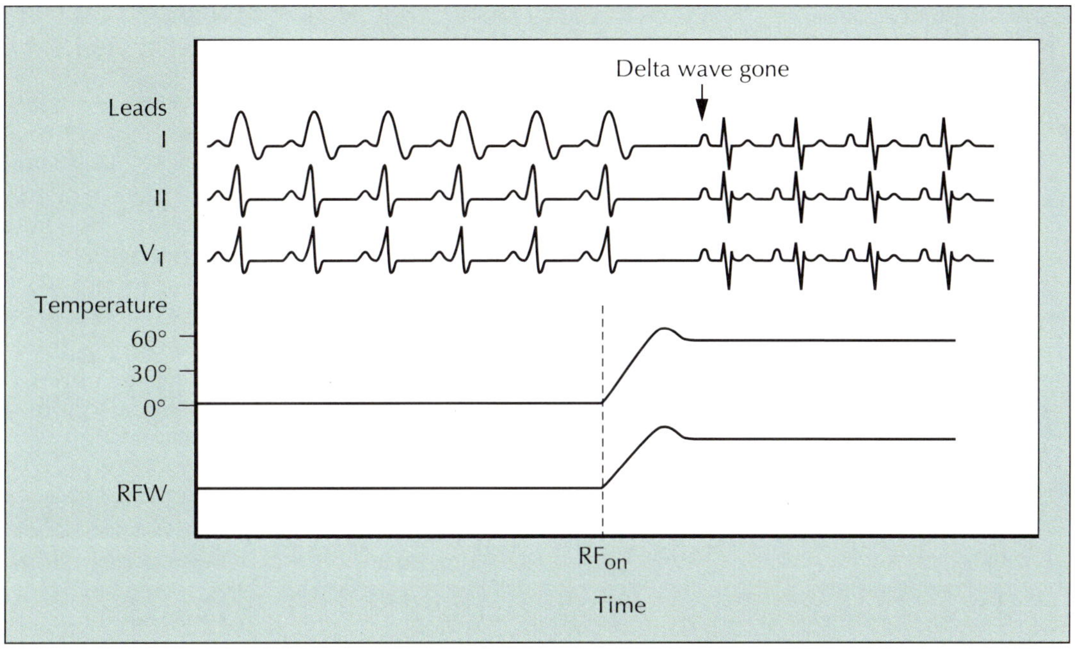

FIGURE 11-3. Temperature monitoring during radiofrequency (RF) ablation. Application of RF energy results in transfer of electrical current to tissue. Tissue temperature rises as a result of current flow through the impedance offered by the tissue. During application of RF energy, blood may become hot enough on the tip of the catheter to form a coagulum, which may break loose and embolize. Transfer of electrical energy (and hence heat) to tissue depends on tissue-catheter contact as well as conductive and convective heat losses. The impedance begins to rise prior to coagulum formation, and in order to continue a constant current, the energy delivered must be increased. Thermistor catheters can sense the rise in temperature at the tip of the catheter. By maintaining a constant temperature, no excess energy is delivered to maintain a constant current, and therefore coagulum formation can be avoided. It is also a means to assess whether there is good contact with the myocardium. RFW—radiofrequency watts.

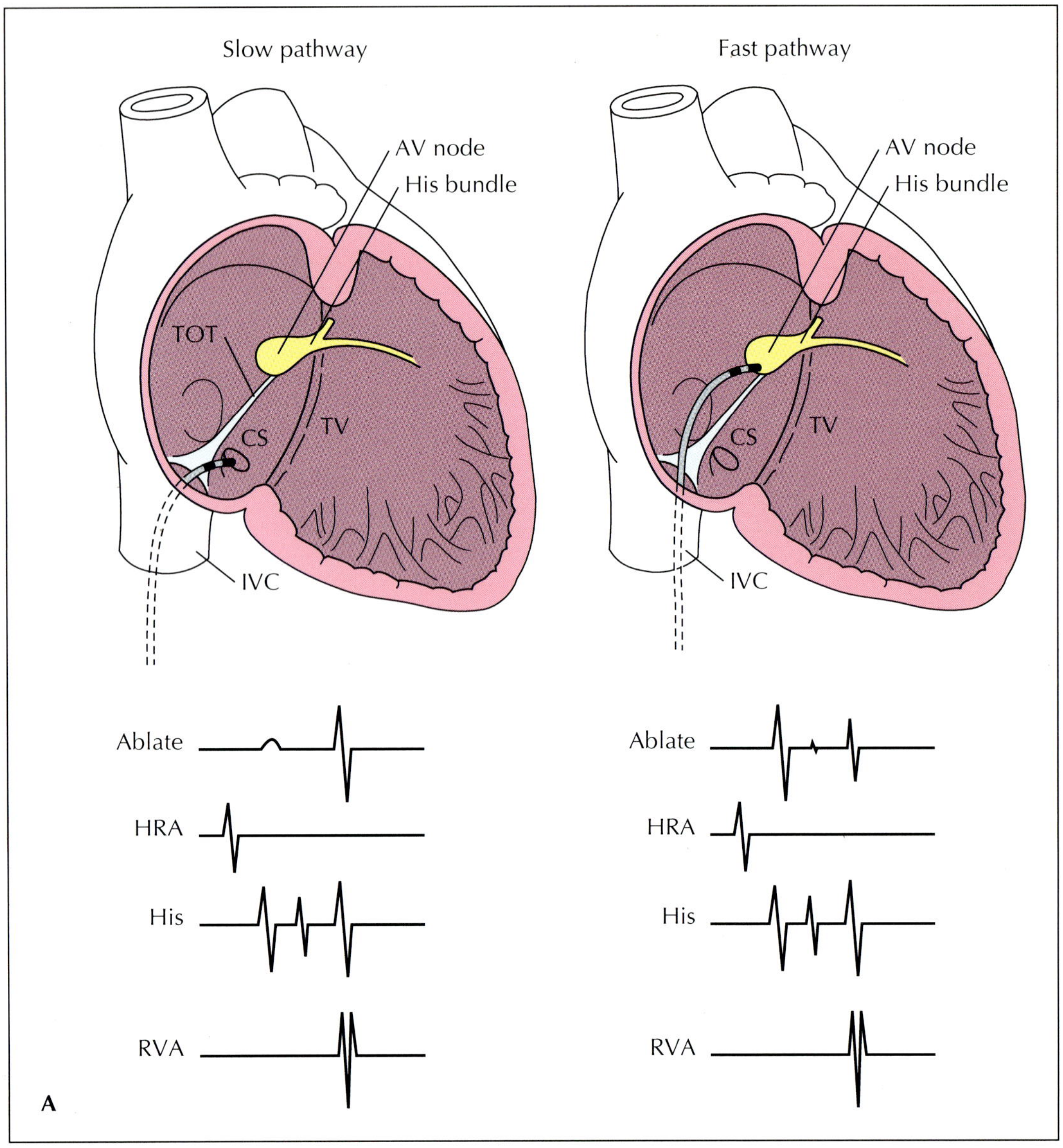

B: SUMMARY OF INTRACARDIAC CATHETER SIGNAL TERMINOLOGY

ABBREVIATION	CATHETER LOCATION
A	Atrium
Abl Dist	Distal tip of the ablation catheter
Abl Prox	Proximal tip of the ablation catheter
CS	Coronary artery sinus
His (Dist, Prox, Mid)	His bundle: distal, proximal, mid
HRA	High right atrium
MAP	Monophasic action potential
ROVE	Ablation catheter used for mapping
RVA	Right ventricular apex
RVOT	Right ventricular outflow tract
TA	Tricuspid annulus
TV	Tricuspid valve
V	Ventricle

Figure 11-4. Atrioventricular (AV) nodal modification. Conduction abnormalities can be reduced or eliminated by means of catheter ablation, a technique that requires knowledge of the conduction pathways. **A**, Slow pathway fibers are thought to travel from the region of the coronary sinus os toward the more anterior and superior AV node. Fast pathway fibers are superior and anterior and therefore closer to the His bundle than slow pathway fibers. Destruction of the fast pathway ("fast pathway modification") (*right side*) results in a long PR interval due to subsequent impulse conduction over the slow pathway and a higher risk of complete AV block (up to 8%). Catheter position is achieved by obtaining a His bundle signal and then pulling the catheter back so that there is a large atrial signal, small to no His signal, and a small ventricular signal. Slow pathway modification (*left side*) can be performed by using the "slow pathway potentials" as a guide [5]), the "midseptal" approach [6]), or the "posterior–mid-anterior" approach [7], which has a more acceptable risk of complete heart block (<1%). The PR interval remains the same because of continued impulse conduction over the fast pathway. Further investigation is needed to clarify whether the mechanism of AV node reentry is truly "intranodal" or requires a portion of the atrium for sustenance of the tachycardia. CS—coronary sinus os; His—His bundle; IVC—inferior vena cava; TOT—tendon of Todaro; TV—tricuspid valve annulus. In **B**, the terminology used in the many electrocardiograms shown in this chapter is explained.

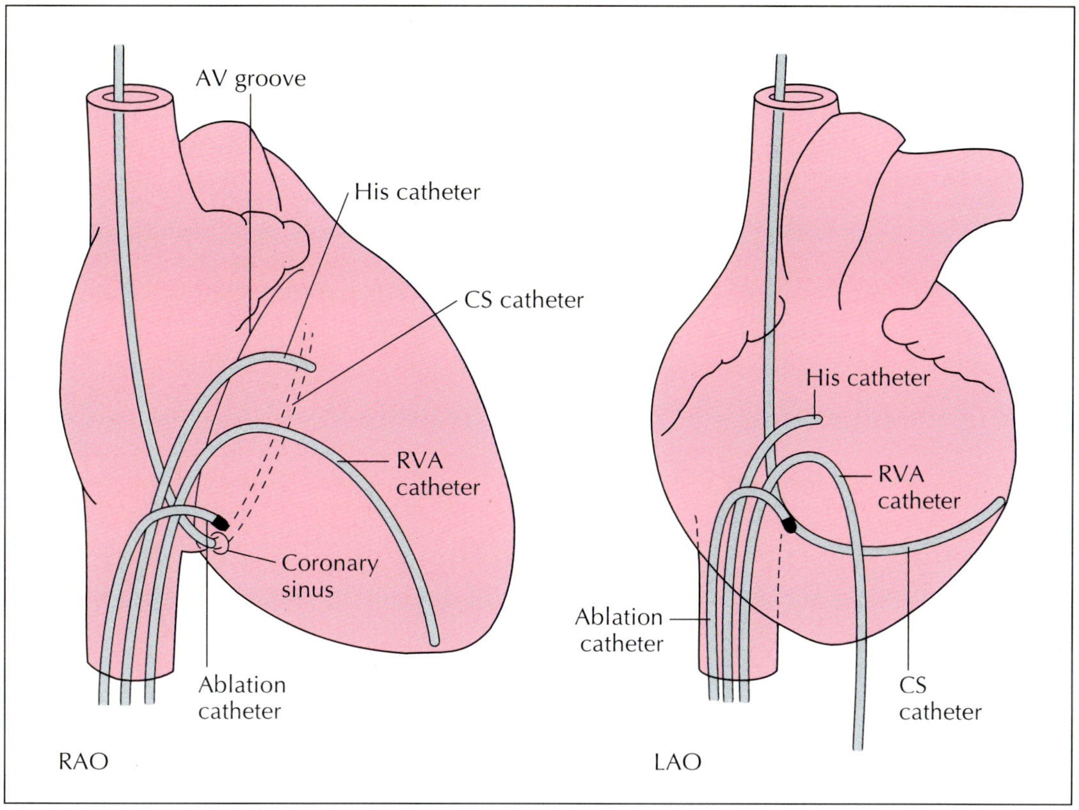

FIGURE 11-5. Right anterior oblique/left anterior oblique views of a slow pathway modification. The atrioventricular (AV) node is found in the apex of the triangle of Koch. The triangle has as its borders the septal leaflet of the tricuspid valve inferiorly, the coronary sinus os posteriorly and laterally, and the tendon of Todaro superiorly. The His bundle is protected by collagenous tissue as it enters into the membranous septum. Catheters: ABL, CS, His, HRA, RVA. (*See* Fig. 11-4B for abbreviations.)

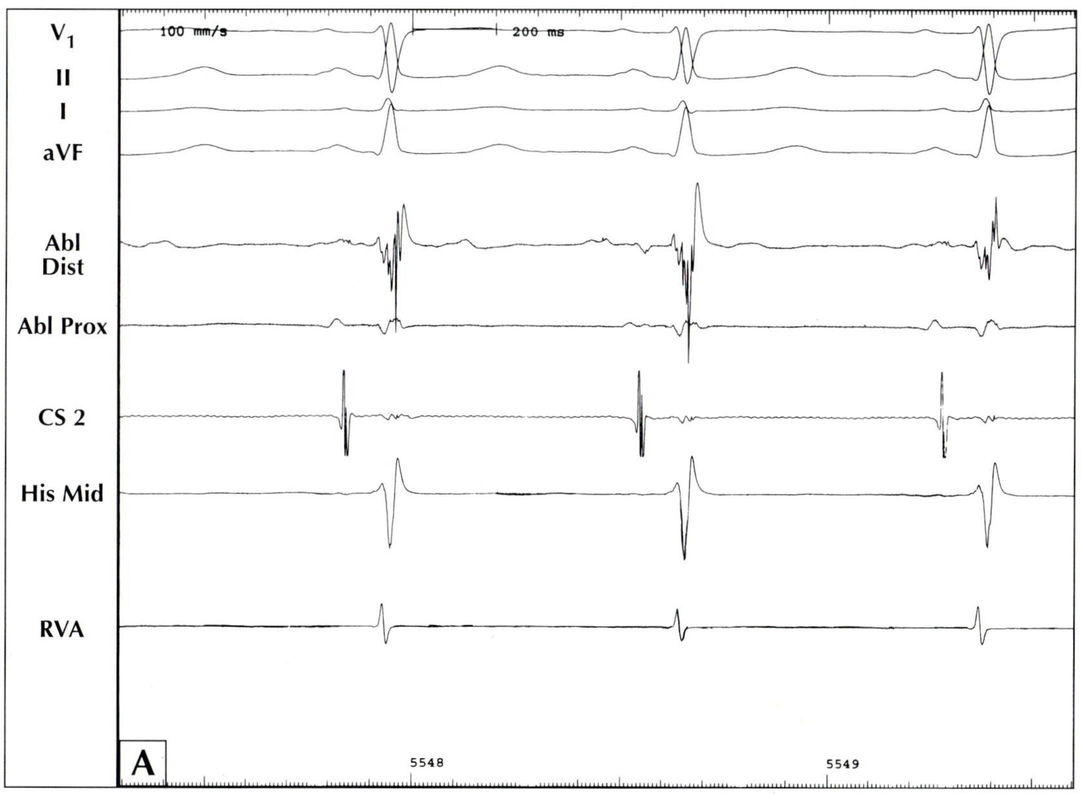

FIGURE 11-6. Electrocardiograms for slow pathway ablation. In **A**, Note that the small atrial electrocardiogram (ECG) compared with the ventricular ECG ratio is < 1 to 5 on the distal tip of the ablation catheter. By ablating toward the ventricular side of the annulus there is less of a chance of atrioventricular block because the His bundle enters into the more protected fibrous sheath in the distal septum (midseptal position). (*continued*)

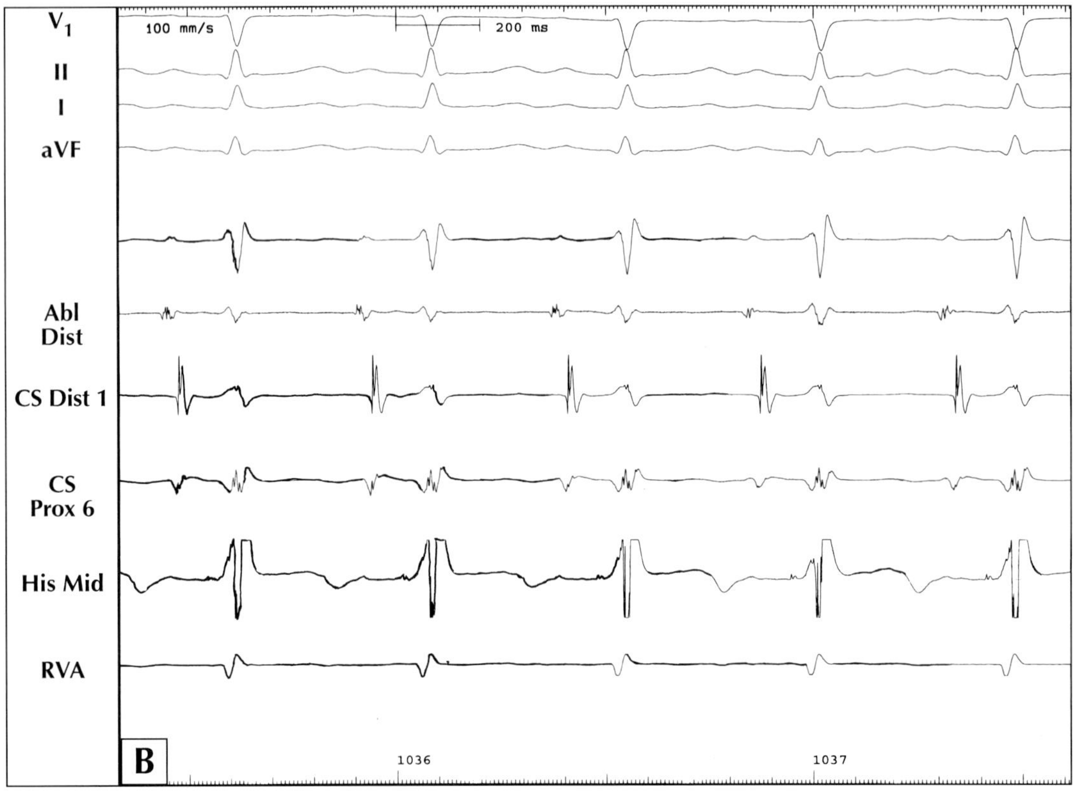

FIGURE 11-6. (*continued*) In many patients, a signal can be obtained near the mouth of the coronary sinus (CS), such as that shown in **B**. On the ablation catheter distal tip, there is a high frequency signal on the atrial ECG, which precedes the atrial ECG from the CS catheter (slow pathway potentials). Surface leads V_1, II, I, and aVF. Intracardiac signals: ABL Dist and Prox, CS, His Mid, and RVA. (*See* Fig. 11-4B for abbreviations.)

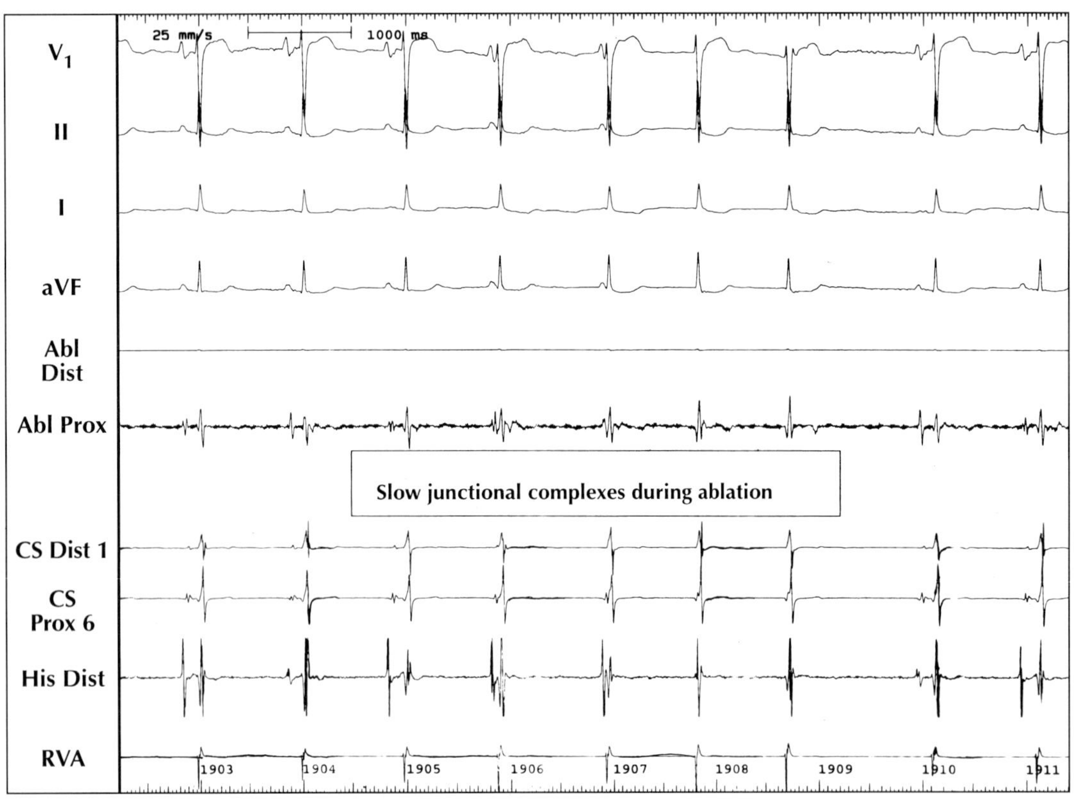

FIGURE 11-7. Slow junctional tachycardia during slow pathway modification. During application of radiofrequency (RF) energy, a slow junctional rhythm (< 120 bpm) is a good indicator of success compared with a fast junctional rhythm (> 120 bpm) or no effect at all. In this figure, surface leads V_1, II, I, and aVF are shown with the intracardiac electrocardiograms of the Abl Dist and Prox, CS Dist and Prox, His Dist, and RVA catheters. The first three beats are sinus beats. Complexes 4 to 7 are junctional complexes with varying PR intervals, rate 100 bpm. Sinus rhythm returns with a normal PR interval, indicating a successful ablation. (See Fig. 11-4B for abbreviations.)

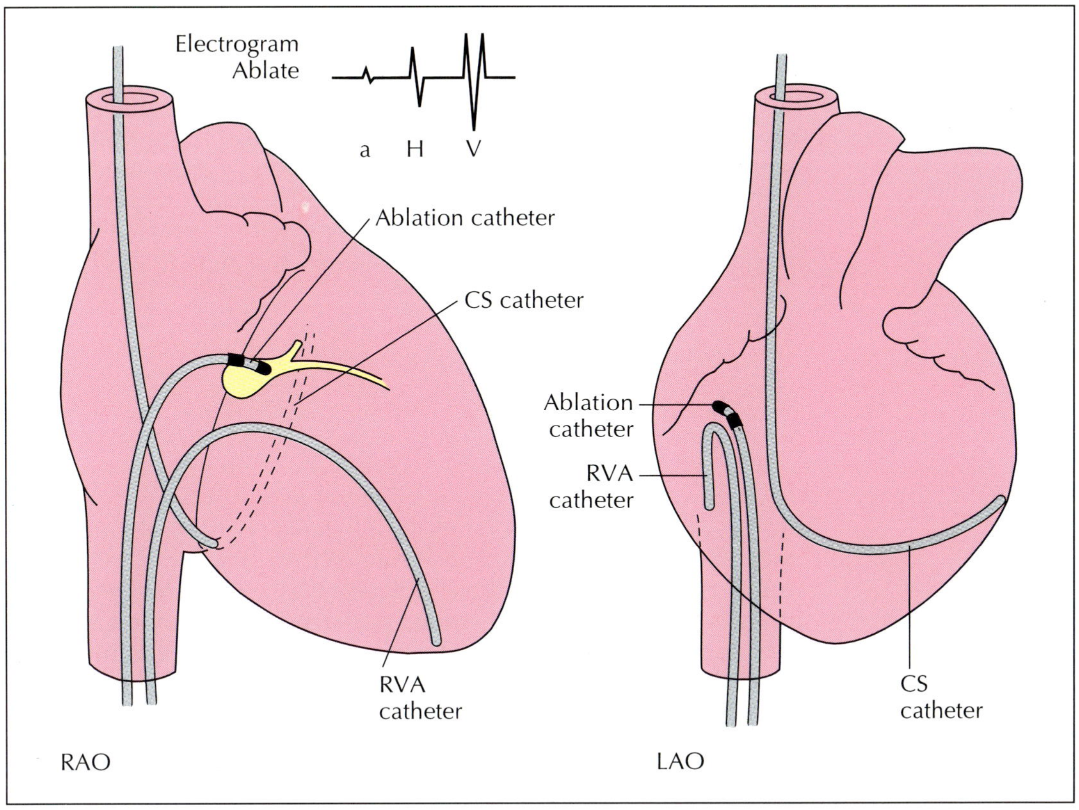

FIGURE 11-8. Right anterior oblique (RAO)/ left anterior oblique (LAO) schematics for an atrioventricular (AV) junctional ablation. Using the femoral approach, the ablation catheter is placed to obtain the largest His and septal atrial signal possible. If the catheter is placed too distally, application of radiofrequency energy will cause right bundle branch block but not complete atrioventricular (AV) block. Therefore, a large atrial signal demonstrates that the proximal His bundle is being recorded. Compared with a slow junctional tachycardia with an AV node modification, there is usually a rapid junctional tachycardia prior to complete heart block. A ventricular electrode catheter is mandatory for pacing after the successful ablation. Although biplane images are shown here, an AV junctional ablation can usually be performed with an anteroposterior image. CS—coronary sinus; His—His bundle; RA—right atrium; RV—right ventricle; TV—tricuspid valve. Catheters: Abl,CS, RVA. (*See* Fig. 11-4B for abbreviations.)

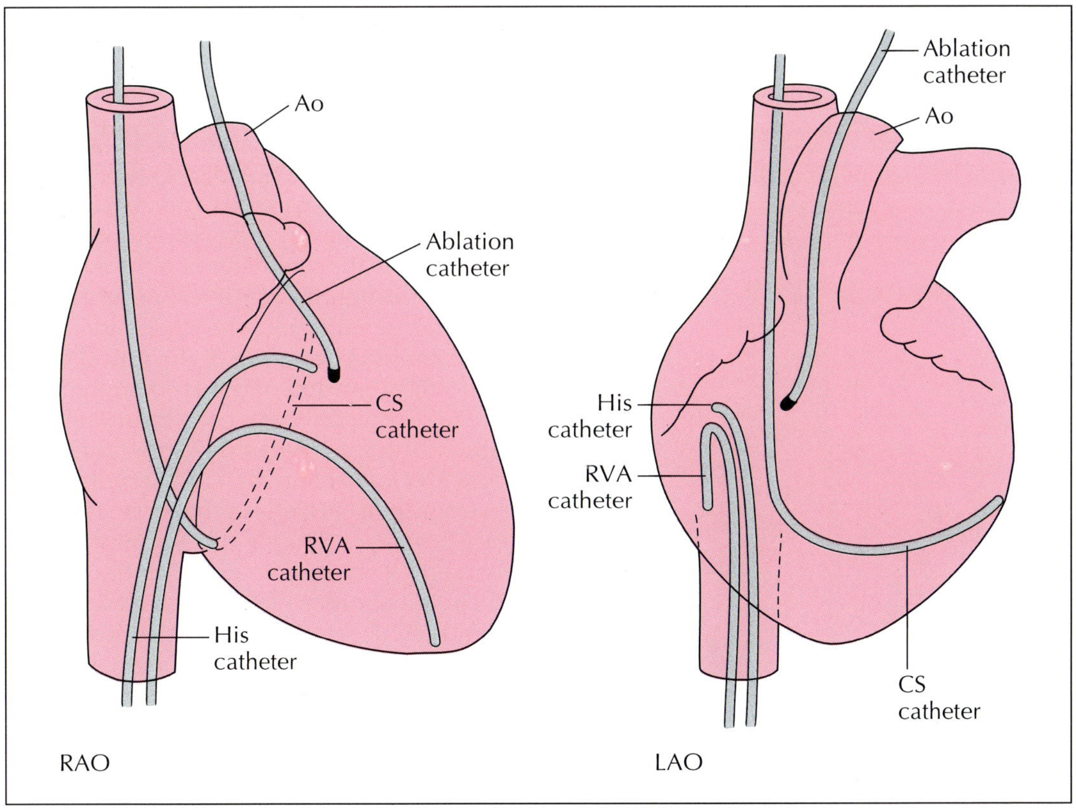

FIGURE 11-9. Right anterior oblique (RAO)/ left anterior oblique (LAO) views of an atrioventricular junctional ablation: left-sided approach. Occasionally, adequate tissue contact cannot be obtained from the right side and it is necessary to approach the His bundle from the left ventricle. A retrograde aortic approach is used with adequate heparinization. The catheter is torqued septally and a His bundle or left bundle branch signal can be elicited just under the aortic valve. Ao—aorta; CS—coronary sinus os; His—His bundle; RA—right atrium; RV—right ventricle; TV—tricuspid valve; Catheters: Abl, AV, CS, RVA, LV (*See* Fig. 11-4B for abbreviations.)

INDICATIONS FOR A COMPLETE AV JUNCTIONAL ABLATION

Atrial fibrillation with rapid ventricular response uncontrolled with medications

Atrial flutter with rapid ventricular response uncontrolled with medications

Atrial tachycardia with rapid ventricular response uncontrolled with medications

Syncope or sudden death due to enhanced AV nodal conduction

FIGURE 11-10. Indications for complete atrioventricular junctional ablation. There are many supraventricular rhythms that use the atrioventricular (AV) node as the "final common pathway" to the ventricle. Despite medications many patients continue to have rapid ventricular responses that cause symptoms. More commonly, they do not tolerate the side effects of these medications. Studies have shown that when the ventricular response is controlled after AV node ablation, patients with depressed ventricular function may show improved systolic function. [8,9,10].

INDICATIONS FOR ELECTROPHYSIOLOGY STUDY/ABLATION IN PATIENTS WITH WPW

Documented atrial fibrillation with syncope or hemodynamic compromise

Syncope of unclear etiology with manifest delta waves

Symptomatic supraventricular tachycardia refractory to medical therapy

Patients desiring a cure without need for lifelong drug therapy.

FIGURE 11-11. Indications for electrophysiology study/ablation in patients with Wolff-Parkinson-White (WPW) syndrome. In a number of large series catheter ablation was applied for treatment of the WPW syndrome. Ablation approaches for left-sided accessory pathways are highly successful with the choice of approach depending on the institution at which the ablation is being performed. Transseptal approaches are highly useful in patients with aortic valve replacements, disease of the aortic arch, or congenital heart disease. Patients with right-sided accessory pathways and Ebstein's anomaly may benefit from coronary artery mapping [1,2,5].

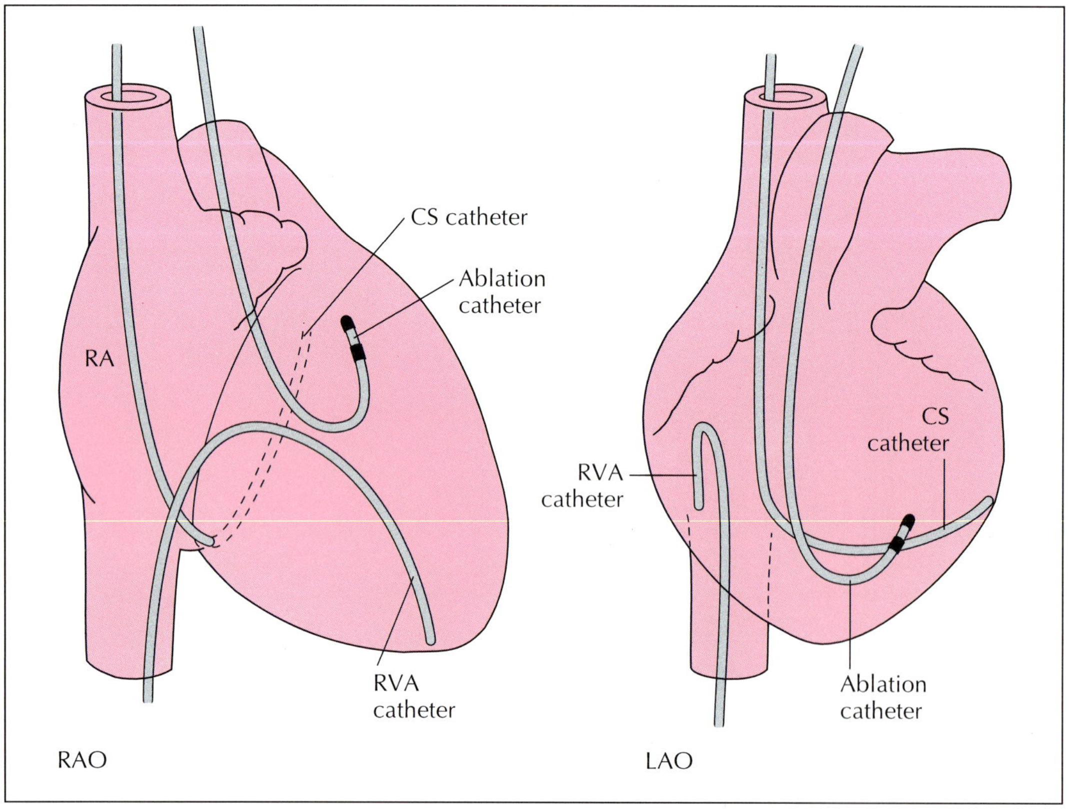

FIGURE 11-12. Right anterior oblique (RAO)/ left anterior oblique (LAO) views of the left-sided accessory pathways (AP). The retrograde aortic approach is demonstrated here. The ablation catheter is placed retrogradely through the aortic valve, and the tip is placed either into the underside of the mitral annulus or on top of the mitral valve on the atrial portion of the atrioventicular groove. The signal from each location is slightly different. When the catheter is below the mitral annulus, the ventricular electrogram is larger and the atrial electrogram is smaller. The signal magnitudes are reversed when the catheter is on the atrial side of the annulus. However, ideally there should be fusion of the atrial and ventricular ECGs with an AP potential on either side of the annulus at the successful site.

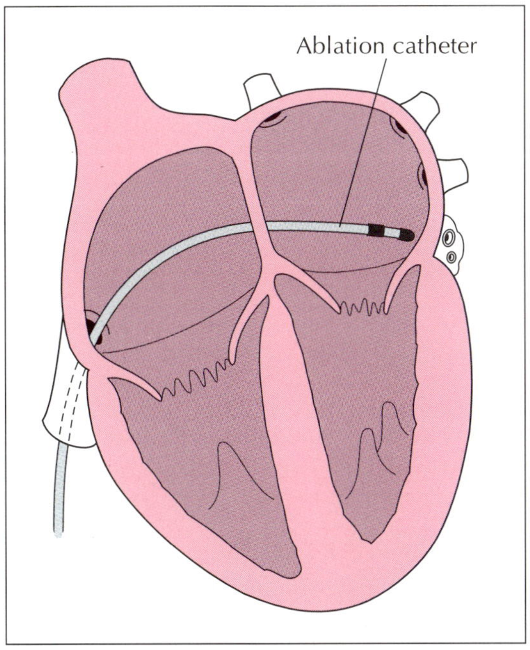

FIGURE 11-13. A left-sided accessory pathway (AP): The transseptal approach is demonstrated here. This technique requires a transseptal approach using a Brockenbrough needle and special sheaths (Mullen or Schwartz). It allows for a sweeping motion for mapping of the atrioventricular groove. If unsuccessful, a retrograde aortic approach can then be attempted without having to reverse anticoagulation.

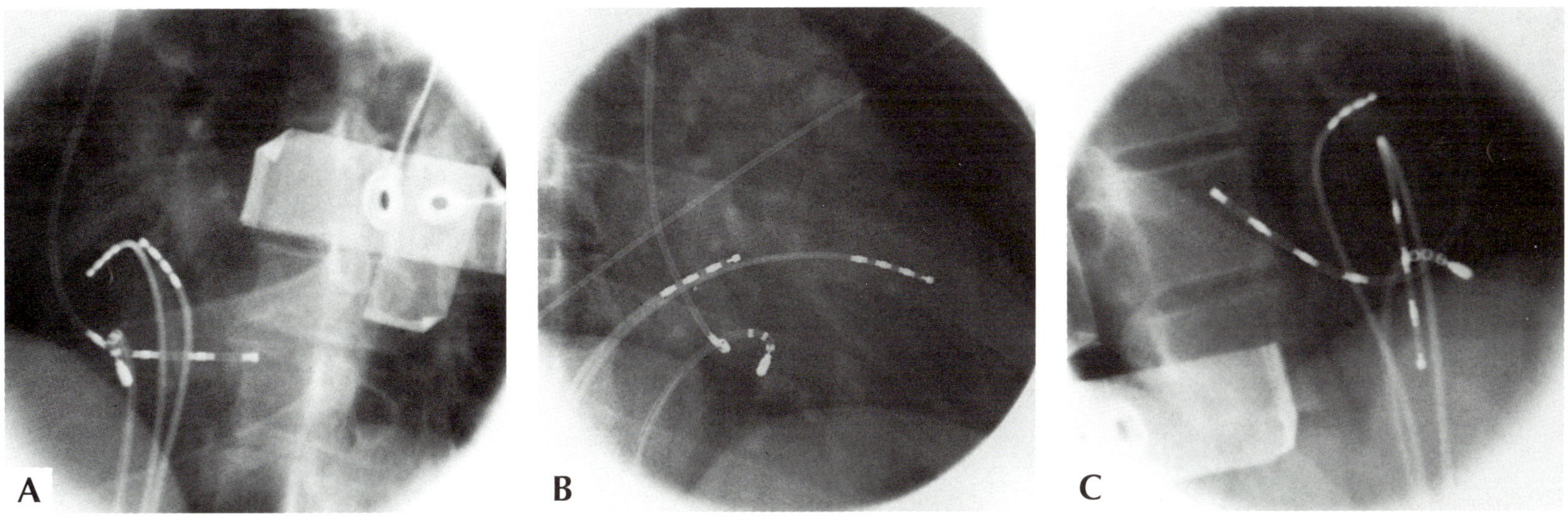

FIGURE 11-14. Left anterior oblique (**A**) and right anterior oblique (**B**) cineradiographic views of a right-sided accessory pathway (AP). **C**, Posterolateral right-sided AP.

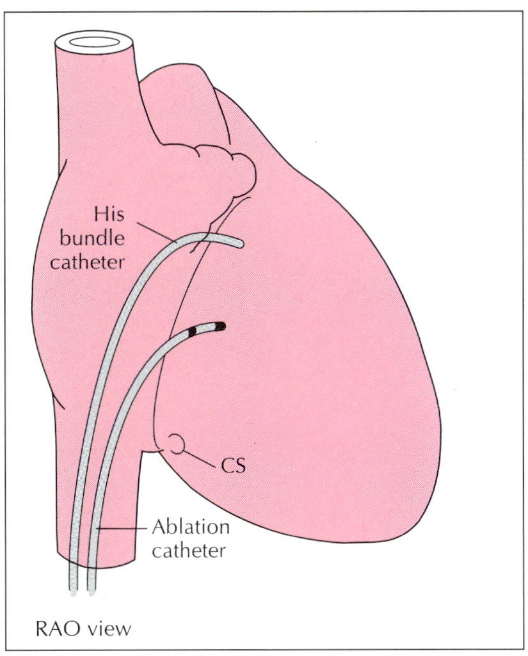

FIGURE 11-15. A right anterior oblique (RAO) view of a midseptal accessory pathway (AP). Midseptal APs are found on the interatrial septum between the coronary sinus (CS) os posteriorly and the atrioventricular (AV) node superiorly. If the accessory pathway is near the AV node, there is a risk of heart block with AP ablation.

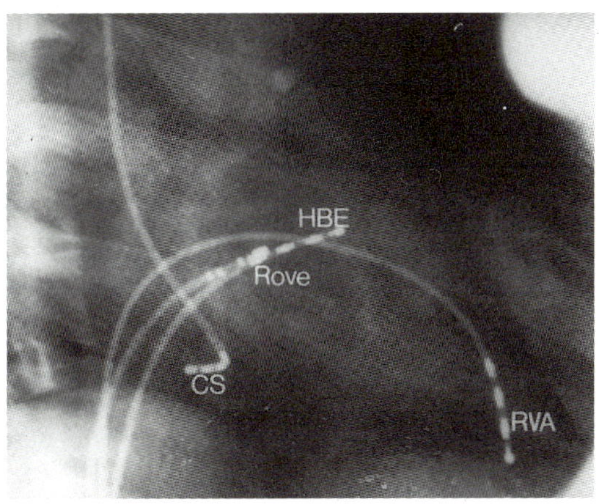

FIGURE 11-16. Right anterior oblique view of an anteroseptal accessory pathway (AP). APs are at the level of the atrioventricular node or more superior along the septum. There is a risk of heart block with AP ablation if the AP is near the His bundle, as with midseptal APs. At times, a better signal or catheter positon can be obtained by placing the ablation catheter from the right internal jugular vein or right subclavian vein rather than from the femoral approach. HBE—His bundle electrode. (*see Fig. 11-4B for other abbreviations.*)

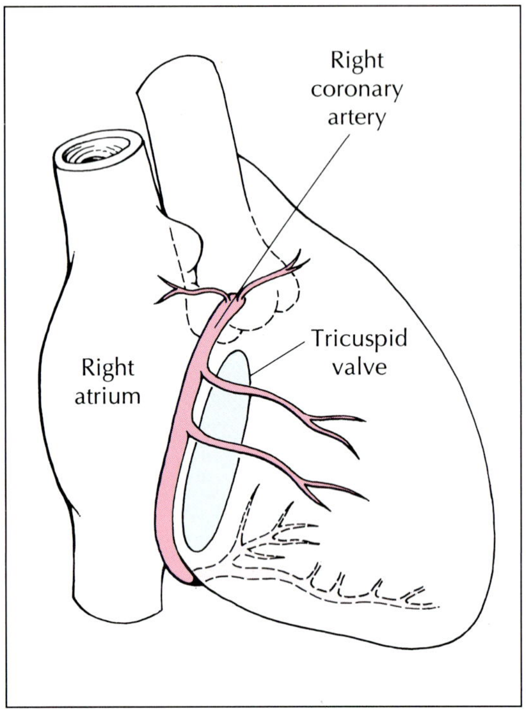

FIGURE 11-17. Relationship of right coronary artery (RCA) and tricuspid valve annulus. The right coronary artery follows the true atrioventricular (AV) groove. Thus, in patients with Ebstein's anomaly in whom the valve is displaced downward, identifying the RCA traces the true AV groove. Electrocardiograms from the right coronary artery can then be used to guide ablation of right-sided accessory pathways.

RIGHT-SIDED ACCESSORY PATHWAY ABLATION

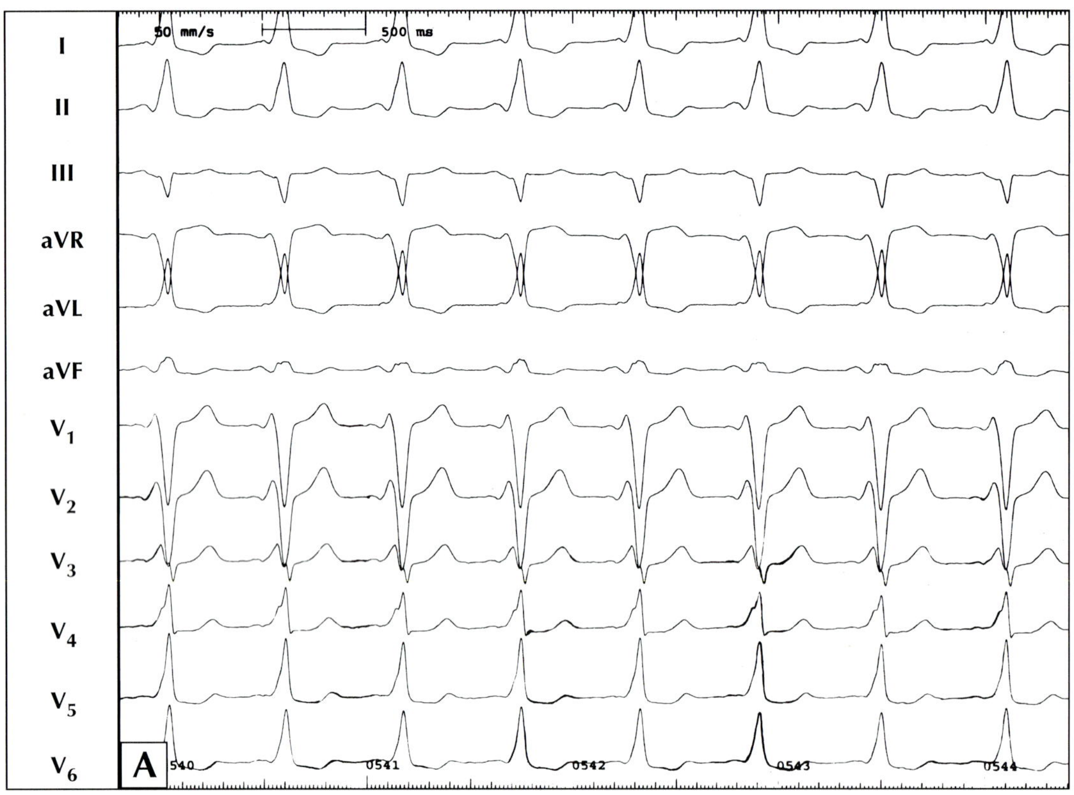

FIGURE 11-18. Electrocardiograms (ECGs) from right-sided accessory pathway (AP) ablation. In **A** through **F**, the surface leads are V_1, I, II, and aVF and the intracardiac signals are Abl, His, and HRA. **A**, A 12-lead ECG with positive delta waves in leads I, II, aVF, and V_3–V_6 and negative delta waves in III. The delta wave in lead V_1 is small. This indicates that the AP is right sided in location. Note that the R-wave transition is in lead V_3, which suggests a right anterior AP. (*continued*)

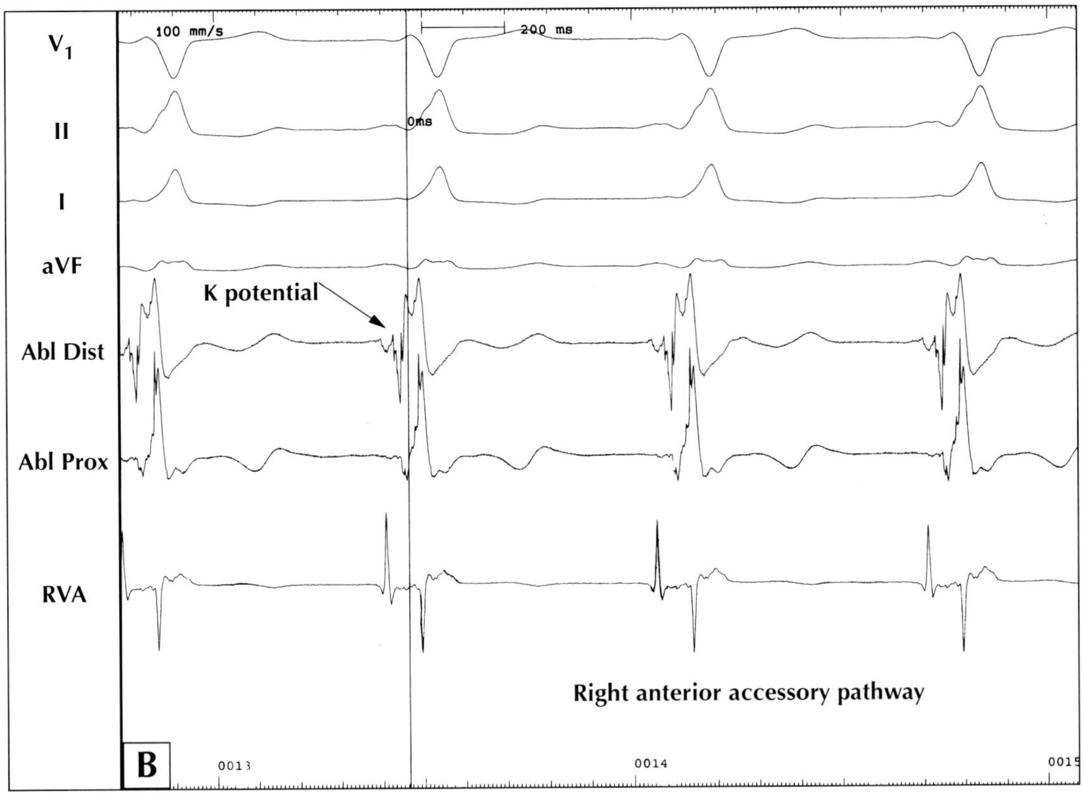

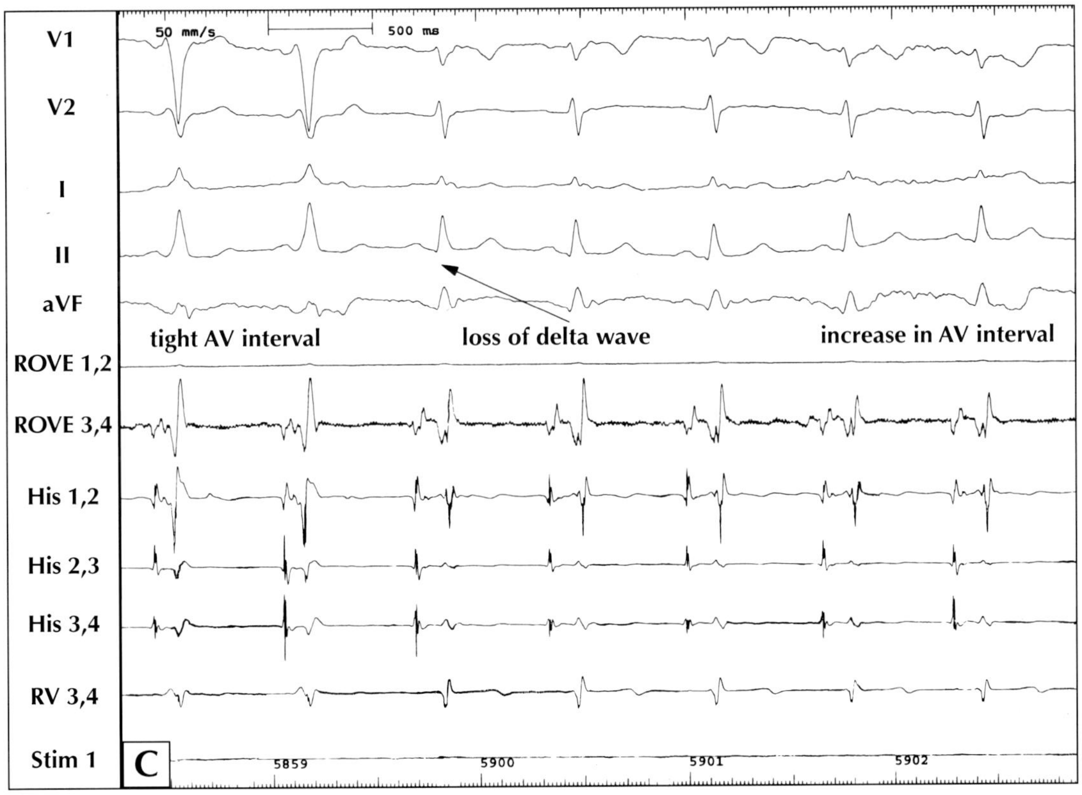

FIGURE 11-18. (*continued*) **B**, At the site of successful ablation, there is a fusion of atrial and ventricular electrical activity on the distal ablation catheter (Abl Dist). The high-frequency signal indicated by the *arrow* is a Kent (K) potential or an accessory pathway potential. It appears prior to the onset of the delta wave.

C, During application of radiofrequency (RF) energy there is loss of the delta wave after two complexes. Note, on the first two complexes there is a short atrioventricular (AV) interval on the surface leads as well as on the intracardiac ECGs, *ie*, the His ECG signal. On the third complex, the delta wave disappears and the AV interval increases. This is due to loss of ventricular preexcitation and AP conduction as well as conduction only over the AV node. The QRS complex is narrow because conduction is over the normal AV node-His Purkinje system. (*continued*)

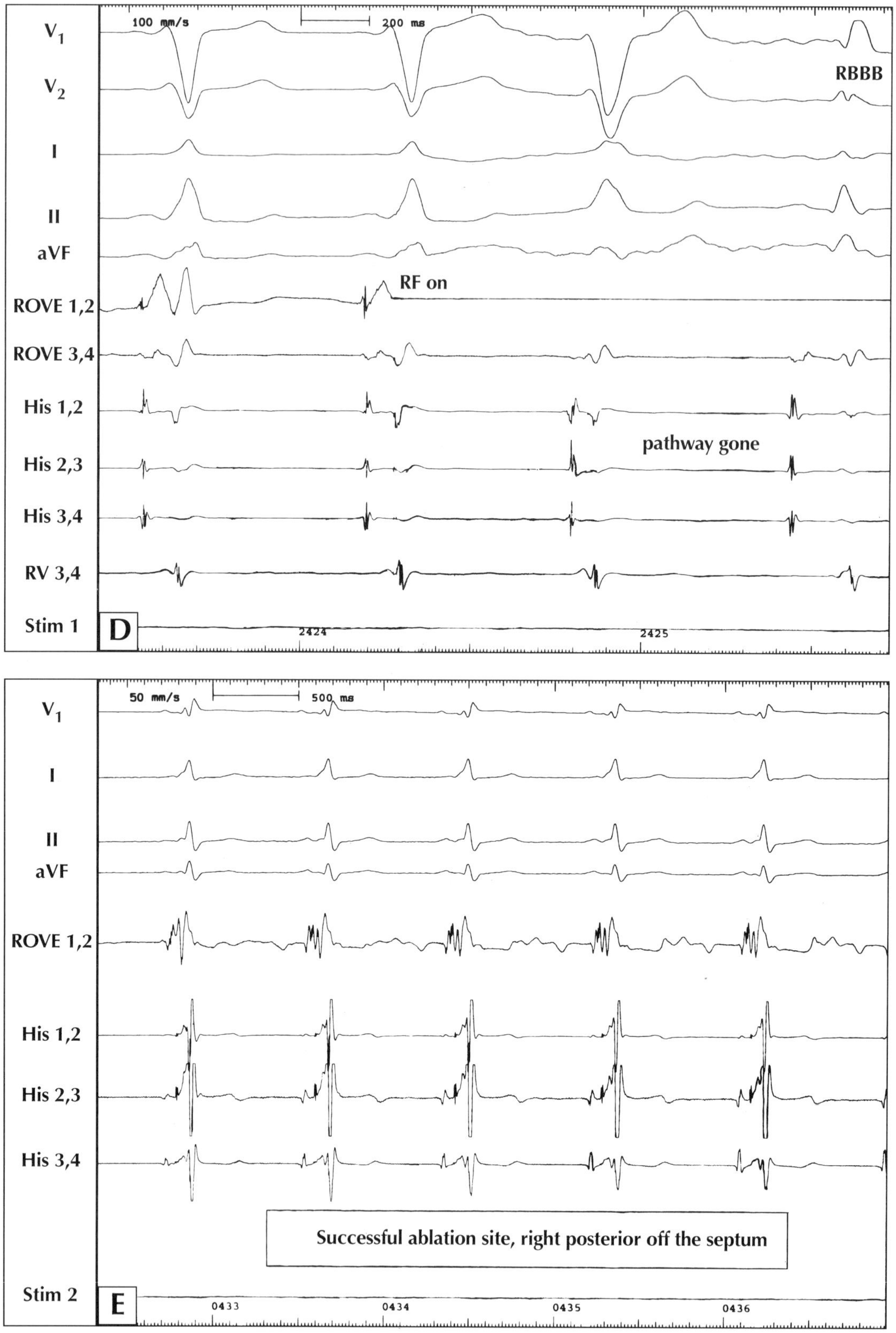

FIGURE 11-18. *(continued)* **D**, After the ablation in C, AP conduction returned. On the subsequent ablation, note the fused electrical activity on the ablation catheter (ROVE 1,2). When RF energy is turned on, the AP is destroyed, the AV interval increases, and there is a right bundle branch block (RBBB) QRS morphology. In this patient, ablation was not near the right bundle, which explains why his ECG demonstrated mostly preexcitation prior to the ablation. There was a right-sided AP, and because of the right-sided conduction delay over the His Punkinje system, preexcitation of the right ventricle occurred over the AP.

In **E**, data from a different patient with an RBBB morphology QRS in lead V1 and isoelectric delta waves in leads II and aVF are shown. This is suggestive of a right posterior AP. The signals are fused on the ROVE catheter, which lies along the right posterior AV groove of the septum, thus indicating a right posterior AP. In a left anterior oblique projection, this would be lateral to the coronary sinus os on the tricuspid annulus. Note, that although the His bundle catheter is also on the right side, the A and V signals are much farther apart than on the ablation catheter. *(continued)*

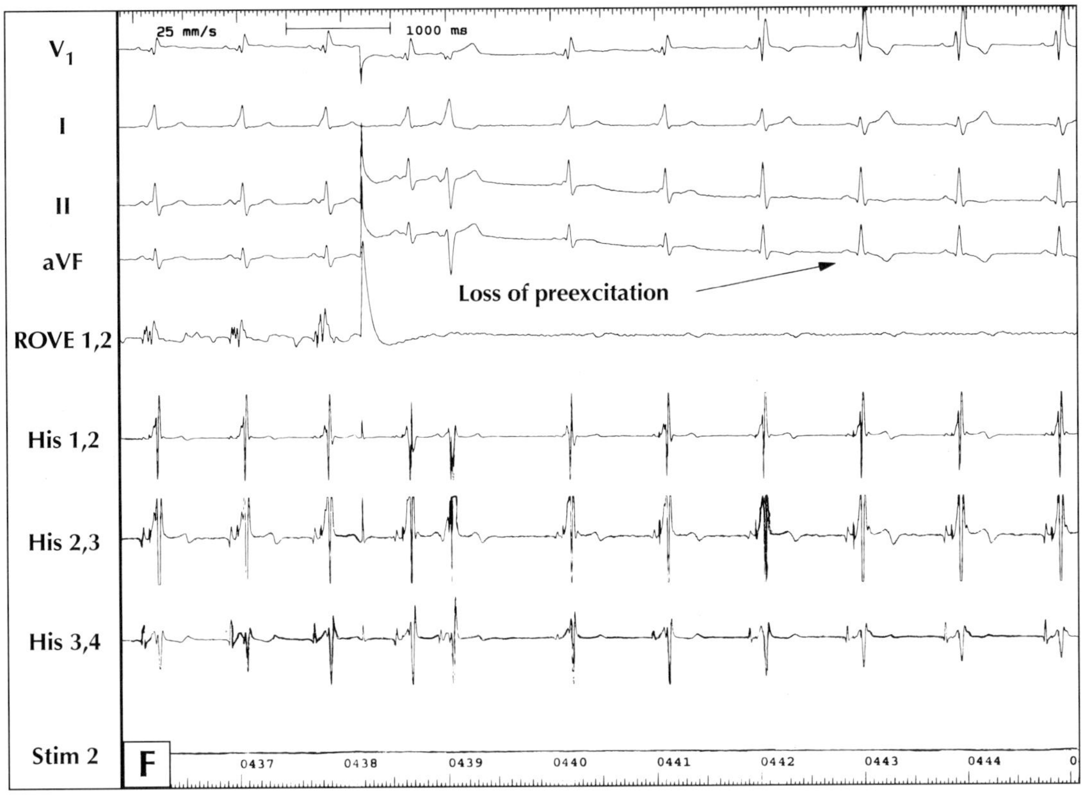

FIGURE 11-18. (*continued*) **F**, Ablation at the site shown in *E*. There is loss of preexcitation on the 8th complex. On the 9th complex the QRS shows a more typical RBBB in lead V_1 with clear His activation prior to ventricular activation on the His catheter. Interestingly, there are T-wave inversions on the surface leads (V_1, aVF). These T-wave changes are thought to be a result of T-wave memory changes and not due to ischemia. (*See* Fig. 11-4*B* for catheter abbreviations.)

Left-Sided Accessory Pathway Ablation

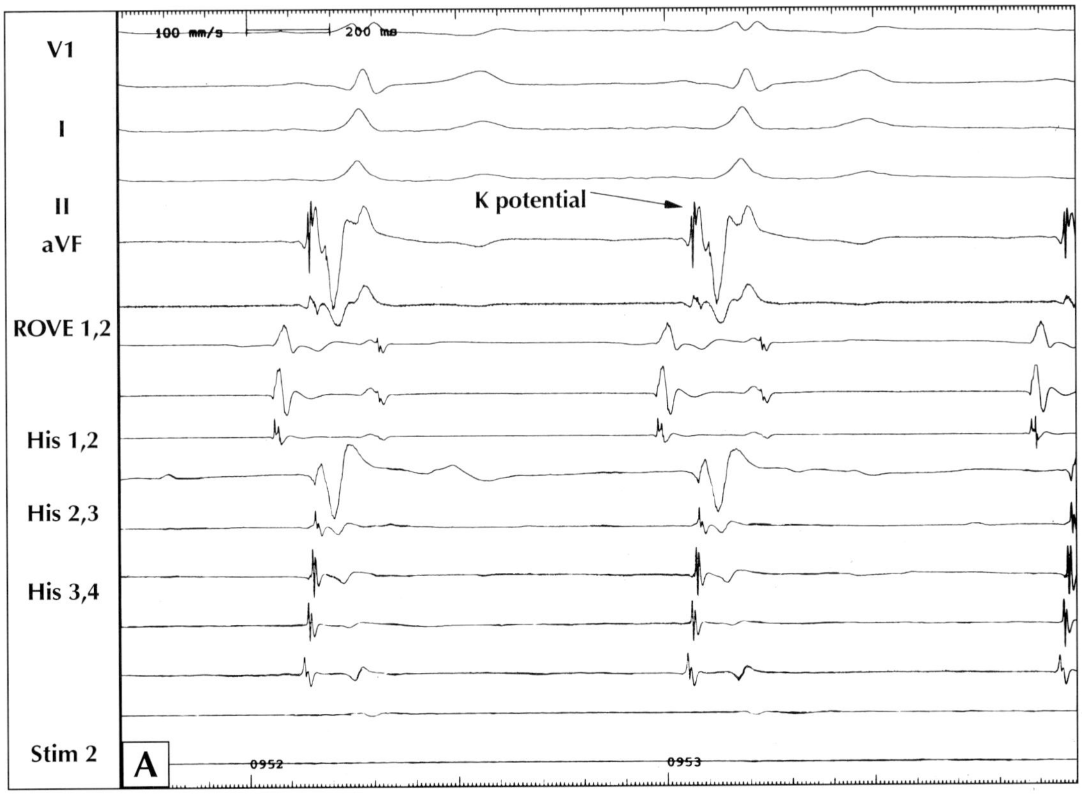

FIGURE 11-19. Electrocardiograms (ECGs) from left-sided accessory pathway (AP). In **A**, the patient has a left-sided AP, as evidenced by a positive delta wave in V_1. The intracardiac ECGs from the coronary sinus (CS) reflects left-sided activation and have a much shorter atrioventricular (AV) interval than those from the His catheter on the right side. As we move proximally to distally along the CS catheter, from the CS os proximally (CS 9,10) to the left free wall (CS 1,2), the AV interval tightens, indicating that the AP is on the left free wall. The ablation (ROVE 1,2) catheter is on the AP. Note the fused atrial and ventricular activity and high frequency Kent (K) potential. This signal was obtained using a transseptal approach. (*continued*)

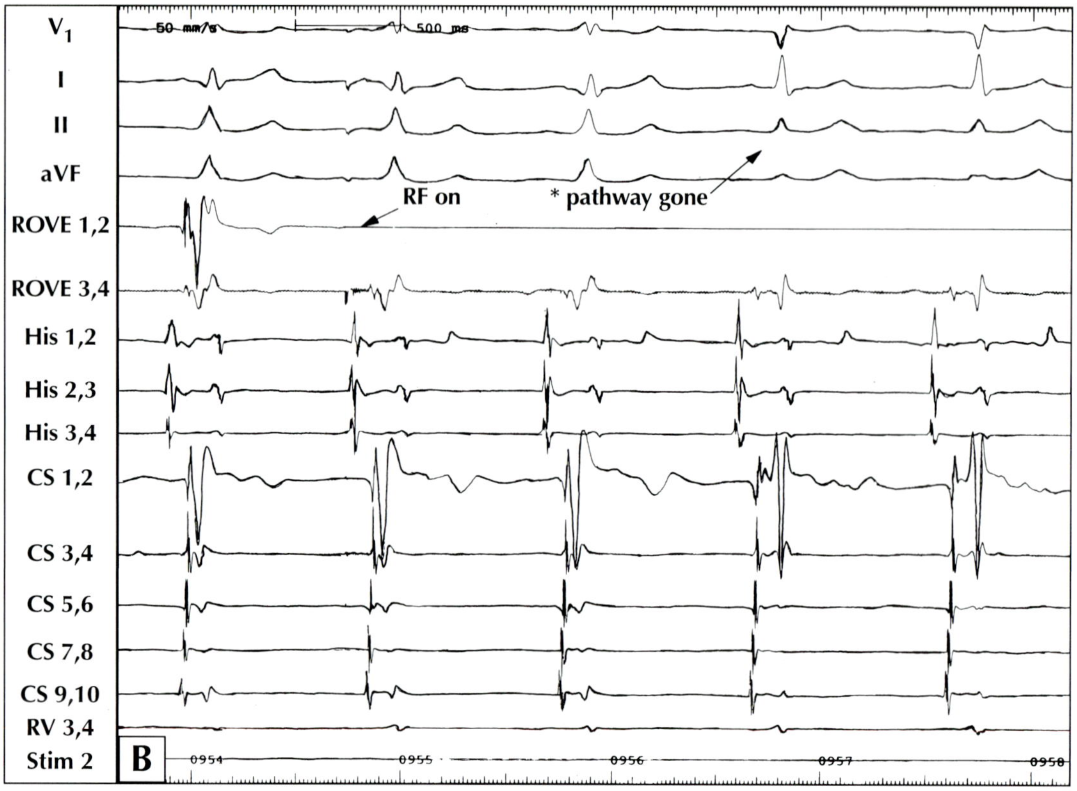

Figure 11-19. (*continued*) **B** demonstrates ablation of the left-sided AP. When radio-frequency (RF) energy is applied to the catheter in the position shown in *A*, the delta wave is gone on the 4th complex. The AV interval now increases at all the coronary sinus locations as well as at the proximal ROVE, because of loss of ventricular preexcitation over the accessory pathway and conduction over the AV node. Note the change in the QRS configuration from the first and second complex to the fourth and fifth complex. The delta wave has disappeared.

Atrial Flutter Ablation

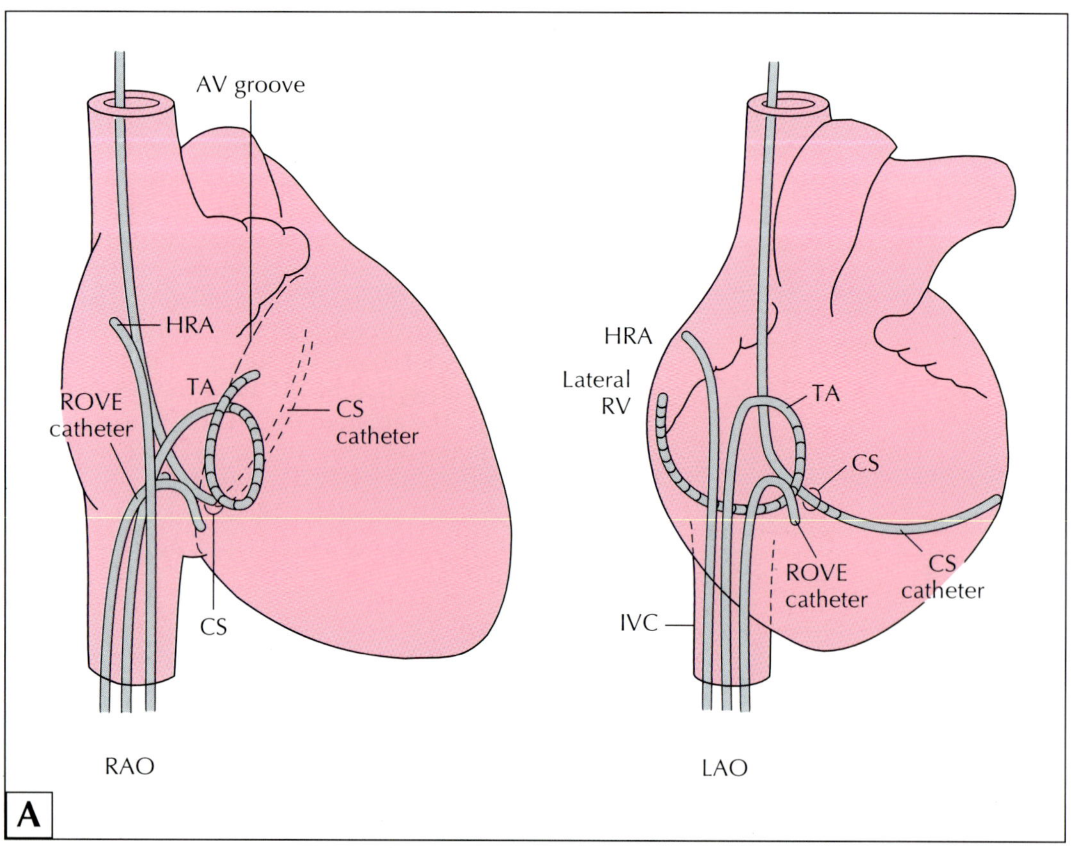

Figure 11-20. Atrial flutter: intracardiac electrograms. **A**, Right anterior oblique (RAO) and left anterior oblique (LAO) projections of catheter placement. The high right atrium (HRA) and coronary sinus (CS) catheters are in their usual positions. The tricuspid annulus (TA) catheter is a 20-electrode catheter with electrodes spanning the distance from the CS os along the tricuspid annulus back toward the lateral right atrium (RA). The steerable catheter (ROVE) is in the posterior region of the RA below the CS os. (*continued*)

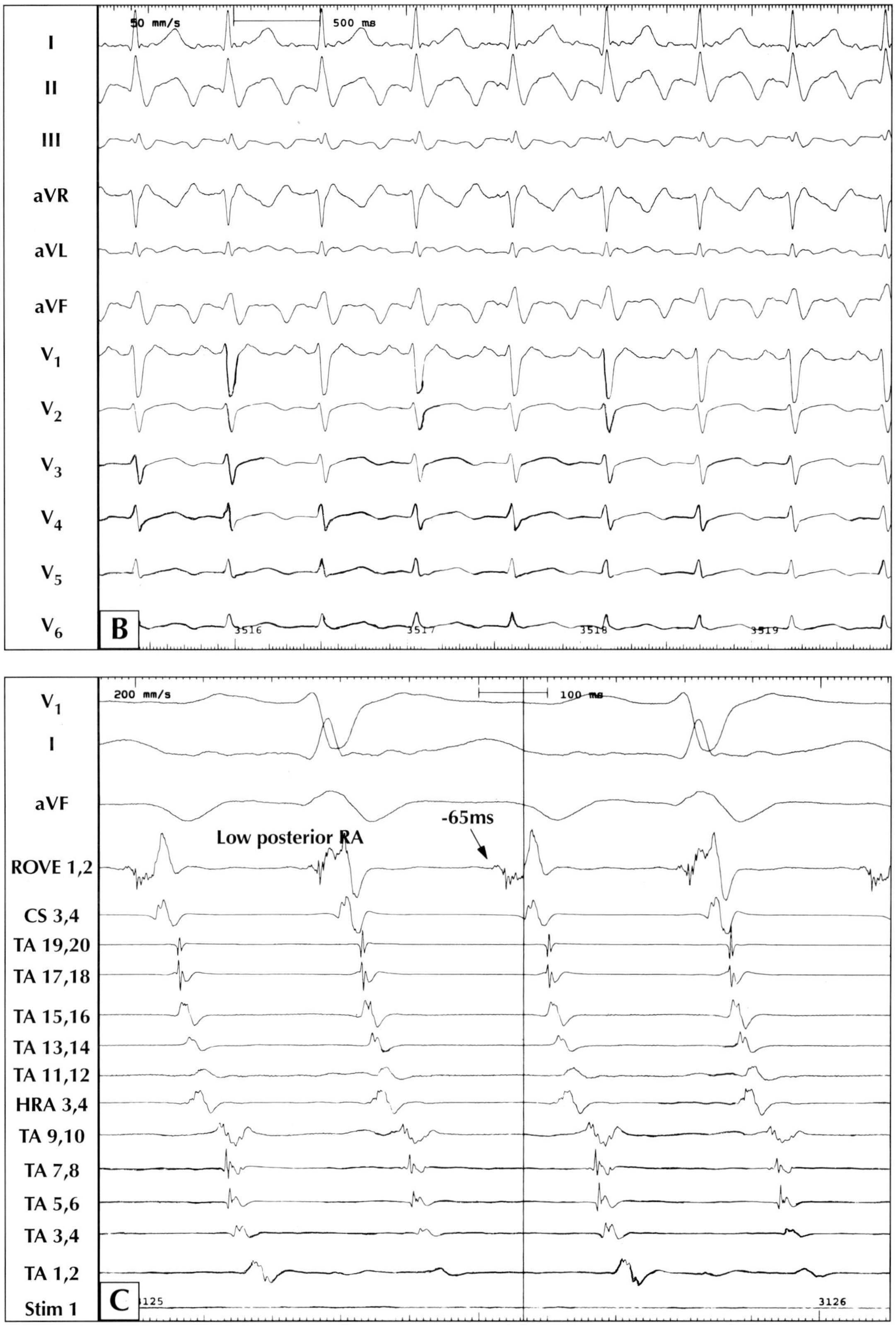

FIGURE 11-20. *(continued)* **B**, In this electrocardiogram (ECG) of atrial flutter, note the negative flutter waves in leads II, III, and aVF, and upright flutter waves in V_1. This is consistent with typical flutter. In **C**, the intracardiac ECGs show the ROVE catheter at the exit site of the slow zone. Conduction travels up the septum, down the lateral right free wall back to the inferior vena cava (IVC) and tricuspid valve leaflet (TVL). The time it takes to travel nearly around the entire atrium is 260 ms, while in the region between the IVC and the TV leaflet until it exits near the CS os is 160 ms. This occurs because the slow zone of conduction is along this region. Note, the beginning of electrical activity at the ROVE catheter, at the exit site of the slow zone, is 65 ms before the beginning of the flutter wave of the ECG. AV—atrioventricular; RV—right ventricle.

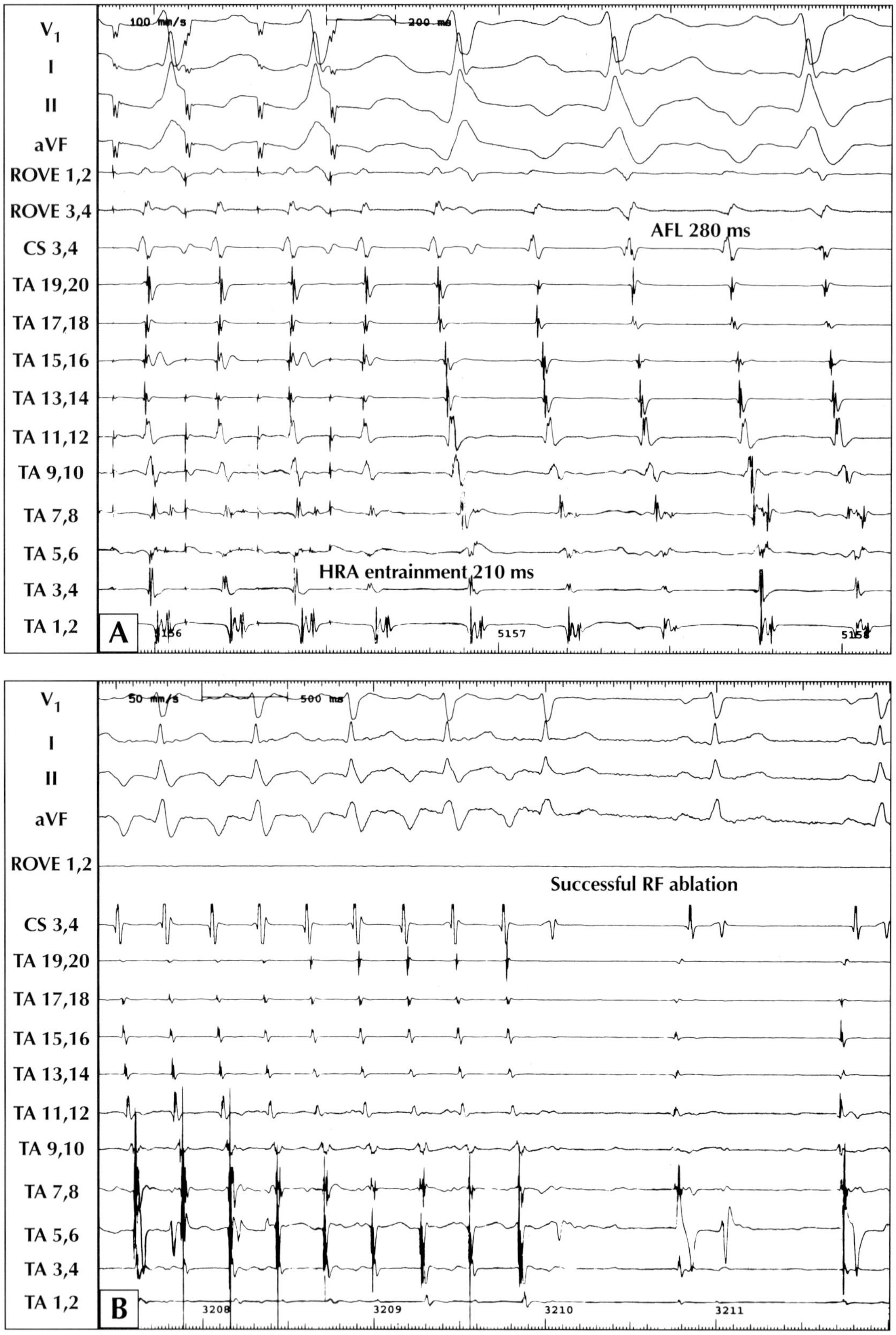

Figure 11-21. In **A**, atrial flutter (AFL) ablation is demonstrated on the electrocardiogram (ECG). Note the entrainment of the atrial flutter circuit. The atrial flutter has a cycle length of 280 ms with a 2:1 ventricular conduction rate. When pacing from the HRA at a faster cycle length (210 ms), the pattern of atrial intracardiac signals changes and the rate increases to the paced cycle length. This is consistent with a reentrant mechanism for atrial flutter. This occurs because the HRA is outside the circuit and the pacing fuses with the reentrant circuit. If the pacing were performed from within the actual atrial flutter circuit, then the ECG sequence would still be faster at the paced rate, but the sequence would not change. This usually occurs in the slow zone of conduction, which is along the posterior right atrium at the junction of the inferior vena cava and tricuspid valve. In **B**, Catheter ablation in the zone of slow conduction results in termination of the atrial flutter circuit. Surface leads: V_1, I, II, and aVF. Intracardiac catheters: Abl, CS, and decapolar tricuspid annulus. (*See* Fig. 11-4B for catheter abbreviations.)

References

1. Lesh MD, *et al.*: Curative percutaneous catheter ablation using radiofrequency energy for accessory pathways in all locations: Results in 100 consecutive patients. *J Am Coll Cardiol* 1992, 19:1303.
2. Jackman WM, *et al.*: Catheter ablation of accessory atrioventricular pathways (WPW syndrome) by radiofrequency current. *N Engl J Med* 1991, 324:1605.
3. Jackman WM, *et al.*: Treatment of supraventricular tachycardia due to atrioventricular nodal reentry by radiofrequency catheter ablation of slow pathway conduction. *N Engl J Med* 1992, 327:313.
4. Williamson BD, Man KC, Daoud E, *et al.*: Radiofrequency catheter modification of atrioventricular conduction to control the ventricular rate during atrial fibrillation. *N Engl J Med* 1994; 331:910–917.
5. Caulkins, *et al.*: Radiofrequency catheter ablation of accessory atrioventricular connections in 250 patients. Abbreviated therapeutic approach to WPW syndrome. *Circulation* 1992, 85:1337.
6. Epstein LM, Scheinman MM, Langberg JJ, Chilson D, Goldberg HR, Griffin JC: Percutaneous catheter modification of the atrioventricular node: a potential cure for atrioventricular nodal reentrant tachycardia. *Circulation* 1989, 80:757–768.
7. Jazayeri MR, Sra JS, Deshpande SS, *et al.*: Electrophysiologic spectrum of atrioventricular nodal behavior in patients with atrioventricular nodal reentrant tachycardia undergoing selective fast or slow pathway ablation. *J Cardiovasc Electrophysiol* 1993, 4:99–111.
8. Langberg JJ, *et al.*: A randomized, prospective comparison of anterior and posterior approaches to radiofrequency catheter ablation of atrioventricular nodal reentry tachycardias. *Circulation* 1993, 87:1551.
9. Langberg JJ, Chin MC, Rosenqvist M, *et al.*: Catheter ablation of the atrioventricular junction with radiofrequency energy. *Circulation* 1989, 80:1527–1535.
10. Guidelines for Clinical Intracardiac Electrophysiological and Catheter Ablation Prodedures. An ACC/AHA report in collaboration with NASPE. *J Am Coll Cardiol* 1995, 26:555–573.

SYNCOPE AND SUDDEN CARDIAC DEATH

12

CHAPTER

Adam Fitzpatrick

SYNCOPE

Syncope is the sudden global loss of cerebral perfusion [1], which generally causes simultaneous loss of consciousness and loss of postural reflexes, causing collapse. It is a very common cause of sudden unexpected loss of consciousness, but it is not the only cause. Syncope is often erroneously believed to be the correct term for any sudden episode of loss of consciousness, but it must be distinguished from other causes of loss of consciousness, and in particular from neurologic causes such as epilepsy.

Typically, syncope causes abrupt loss of consciousness with little or no aura and a collapse, the body falling with gravity if it is not supported. This may sometimes produce significant injury, even when the cause of syncope is benign. There is usually a rapid return of cognitive functions after the return of cerebral perfusion and consciousness. In contrast, epilepsy causes loss of consciousness that may be preceded by an aura, movement abnormalities, and results in a postictal syndrome with confusion. One *crucial* distinguishing feature is facial pallor during an episode, which occurs in syncope due to loss of perfusion of facial skin but not in epilepsy because perfusion of the head is maintained. During a seizure, unconsciousness results from chaotic depolarization of cerebral neurons. Some of the abnormalities of neuronal depolarization can be seen in epileptic patients, even when there is no seizure, by recording the electroencephalogram. Syncope accounts for 1% to 6% of the 20 to 25 million hospital admissions a year in the United States [2,3].

The mechanisms of syncope involve both cardiac and vascular disturbances. Typical cardiac causes are hypotension due to an arrythmia or due to central obstruction of blood flow, such as that which occurs in aortic valvular stenosis. Typical vascular causes are due to effective hypovolemia, such as occurs with postural hypotension. Many patients with syncope remain undiagnosed after prolonged investigation [2,3] because it is unusual for a syncopal episode to occur while a patient is being supervised or monitored in or out of the hospital. Usually the patient presents after an episode is over, and the cause may remain obscure. Many patients with syncope are otherwise healthy, and have a good long-term outcome, largely determined by the extent and severity of underlying heart disease [2].

Effective hypovolemia is any situation in which circulating blood volume becomes inadequate for the size of the arterial compartment. Since hypovolemia results in a fall in cardiac output, and blood pressure is the product of cardiac output and resistance to blood flow, a fall in cardiac output results in a fall in blood pressure. If this is severe enough, it will cause cerebral hypoperfusion and syncope. The most common cause of effective hypovolemia is vasovagal syncope in which sudden vasodilatation results in hypotension and syncope. In this situation venous return to the heart falls, causing a fall in cardiac output, but there is also a sudden fall in peripheral resistance. This is believed to be the result of paradoxical triggering of stretch receptors that are found throughout the left ventricle and normally contribute to baroreceptor control of blood pressure and heart rate [4]. Normally, an increase in ventricular stretch, for example due to a sudden increase in venous return, results in a fall in blood pressure mediated by a fall in peripheral resistance and heart rate, a so-called Bezold-Jarisch reflex. During paradoxical stimulation, receptor stimulation leads to bradycardia and vasodilatation when the left ventricle is underfilled. This combination of falling cardiac output and falling peripheral resistance rapidly results in hypotension and syncope. Much less common is syncope in patients who have suffered a brisk gastrointestinal hemorrhage, particularly when they stand up [5]. Here, as in postural hypotension, vasoconstrictor reflexes are inadequate to maintain blood pressure but, in this case, it is because they cannot compensate fully for blood loss.

In any patient with syncope, but particularly young patients, especially if there is a history of sudden death in the family, a careful search must be made for evidence of long QT syndrome. Syncope in this syndrome is due to nonsustained episodes of polymorphic ventricular tachycardia (VT) [6].

Sudden Cardiac Death

Sudden cardiac death is defined as natural, unexpected death, occurring instantaneously, during sleep or within minutes after development of symptoms. VT or ventricular fibrillation (VF) is responsible for approximately 80% of sudden cardiac deaths, particularly in patients with ischemic heart disease [7]. Sudden cardiac death is most prevalent in patients with structural heart disease. The most commonly associated condition is ischemic heart disease [7,8]. Most studies have focused on various risk factors associated with sudden death, and there is evidence to suggest that this mode of death may be triggered by ischemia, autonomic abnormalities (i.e., increased sympathetic and decreased parasympathetic tone), and premature ventricular contractions. All of these triggers play upon the appropriate substrate which, for patients with myocardial infarction, represents a scar due to prior infarction. We can divide populations at risk into categories depending on whether structural cardiac disease is present or absent. In addition, sudden death may not be associated with known structural disease. Specific examples of each category are discussed in this chapter. The challenge for clinicians is to recognize the risk factors that have been associated with sudden cardiac death, particularly in post myocardial infarction patients.

Left ventricular ejection fraction has been recognized as an independent risk factor for sudden death, but the predictive accuracy of a left ventricular ejection fraction of less than 40% is only 25%. Hence, a stepwise logistic regression using multiple risk factors has been suggested to improve the predictive accuracy. These factors include high-density premature ventricular complexes (or nonsustained ventricular tachycardia) [8], abnormal signal-averaged electrocardiogram (ECG) [9], heart rate variability [10], baroreceptor sensitivity [11], or invasive electrophysiologic testing [12,13]. To date, studies have shown that nonsustained VT, poor ejection fraction (< 40%), and an abnormal signal-averaged ECG is predictive of 50% of patients having an episode of either sustained VT, VF, or sudden death after infarction.

Probably much less important as a cause of sudden death are bradyarrhythmias, such as paroxysmal complete heart block or sinus node arrest. However, these arrhythmias are very important causes of syncope [2].

Obstruction to central blood flow may result in syncope or death. Common causes are aortic valvular stenosis and acute massive pulmonary embolism. Rarely, sudden death occurs as a result of drug side effects or metabolic disturbance, although usually such patients have underlying structural heart disease. Some patients with Wolff-Parkinson-White syndrome may experience atrial fibrillation, which may be conducted rapidly over an accessory pathway resulting in VF [14], but this appears to be rare. Occasionally, patients with supraventricular tachycardias present with sudden death, usually in the setting of very rapid heart rates due to accelerated atrioventricular nodal conduction.

Patients who survive an episode of sudden cardiac death should undergo detailed electrophysiologic studies. These studies are designed to exclude the presence of "curable" causes of sudden death. The latter include bundle branch reentrant tachycardia and rapid supraventricular tachycardias, including those associated with anomalous bypass tracts. If a sustained ventricular arrythmia is provoked, then the patient may undergo serial electropharmacologic testing. The most effective drugs in these patients are sotatol (class III and beta blocker activity) and amiodarone (class I, II, III, IV activities).

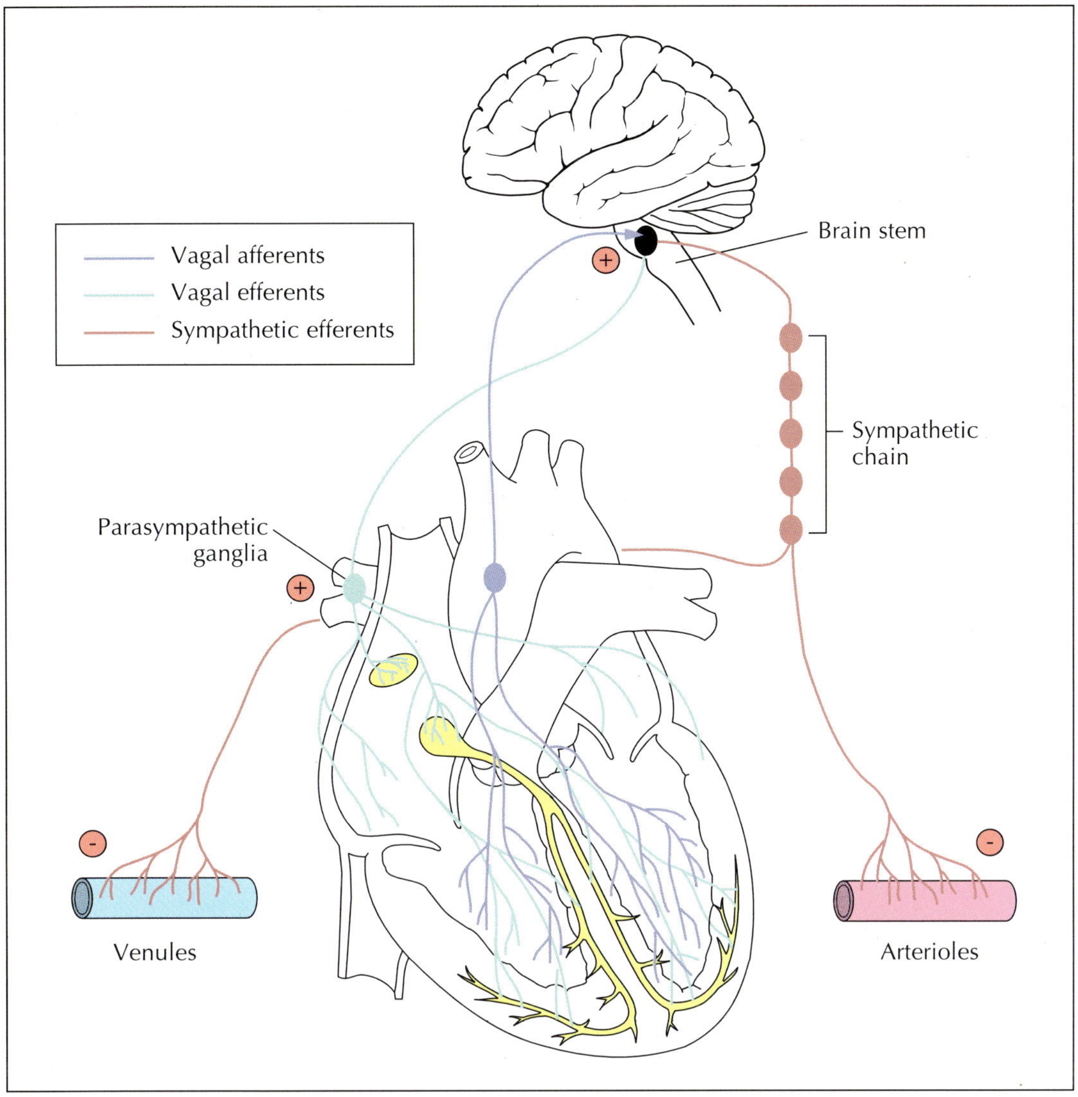

FIGURE 12-1. Mechanisms of vasovagal syncope. During vasovagal syncope, left ventricular (LV) stretch receptors may be triggered. These receptors normally respond to LV stretch by sending vagal afferent activity to the brain stem to reduce (*minus sign*) arteriolar vasoconstriction (mediated by sympathetic outflow to these resistance vessels), and heart rate (mediated by increased [*plus sign*] vagal outflow to the cardiac plexi that innervate sinoatrial and atrioventricular nodes). It appears that a vasovagal attack may result from inappropriate or paradoxical triggering of these receptors when LV stretch is not increased but reduced as a result of a sharp fall in venous return.

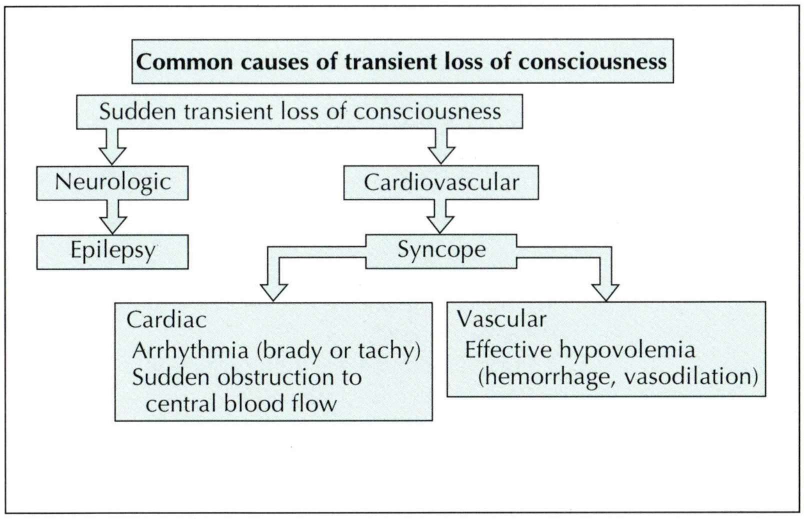

FIGURE 12-2. Common causes of transient loss of consciousness. Syncope is not the only cause of sudden temporary loss of consciousness; many other causes exist. Syncope is frequently mistaken for epilepsy, since abnormal movements are often witnessed, leading to a mistaken diagnosis. The most common *neurologic* cause of sudden loss of consciousness is epilepsy. Syncope is a cardiovascular cause of sudden loss of consciousness, and both cardiac and vascular causes exist. Common *cardiac* and *vascular* causes of syncope are shown in this figure. Any arrhythmia may give rise to syncope, including supraventricular tachycardias, ventricular tachyarrhythmias, and asystolic pauses with abnormalities of sinoatrial and atrioventricular conduction. Syncope may occur when such pauses last more than a few seconds. Obstruction to the flow of blood out of the heart may cause syncope. This can occur with stenosis of the aortic valve, with large pulmonary emboli, and with left (and rarely right) atrial tumors. These obstructions include myxomas and ball-valve thrombi associated with mitral valve stenosis.

Syncope

COMMON CARDIAC CAUSES OF SYNCOPE

CARDIAC BRADYARRHYTHMIAS

SA disease with pauses due to
- Sinus arrest
- SA block
- Tachy-brady syndrome

Atrioventricular conduction disease
- Second or third-degree heart block

TACHYARRHYTHMIAS

Supraventricular tachycardias
- Junctional reciprocating tachycardias with rapid rates
  - AV reentry
  - AV reciprocating tachycardia
- Atrial arrhythmias with supranormal AV conduction

Ventricular tachycardia

VASCULAR CAUSES

Vasovagal syncope

Postural hypotension

Figure 12-3. Common cardiac causes of syncope. Asystolic pauses may occur with abnormalities of sinoatrial (SA) and atrioventricular (AV) conduction. Syncope may occur when such pauses last more than a few seconds. Supraventricular tachycardias may cause syncope if heart rates are very fast and cardiac output falls sufficiently. Ventricular tachyarrhythmias may cause syncope even when heart rates are not excessive, because patients with ventricular arrhythmias commonly have impaired ventricular function and limited reserve with which to maintain cardiac output during tachycardia.

When a person moves from a lying to an upright position, there is a shift of central blood volume to the lower extremities with the force of gravity. This shift results in a fall in venous return to the heart and a consequent fall in cardiac output. This fall would result in a fall in blood pressure and a risk of inadequate cerebral perfusion if peripheral resistance did not rise to compensate for the fall. The vasomotor center in the brain stem responds to a reduction in firing from arterial and cardiopulmonary baroreceptors and increases sympathetic outflow from the hypothalamus to skeletal muscle arterioles. This increase results in an increase in peripheral resistance, thereby maintaining blood pressure with as little change as possible. In postural hypotension, there is a defect in the reflexes that cause the increase in sympathetic outflow to compensate for falling venous return. As a consequence, a change in posture reliably causes a fall in blood pressure, often resulting in dizziness or syncope.

In vasovagal syncope, there may be no postural hypotension. Episodes of syncope occur periodically, sometimes in predictable circumstances, but often without warning. There is inappropriate bradycardia and vasodilatation during these episodes.

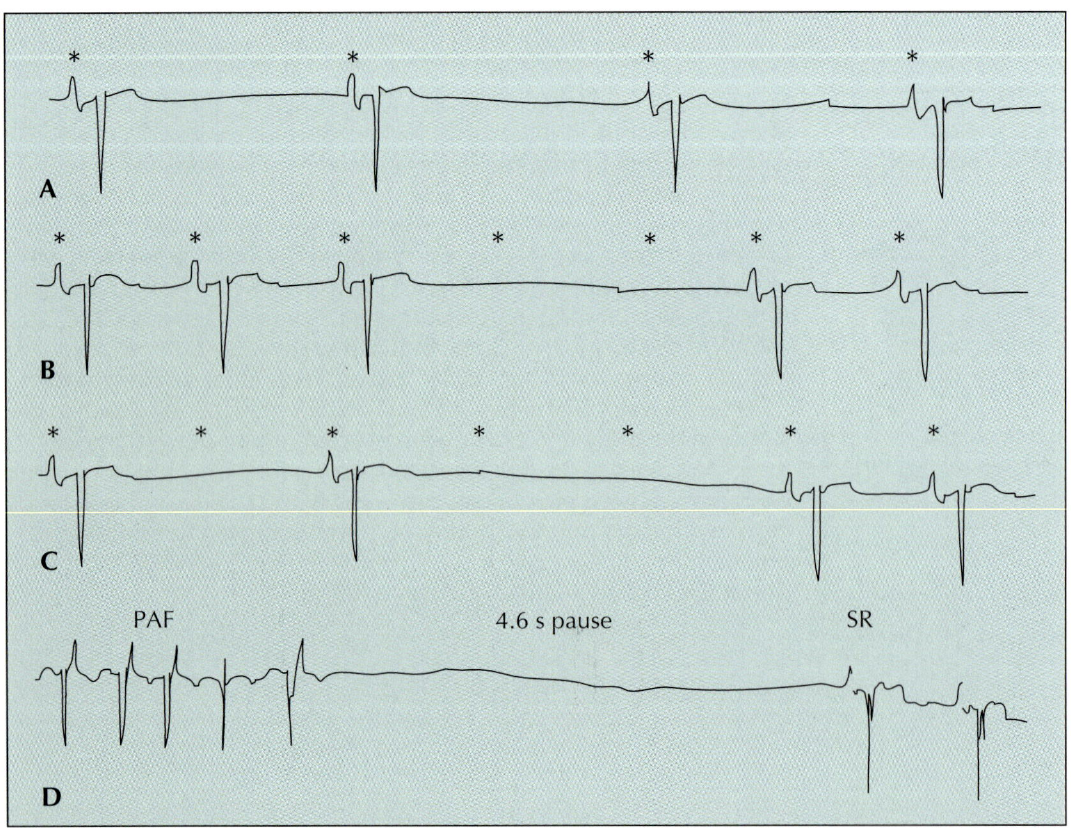

Figure 12-4. Sinoatrial (SA) node disease. Four electrocardiographic (ECG) recordings depicting typical manifestations of SA node disease. *Asterisks* indicate the time of activation, or expected activation of the sinus mechanism, in all strips. **A**, A persistent sinus bradycardia. **B**, A pause caused by sinus arrest. **C**, Pauses caused by SA node block. SA node block is distinguished from sinus arrest by the finding that any pause is a multiple of the basic sinus cycle length and is caused by firing of the sinus node that fails to capture the atrium due to exit block. Sinus arrest is caused by failure of the sinus mechanism to depolarize, and therefore it does not typically produce a pause that is a multiple of the basic cycle length. **D** depicts so-called tachy-brady syndrome. This commonly occurs in SA node disease and is manifested by an episode of atrial tachycardia, typically atrial fibrillation, with a prolonged pause immediately after spontaneous termination of the tachycardia.

Any of these manifestations of SA node disease may give rise to prolonged asystolic pauses with resultant syncope. PAF—paroxysmal atrial fibrillations; SR—sinus rhythm.

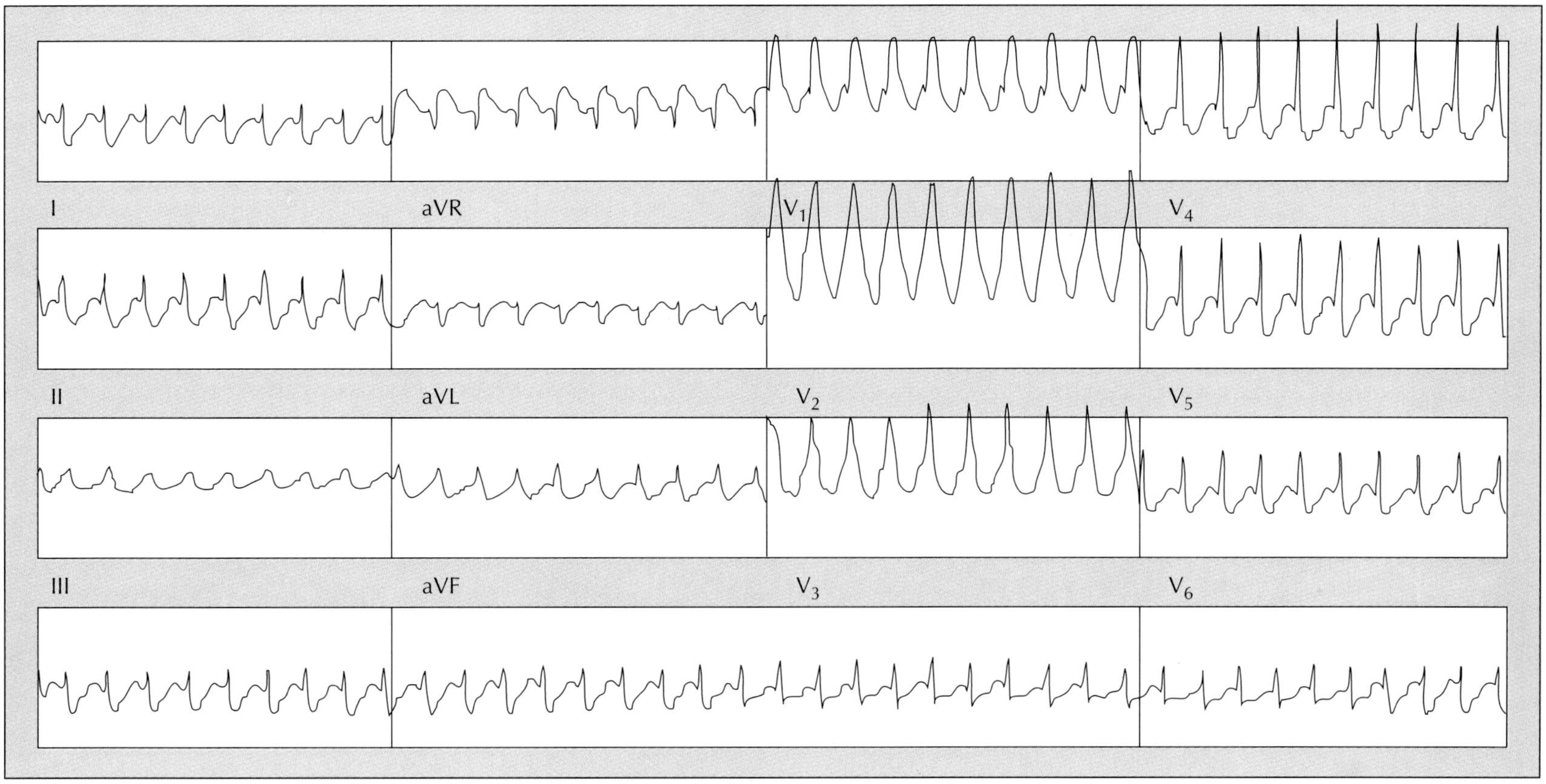

FIGURE 12-5. Supraventricular tachycardia with syncope. Despite the alarming appearance of this 12-lead electrocardiogram from a 25-year-old man with syncope, close inspection reveals that the diagnosis was one of supraventricular tachycardia with aberrant atrioventricular (AV) node conduction, (right bundle branch block). The patient underwent electrophysiologic study during which AV nodal reentrant tachycardia was induced, associated with a very rapid ventricular rate, right bundle branch block, and near-syncope. He underwent successful AV nodal radiofrequency catheter modification and remains cured.

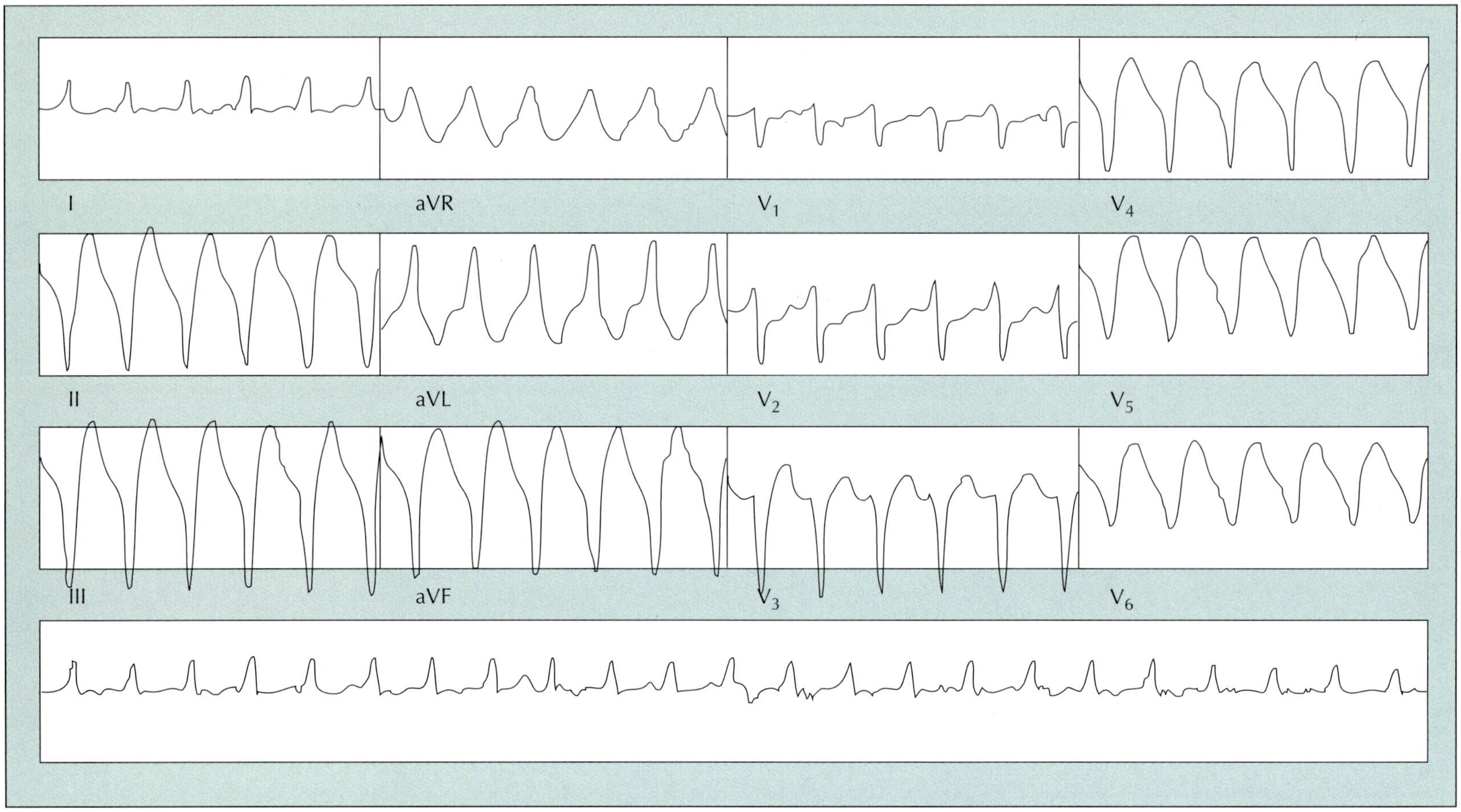

Figure 12-6. Ventricular tachycardia with syncope. A 12-lead electrocardiogram from a 65-year-old woman with a history of syncope, previous myocardial infarction, and poor left ventricular function. During electrophysiologic testing using programmed ventricular stimulation, rapid ventricular tachycardia was reproducibly induced with hypotension and near-syncope. Antiarrhythmic drug testing was unsuccessful, and she received an implanted cardioverter defibrillator.

Treatment with antiarrhythmic drugs fails in many patients being investigated for sudden cardiac death associated with ventricular arrhythmias. Some patients are suitable for treatment by catheter or surgical ablation, but at the present time, many receive implantable cardioverter defibrillators.

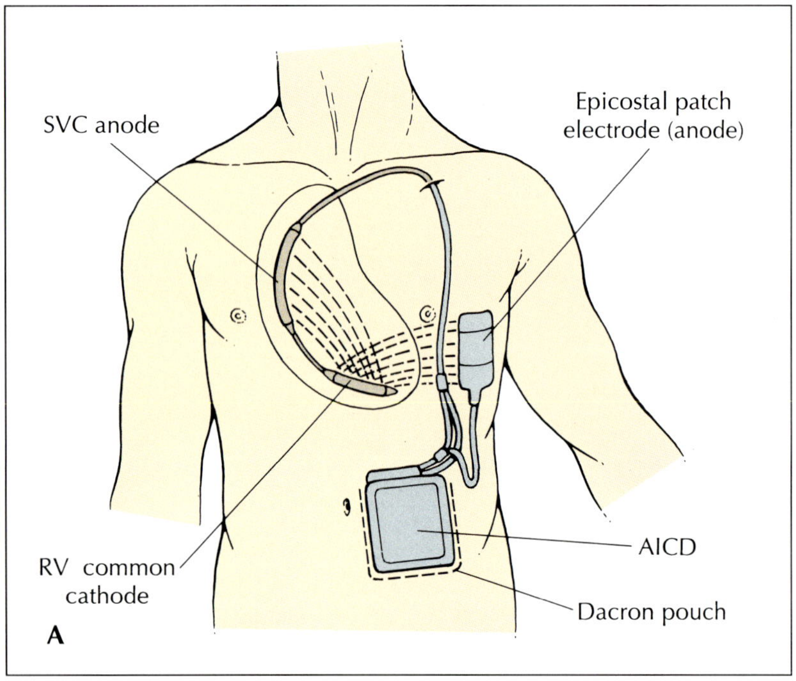

Figure 12-7. An implantable cardioverter defibrillator (*see also* Chapter 9). This device is placed subcutaneously in the electrophysiologic laboratory under general anesthesia (**A**). A tripolar sensing, pacing, and shocking electrode is passed transvenously via the left subclavian vein to the right ventricle (RV). A patch electrode is placed in the left axillary region, and the leads are tunneled to an implanted pulse generator lying subcutaneously in the abdomen. (*continued*)

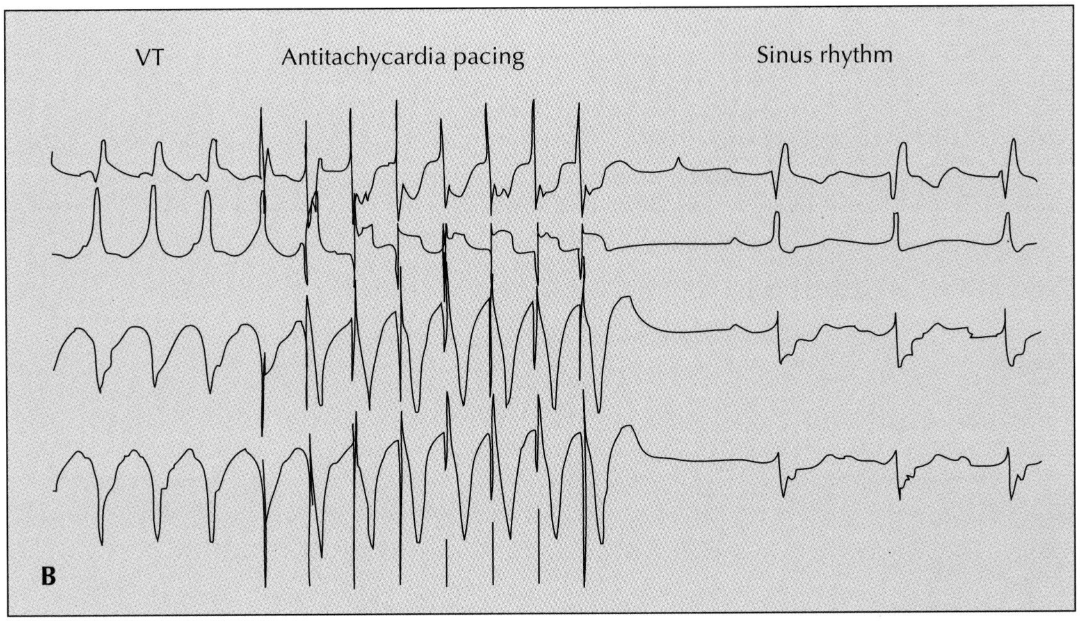

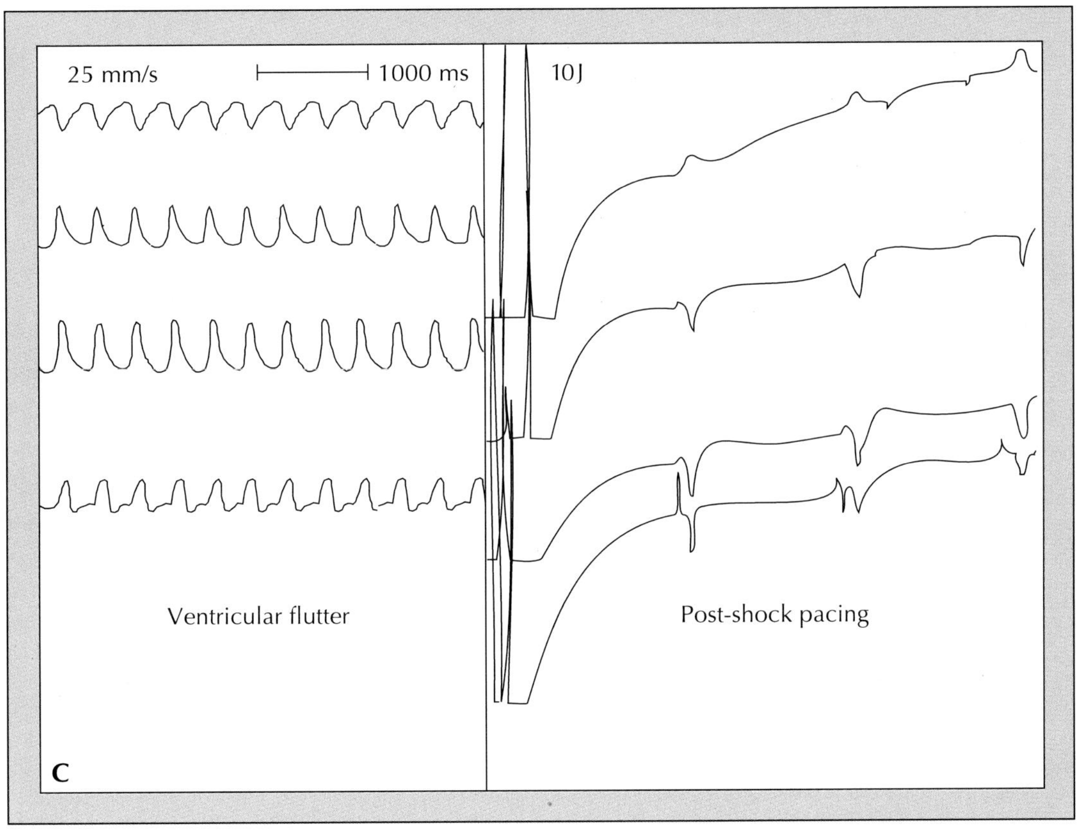

FIGURE 12-7. (*continued*) Detection of a rapid heart rate by the device (above a programmable rate cut-off) initiates a programmable series of therapies ranging from antitachycardia pacing (**B**), through low energy cardioversion to high energy defibrillation (**C**). AICD—automatic implantable cardioverter/defibrillator; SVC—superior vena cava; VT—ventricular vena cava.

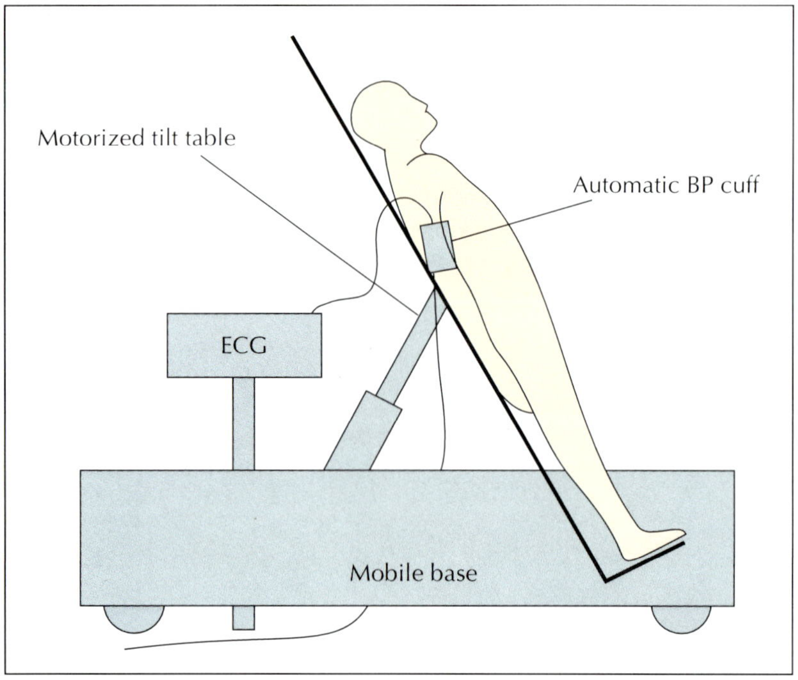

Figure 12-8. Tilt table. A diagram of the equipment used for tilt-table testing for unexplained syncope. Usually some form of motorized table is employed that can rapidly elevate and lower the patient to 60°. An electrocardiograph (ECG) is required to monitor heart rate and rhythm, and an automatic blood pressure cuff (or better, a Finepress [Ohmeda, Utah]) digital plethysmograph, which gives continuous noninvasive phasic blood pressure) is used to monitor blood pressure. BP—blood pressure.

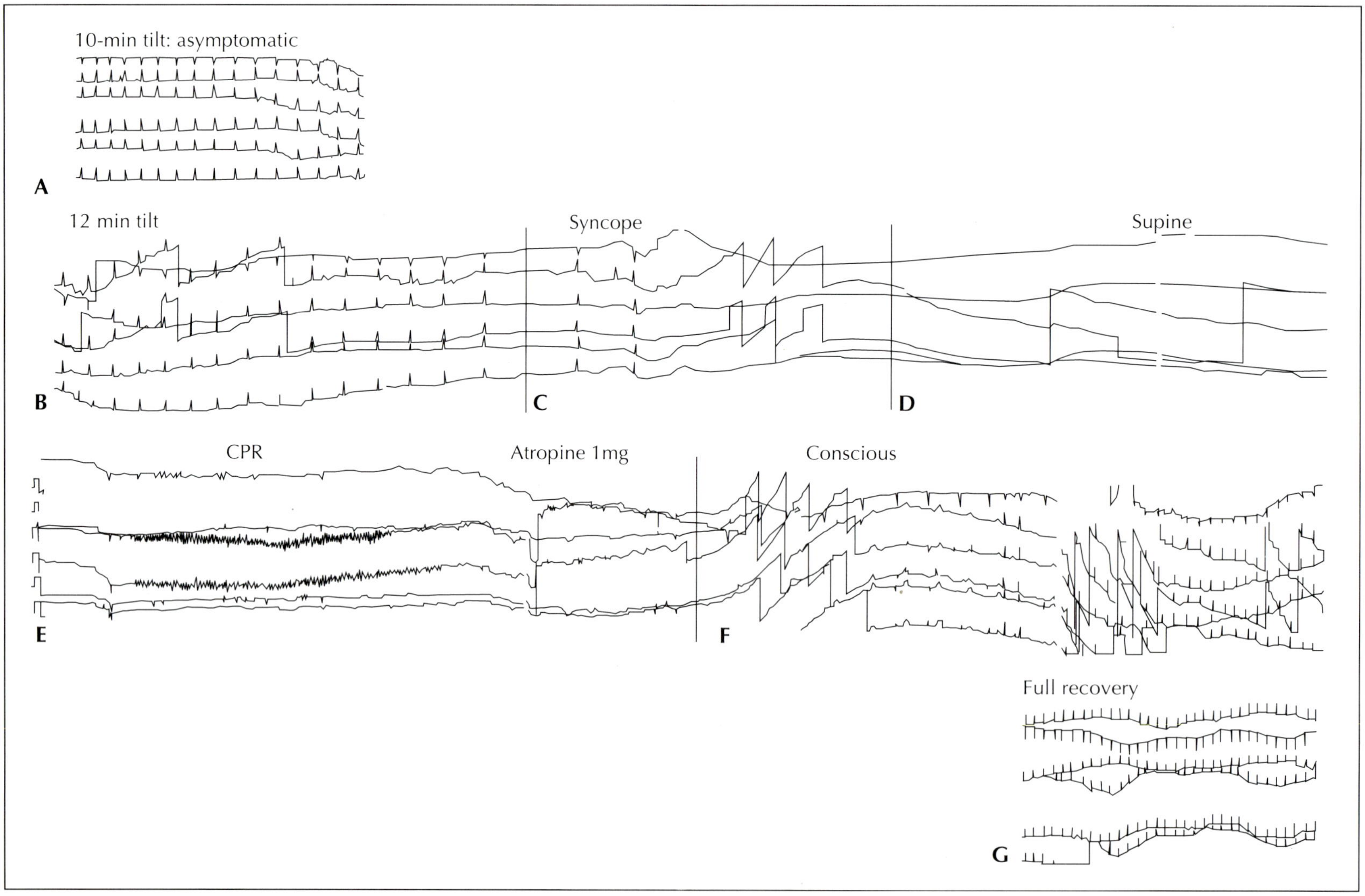

Figure 12-9. Vasovagal syncope occurring during head-up tilt testing. A montage of a continuous 6-lead electrocardiographic recording during 60° head-up passive tilt in a 22-year-old woman with recurrent syncope. At 12 minutes of tilt she was asymptomatic. A few seconds later she developed hypotension associated with sinus bradycardia, atrioventricular block, and then asystole, which lasted for 50 seconds. Cardiopulmonary resuscitation (CPR) was initiated and she received intravenous atropine. A few seconds later she became conscious again, and after a few minutes she was able to get up and walk away. Tilt testing has become a very useful tool in the assessment of patients with unexplained syncope. By reproducing symptoms in the presence of a medical witness, a diagnosis may be made with confidence.

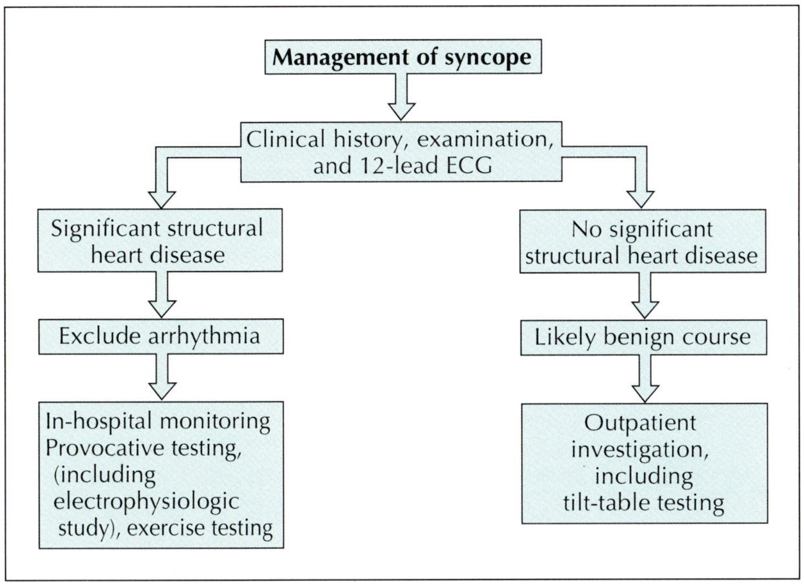

FIGURE 12-10. Algorithm for management of syncope. Syncope may occur in patients with structurally normal hearts or structurally diseased hearts. When the heart is normal, syncope may be troublesome and distressing, but the prognosis is generally good. When there is significant structural heart disease, the more severe the disease, the worse the prognosis. Simple investigations usually allow the physician to determine if significant stuctural heart disease is present. These investigations should not exclude a careful clinical evaluation, a 12-lead electrocardiogram (ECG), and often an echocardiogram as well. Absence of any obvious abnormality in these evaluations indicates that outcome will likely be good. Patients may have severe symptoms, nevertheless, and often an outpatient tilt-table test is indicated, since vasovagal or "neurally mediated" syncope is the likely cause. When structural heart disease is present, a search for an arrhythmic cause of syncope is indicated. In this case the prognosis may be poor, but an accurate diagnosis and the correct treatment may improve it significantly.

SUDDEN DEATH

CAUSES OF SUDDEN CARDIAC DEATH

STRUCTURAL	FUNCTIONAL
Coronary artery disease	Hypoxia, electrolytes, abnormalities
Cardiomyopathy	Long QT syndromes
Hypertrophic	Congenital
Dilated	Acquired
Restrictive	Coronary artery spasm
Valvular heart disease	Catecholamine induced
Aortic stenosis	Polymorphous ventricular tachycardia
Pulmonic stenosis	Right ventricular outflow tract
Congenital	
Right ventricular dysplasia	
Status post correction of Tetralogy of Fallot	
VSD, transposition of the great vessels	

FIGURE 12-11. Causes of sudden cardiac death. VSD—ventricular septal defect.

RISK FACTORS FOR SUDDEN CARDIAC DEATH POST MYOCARDIAL INFARCTION*

MYOCARDIAL INFARCTION	RISK
Nonsustained ventricular tachycardia Depressed left ventricular ejection fraction Abnormal signal-averaged ECG	17-fold
Abnormal heart rate variability [10]	5-fold
Abnormal baroreceptor hypersensitivity [11]	—

*A combination of finding the first three factors defines a population at 17-fold increased risk compared with those without these parameters. Similarly, abnormal heart rate variability is associated with a 5-fold increased risk.

FIGURE 12-12. Risk factors for sudden cardiac death post myocardial infarction. ECG—electrocardiogram.

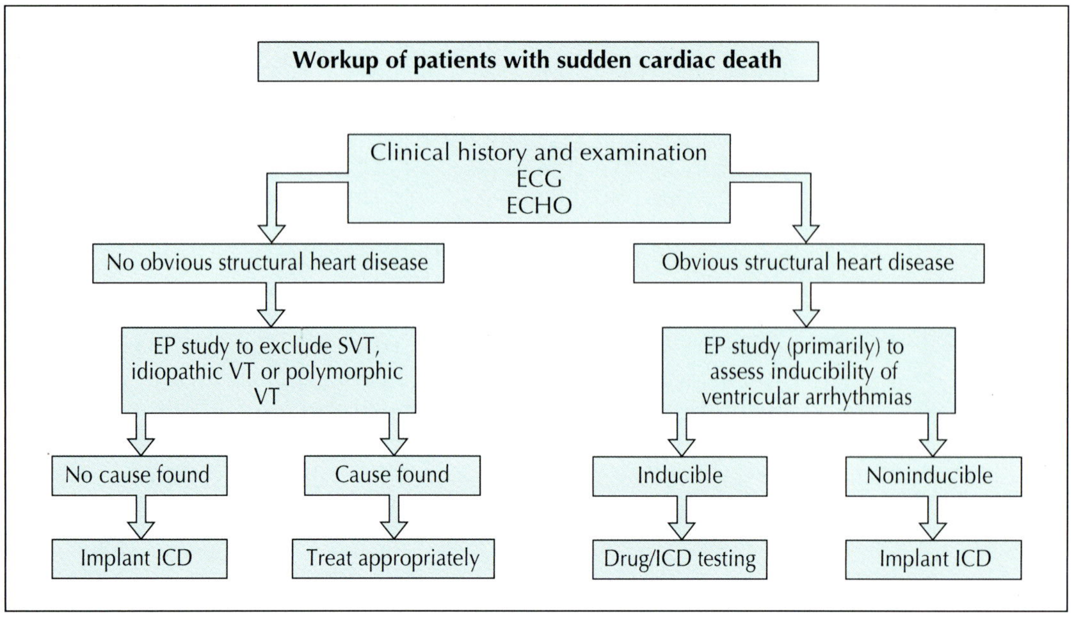

FIGURE 12-13. Diagnostic work-up in patients with aborted sudden cardiac death. ECG—electrocardiogram; ECHO—echocardiogram; EP—electrophysiology; ICD—implantable cardioverter defibrillator; SVT; supraventricular tachycardia; VT—ventricular tachycardia.

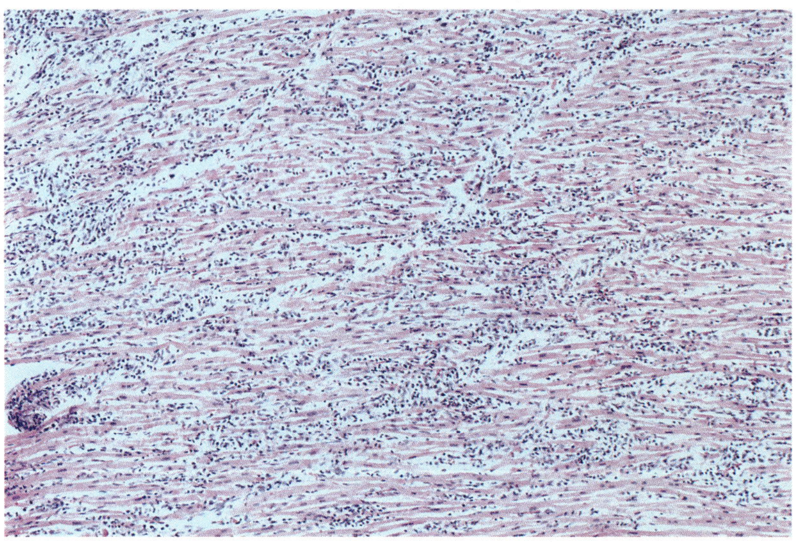

FIGURE 12-14. Sudden death in a child with acute myocarditis. A high-power photomicrograph of a conventional hematoxylin and eosin–stained section of ventricular myocardium from a 5-year-old child who died suddenly, 3 weeks after suffering a mild parvovirus infection. The section shows striking inflammatory cell infiltration with myocyte damage, indicating an active myocarditis. The child is presumed to have died as result of a fatal ventricular arrhythmia.

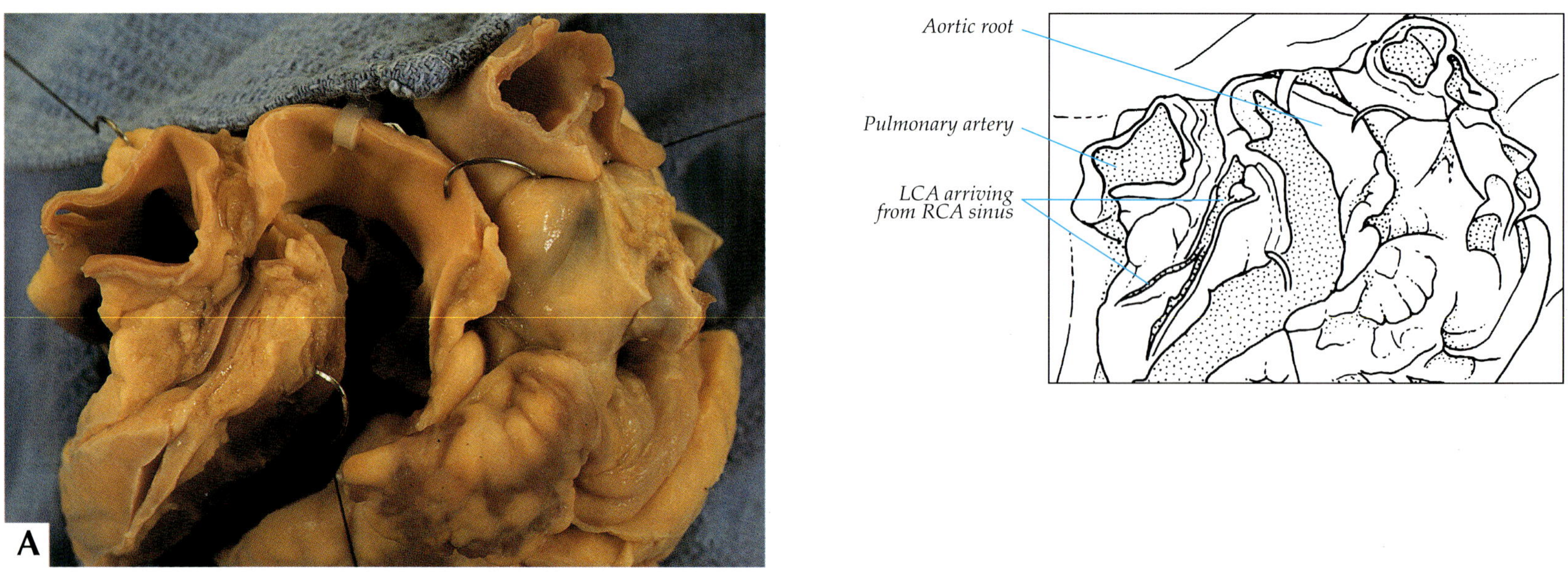

FIGURE 12-15. Sudden death in a patient with coronary artery anomalies. **A**, A gross pathology specimen, with accompanying line drawing, showing the location and course of an aberrant left coronary artery (LCA) arising from the right coronary sinus of Valsalva and running between the aortic root and the main pulmonary artery in a patient who had suffered sudden cardiac death during exercise. The artery runs between the great arteries and is thought to be constricted (or kinked at its origin) by them during exercise, leading to severe myocardial ischemia, ventricular fibrillation, and death. *(continued)*

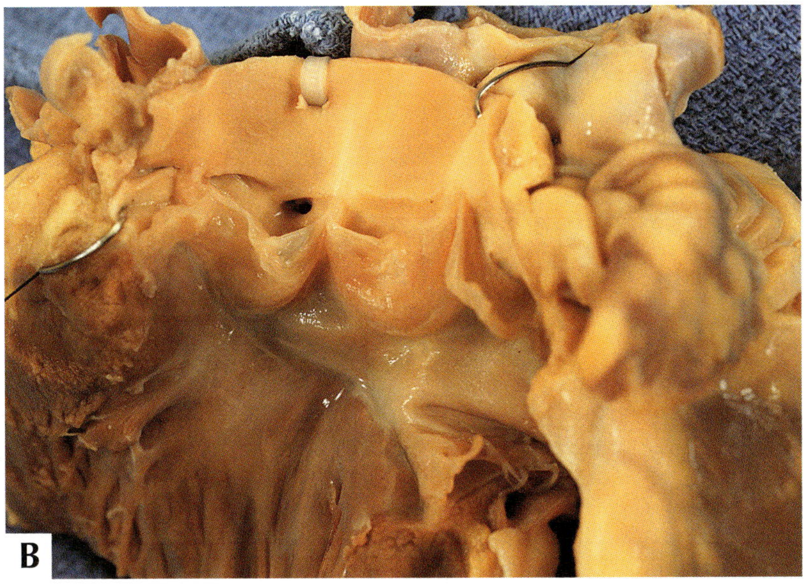

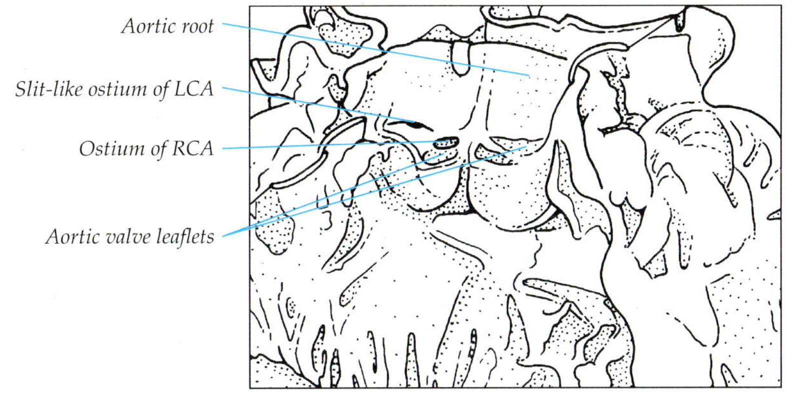

FIGURE 12-15. (*continued*) **B**, Alternative view of the gross anatomy of an aberrant LCA, showing a "slit-like" LCA orifice, next to the right coronary artery orifice, lying in the right coronary sinus of Valsalva. RCA—right coronary artery.

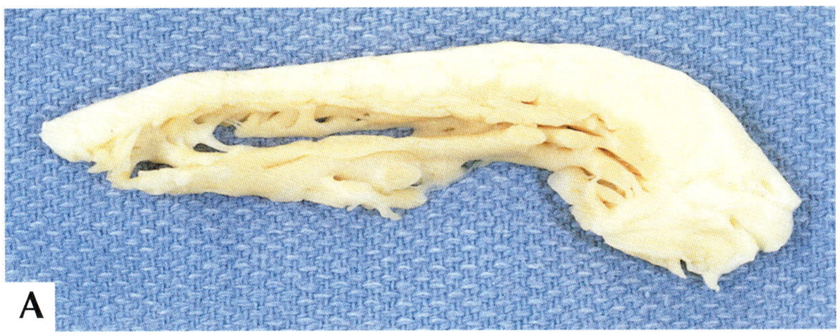

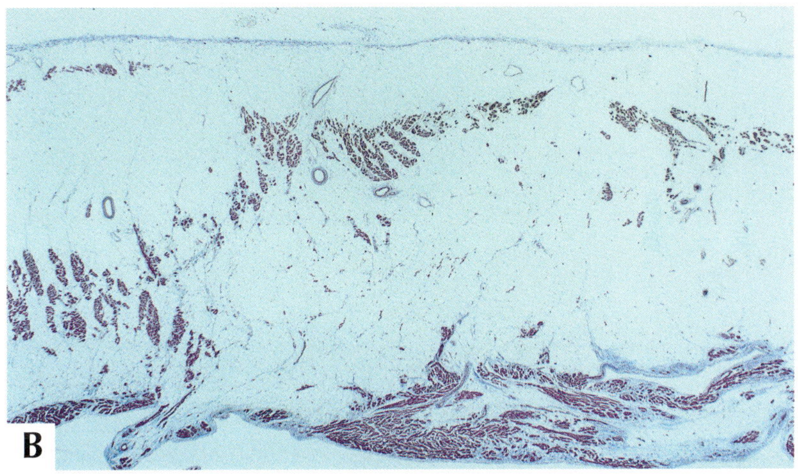

FIGURE 12-16. Histologic appearances in a patient with sudden cardiac death associated with right ventricular (RV) dysplasia. **A**, A gross histopathologic specimen showing typical appearances of RV dysplasia (in a severe form sometimes referred to as Uhl's anomaly). Replacement of the RV free wall myocardium with fibro-fatty tissue is the hallmark of this disease. It may be familial and can be associated with sudden cardiac death due to the development of ventricular arrhythmias. **B**, Light microscopic specimen from the same patient. Between the epicardium above and the endocardium below, the myocardium of the RV free wall is grossly infiltrated and replaced by adipose tissue.

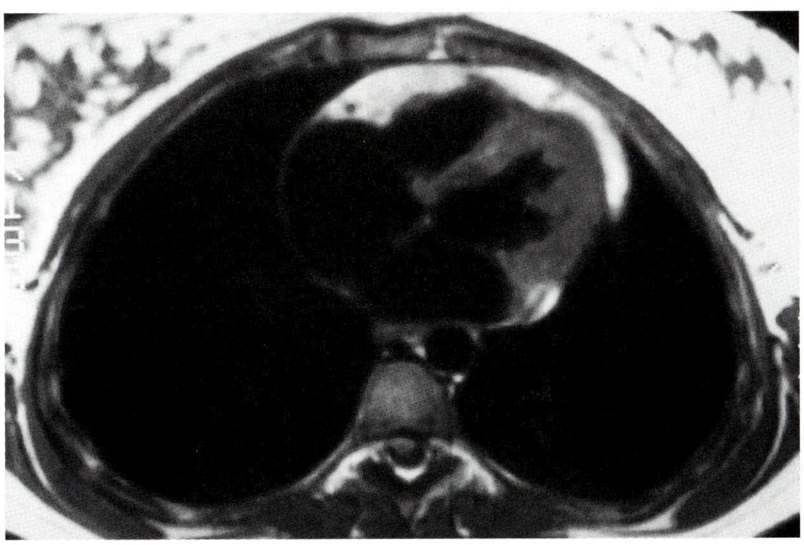

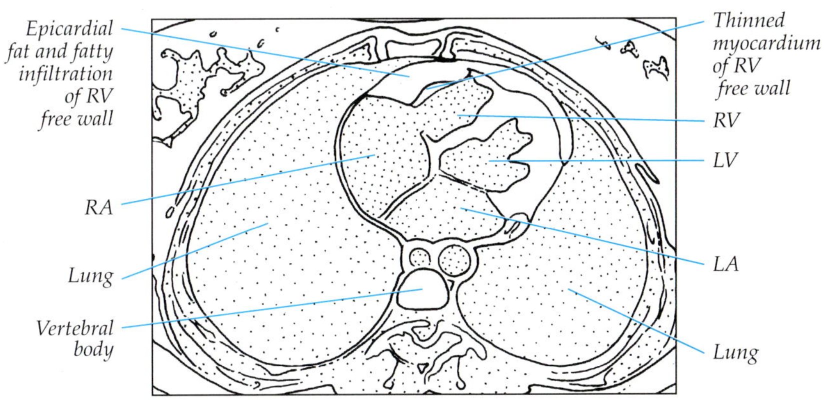

FIGURE 12-17. Magnetic resonance image of right ventricular (RV) dysplasia. This image was acquired from a patient with a history of ventricular tachycardia of RV origin, showing replacement of normal myocardium by fatty tissue. LA—left atrium; LV—left ventricle; RA—right atrium.

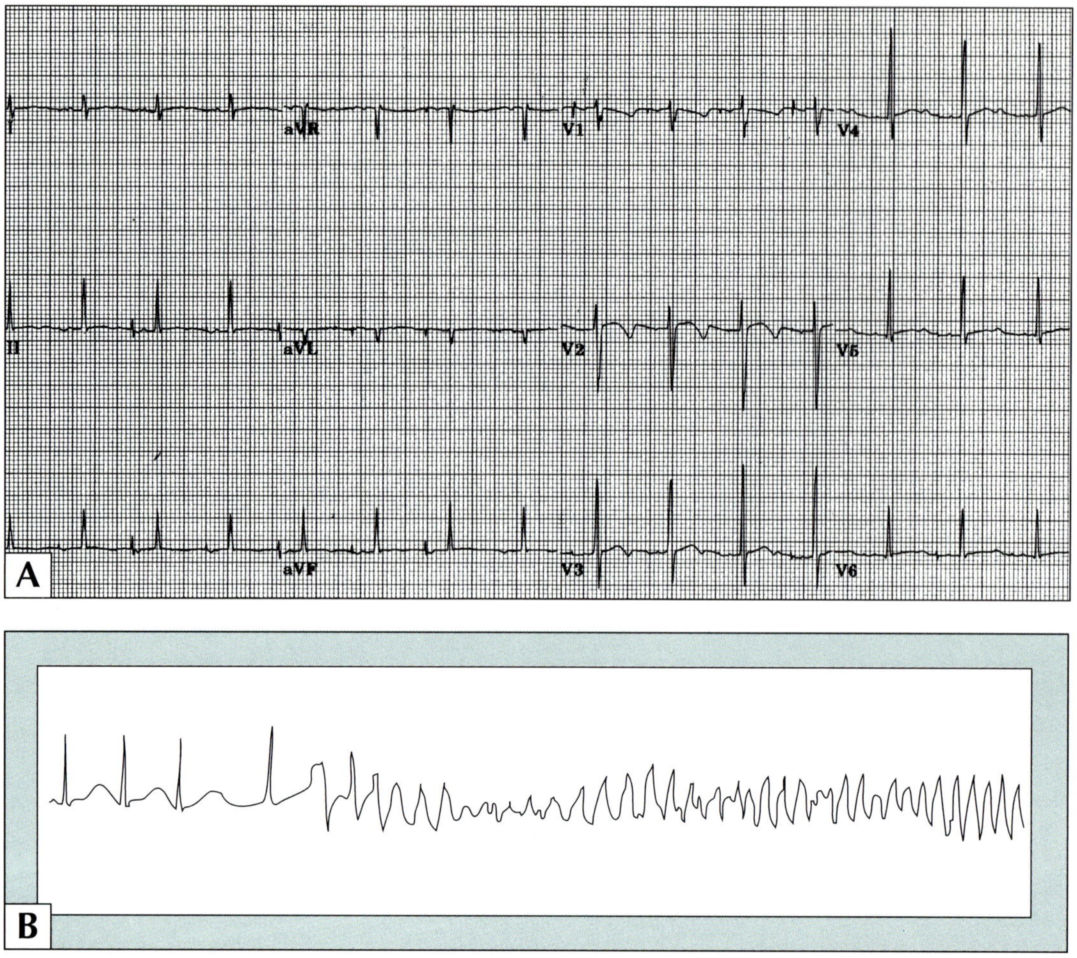

FIGURE 12-18. The long QT syndrome. **A**, 12-lead electrocardiographic (ECG) tracings from an 11-year-old girl with an episode of sudden cardiac death showing a prolonged QTc (Qt-interval corrected for heart rate). **B**, ECG from the same child showing the initiation of torsades de pointes by short-long R-R cycles caused by an episode of sinus arrest during sinus tachycardia. In the presence of QT prolongation, and the underlying abnormality of repolarization implied by it, after-depolarizations may reach threshold, leading to a further premature action potential and cell membrane depolarization. (*see* Chapter 7).

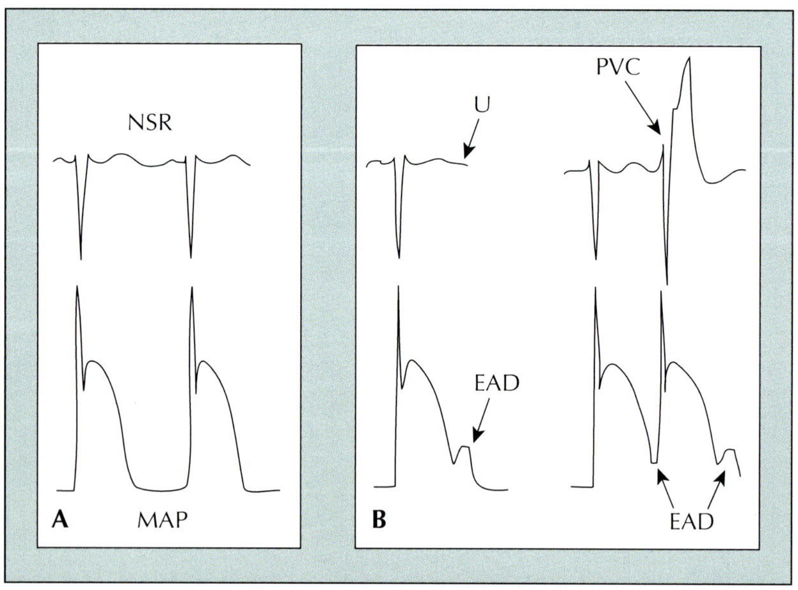

FIGURE 12-19. **A**, Normal simultaneous surface ECG complexes, *ie*, normal sinus rhythm (NSR) and endocardial catheter monophasic action potential (MAP) recordings. **B**, A typical abnormal QRSTU complex in long QT syndrome with the prolongation of repolarization in the surface ECG reflected in a prominent early after-depolarization (EAD) recorded by the MAP catheter. On the right is shown the effect of an EAD reaching membrane potential and triggering a premature ventricular depolarization (*ie*, premature ventricular contraction [PVC]). Torsade de pointes occurs when EADs repetitively cause ventricular depolarization from widespread foci in the ventricular myocardium. The result is a rapid disorganized, or polymorphic, ventricular tachycardia that may degenerate into ventricular fibrillation, resulting in death.

DRUG DOSING FOR PATIENTS WITH ABORTED SUDDEN CARDIAC DEATH

AMIODARONE

Loading dose of 10–12g (over two weeks)

Intravenous dosing for recurrent life-threatening ventricular tachycardia or ventricular fibrillation, 5 mg/kg, over 20–30 min as loading dose, followed by infusions of 1 g/d for at least 3 d.

Chronic dose of 200–400 mg/d.

SOTALOL

Test dose of 80 mg

Chronic dose of 320–640 mg/d

FIGURE 12-20. Management of patients after resuscitation from cardiac death. The advantages of sotalol therapy include a shorter duration of monitoring before retesting is performed and a lower incidence of side effects. Disadvantages include restrictions in use for those who cannot tolerate beta-blocker therapy and the risk of serious proarrythmia (*i.e.*, torsade de pointes). Sotalol cannot be used in patients with severe depression of the left ventricular ejection fraction (< 25%). Amiodarone has the advantage of being effective and safe for patients with congestive heart failure, and the prolonged half-life allows for once per day dosing. The disadvantages are multiple organ toxicity, including lung, liver, skin, eyes, and thyroid, and hypotension with intravenous administration. If there is no inducible arrhythmia, or if no drug is found to be effective, then an automatic defibrillator is the best therapy.

References

1. Kapoor W: Chapter 30: Hypotension and syncopy. In *Heart Disease: A Textbook of Cardiovascular Medicine*, ed. 4. Edited by Braunwald E. Philadelphia: WB Saunders; 1992:890.
2. Kapoor WN, Karpf M, Weant S, *et al.*: A prospective evaluation and follow-up of patients with syncope. *N Engl J Med* 1983, 309:197–203.
3. Day SC, Cook EF, Funkenstein H, Goldman L: Evaluation and outcome of emergency room patients with transient loss of consciousness. *Am J Med* 1982, 73:15–23.
4. Thoren P: Characteristics of left ventricular receptors with nonmedullated vagal afferents. *Circ Res* 1977, 40:415–421.
5. Schwartz TW: Vagal slowing of the heart during haemorrhage: observations from 20 consecutive patients. *BMJ* 1986, 292:364–366.
6. Eldar M, Griffin JC, Van Hare GF, *et al.*: Combined use of beta-adrenergic blocking agents and long-term cardiac pacing for patients with the long QT syndrome. *J Am Coll Cardiol* 1992, 20:830–837.
7. Kannel WB: Sudden death: lessons from subsets in population studies. *J Am Coll Cardiol* 1985, 5:141–149.
8. Mukarji J, Rude RE, Poole WK, and the MILIS Study Group: Risk factors for sudden death after MI: two-year follow up. *Am J Cardiol* 1984, 54:31–36.
9. Odemuyiwa O, Malik M, Farrell T, *et al.*: Comparison of the predictive characteristics of heart rate variability index and left ventricular ejection fraction for all-cause mortality, arrythmic events, and sudden death after acute myocardial infarction. *Am J Cardiol* 1991, 68:434–439.
10. Kleiger RE, Miller JP, Bigger JT Jr, Moss AJ, and the Multicenter Post Infarction Research Group: Decreased heart rate variability and its association with increased mortality after acute myocardial infarction. *Am J Cardiol* 1987, 59:256–262.
11. Farrell TG, Cripps TR, Malik M: Baroreflex sensitivity and electrophysiological correlates in patients after acute myocardial infarction. *Circulation* 1991, 83:945–952.
12. Camm AJ, Fei L: Risk stratification after myocardial infarction. *PACE* 1994, 17:401–409.
13. Farrell TG, Bashir Y, Cripps T: Risk stratification for arrythmic events in postinfarction patients based on electrocardiogram. *J Am Coll Cardiol* 1991, 18:687–697.
14. Klein GJ, Bashore TM, Sellers TD, *et al.*: Ventricular fibrillation in the Wolff-Parkinson-White syndrome. *N Engl J Med* 1979, 301:1080–1085.

Cardiopulmonary Resuscitation

13

CHAPTER

Todd J. Cohen

Early cardiopulmonary resuscitation (CPR) is a critical component of a successful outcome from cardiac arrest. The purpose of CPR is to promptly resuscitate the victim without myocardial or cerebral damage. This can effectively be accomplished because of the rapid and wide availability of this technique. However, despite its effectiveness, less than 20% of patients who receive standard CPR survive to hospital discharge. Basic and advanced cardiac life support (BCLS and ACLS) provide the means to administer resuscitative efforts that include CPR, pharmacologic agents, and defibrillation. BCLS includes early activation of the emergency medical system and early CPR. ACLS encompasses more advanced therapies, including pharmacologic support, pacing, cardioversion, and defibrillation. Together, BCLS and ACLS provide critical links in the chain of survival. These principles have been widely spread by the American Heart Association and the American Red Cross to medical, paramedical, and lay personnel.

Since CPR was first described in 1960 by Kowenhoven [1], little has changed relative to the universal applicability of this technique. Part of the reason for the wide acceptance of standard manual CPR is its simplicity and cost. This technique is the cornerstone for successful resuscitation of cardiac arrest victims. This method is taught throughout the United States by the American Heart Association and American Red Cross and in Europe by the European Resuscitation Council.

Recently, several alternatives have been shown to improve cardiopulmonary circulation in both animal and human models.

In the United States alone, sudden cardiac death from ventricular arrhythmias accounts for at least 350,000 deaths per year. CPR and early defibrillation have been shown to be effective in reducing the mortality from these episodes. The practical application of newer techniques to a large cardiac arrest population remains to be seen. Some newer resuscitation methods include interposed abdominal counterpulsation CPR, circumferential pneumatic vest CPR, and active compression-decompression CPR. In addition, rescue defibrillation can be administered in a variety of settings. This chapter reviews the history of CPR, BCLS and ACLS, defibrillation, and recent advances in both the field of CPR and of defibrillation. In addition, appropriate electrical and pharmacologic management of cardiac arrest victims is discussed.

The Chain of Survival

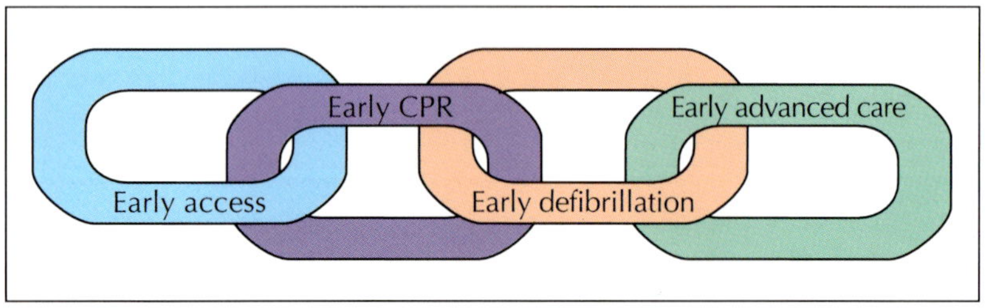

Figure 13-1. The chain of survival of cardiopulmonary resuscitation (CPR) links the four most important aspects of a successful outcome. These links include (in sequential order) early access to the emergency medical system, CPR, and defibrillation, followed by advanced care. If one link is broken, survival rates are severely impaired. (*Adapted from* Cummins and coworkers [2]; with permission.)

PRINCIPAL ETIOLOGIES OF SUDDEN CARDIAC DEATH

- Coronary artery disease
- Outflow tract obstruction
  - Valvular
  - Hypertrophic cardiomyopathy
- Cardiomyopathies
  - Idiopathic
  - Drug induce
  - Infiltrative
- Primary electrical disorders
  - Congenital long QT syndrome
- Drug induced
  - Type IA antiarrhythmic drugs

Figure 13-2. The principal etiologies of sudden cardiac death, (which is also termed *aborted sudden death*). Mortality rates from cardiovascular disease have been declining over the past decades, but it still accounts for nearly 50% of all deaths. Two thirds of cardiac deaths occur in an out-of-hospital setting, thus placing sudden cardiac death as the primary medical emergency in the United States [3–7].

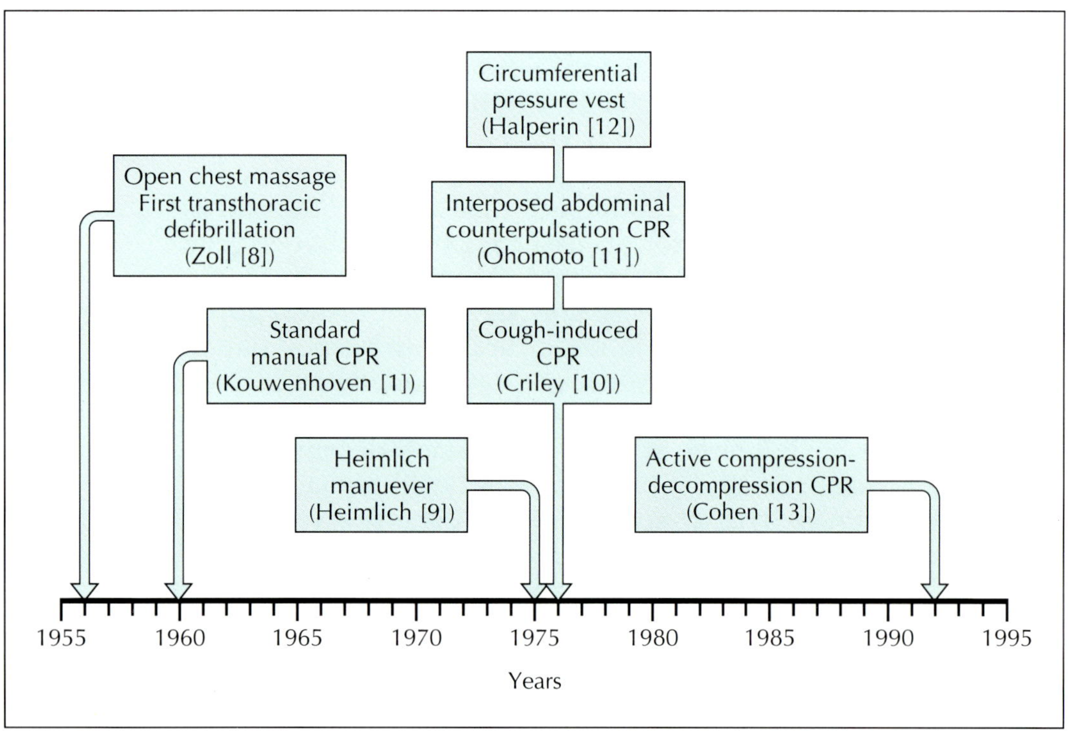

Figure 13-3. Major advances in CPR. Only recently have CPR techniques been widely used in out-of-hospital as well as in-hospital clinical settings. Kowenhoven *et al.* introduced external manual CPR in 1960, which revolutionized the care of victims of sudden cardiac arrest [1]. This method is widely taught throughout the world today by the American Heart Association and American Red Cross. Since 1960, investigators have been developing new methods of resuscitation to improve circulation and neurologic outcome [14].

ASSESSMENT OF RESPONSIVENESS AND PREPARATION FOR CPR

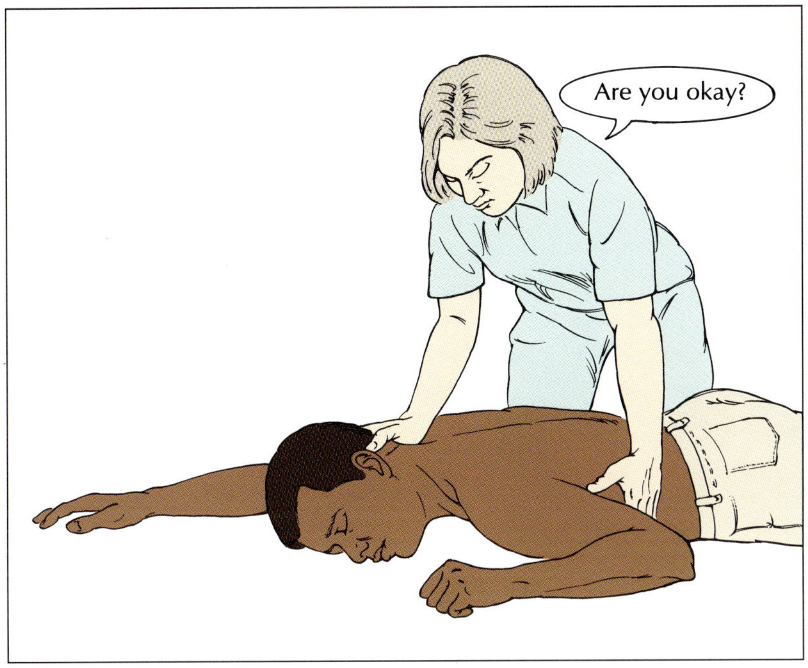

FIGURE 13-4. Basic cardiac life support (BCLS) is the first component in the chain of survival. This component of resuscitation includes both early access to the emergency medical system and early CPR. The initial step in BCLS is to evaluate the victim's level of responsiveness. This is performed by gently shaking the person, asking "Are you okay," and observing whether there is any movement. If the person is unresponsive, the rescuer should activate the emergency medical service system by directing the closest person to dial 911. If no one else is around, the rescuer places the call. BCLS includes CPR and airway management, including the Heimlich maneuver. (*Adapted from* American Heart Association [14]; with permission.)

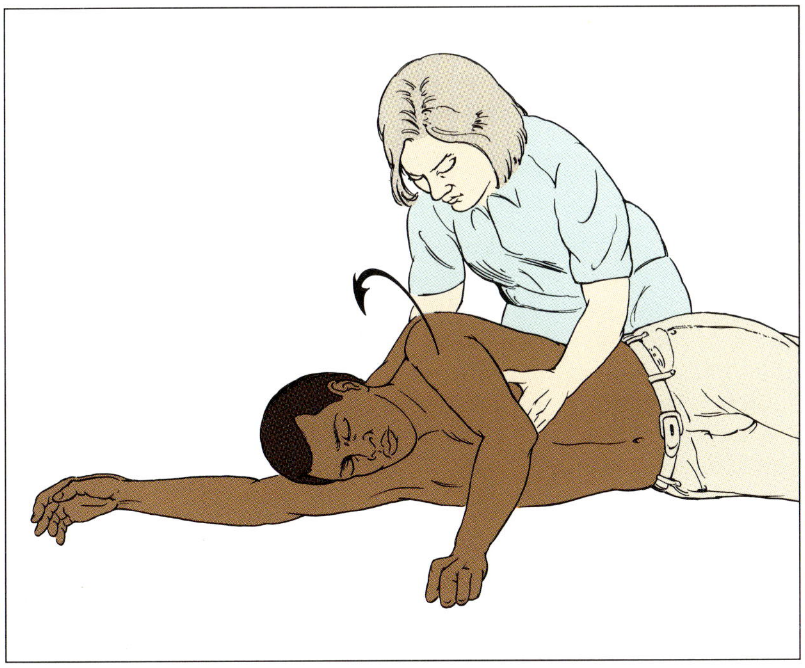

FIGURE 13-5. Positioning for CPR. Before CPR can be performed, the cardiac arrest victim must be positioned face-up on a hard, flat surface. This will permit efficient and effective performance of manual compressions during CPR. (*Adapted from* American Heart Association [14]; with permission.)

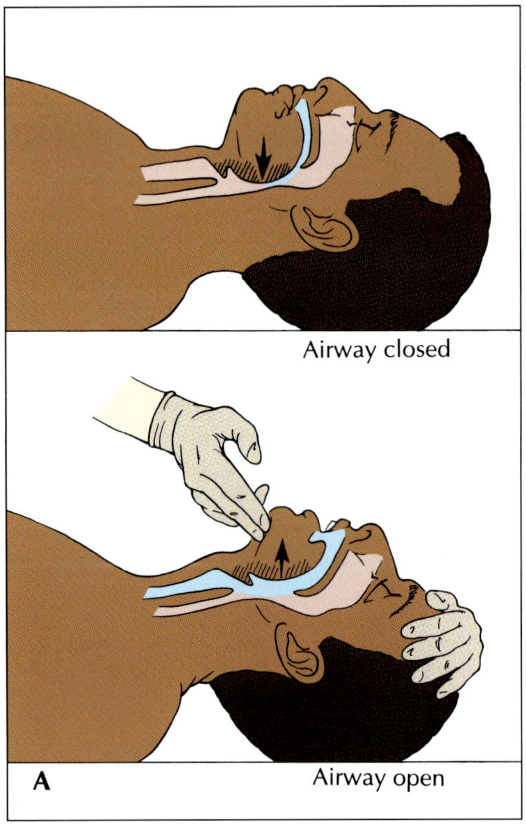

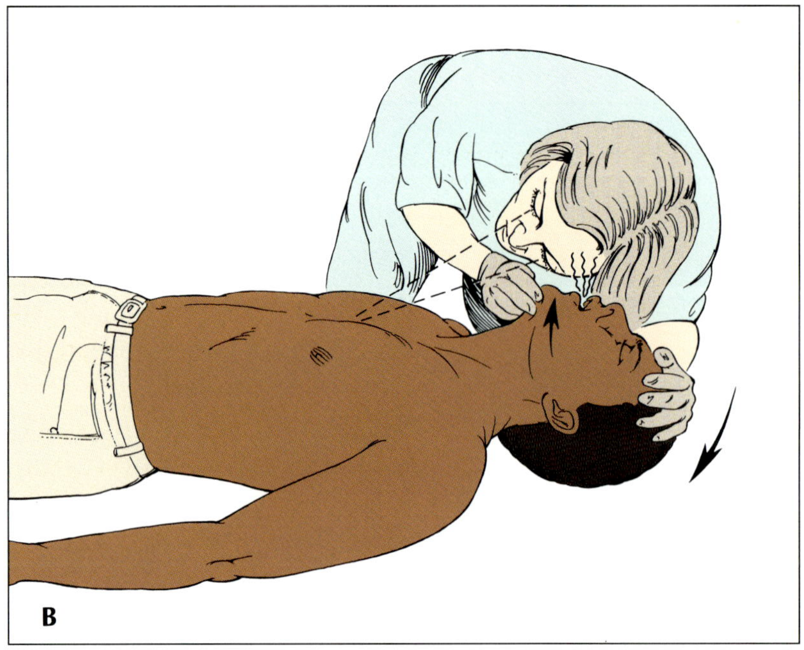

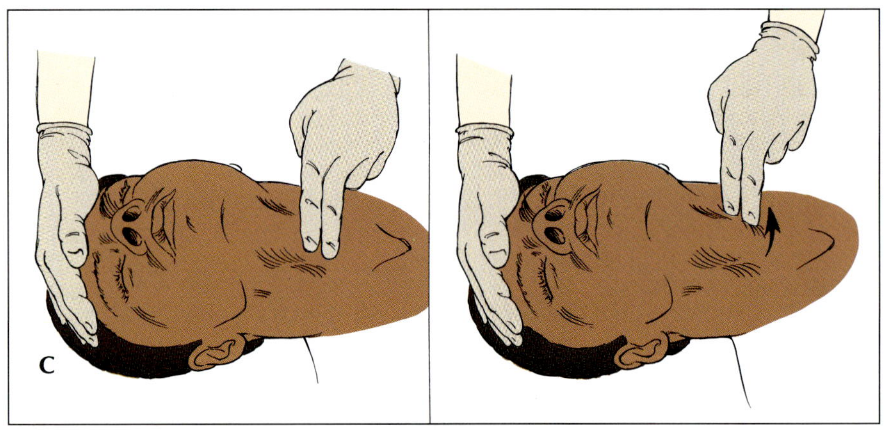

FIGURE 13-6. The ABCs of basic life support, airway, breathing, and circulation, must be assessed when a victim is found unresponsive [14,15]. **A,** Airway. The head tilt/chin lift is the first maneuver that is performed in order to open the airway. With the rescuer positioned on the victim's right side, the rescuer's left hand is placed on the forehead with two fingers from the right hand below the chin. The head is then pivoted backward and the two fingers lift the chin to open the airway and relieve obstruction by the epiglottis and tongue. **B,** Breathing is assessed by looking for chest expansion, listening for respirations and actually feeling the exhalation. In essence the rescuer *looks*, *listens*, and *feels*. The observation of chest expansion without feeling exhalation suggests a bronchopulmonary obstruction. In this case, circulation may be intact. **C,** To check circulation, the index and middle fingers of the right hand are used to palpate pulsation in the carotid artery. These fingers are slid down from below the chin toward the trachea and then laterally along the neck muscles. The presence and quality of pulsation will determine the urgency to perform CPR. For example, with the absence of a palpable carotid pulse, even with the presence of electrical activity from the heart, CPR should be initiated. (*Adapted from* American Heart Association [14]; with permission.)

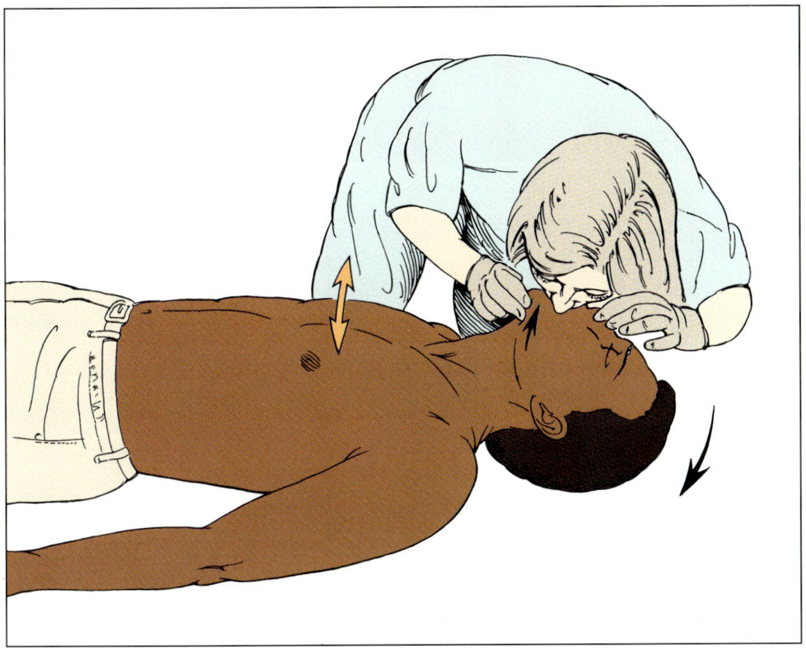

Figure 13-7. Mouth-to-mouth resuscitation, an important component of CPR, is performed by maintaining the head tilt/chin lift and making an airtight seal against the victim's mouth. Alternatively, mouth-to-nose and mouth-to-stoma resuscitation can be performed where appropriate. This form of ventilation can be performed without chest compressions when a palpable carotid pulse is felt without evidence of respiration. (*Adapted from* American Heart Association [14]; with permission.)

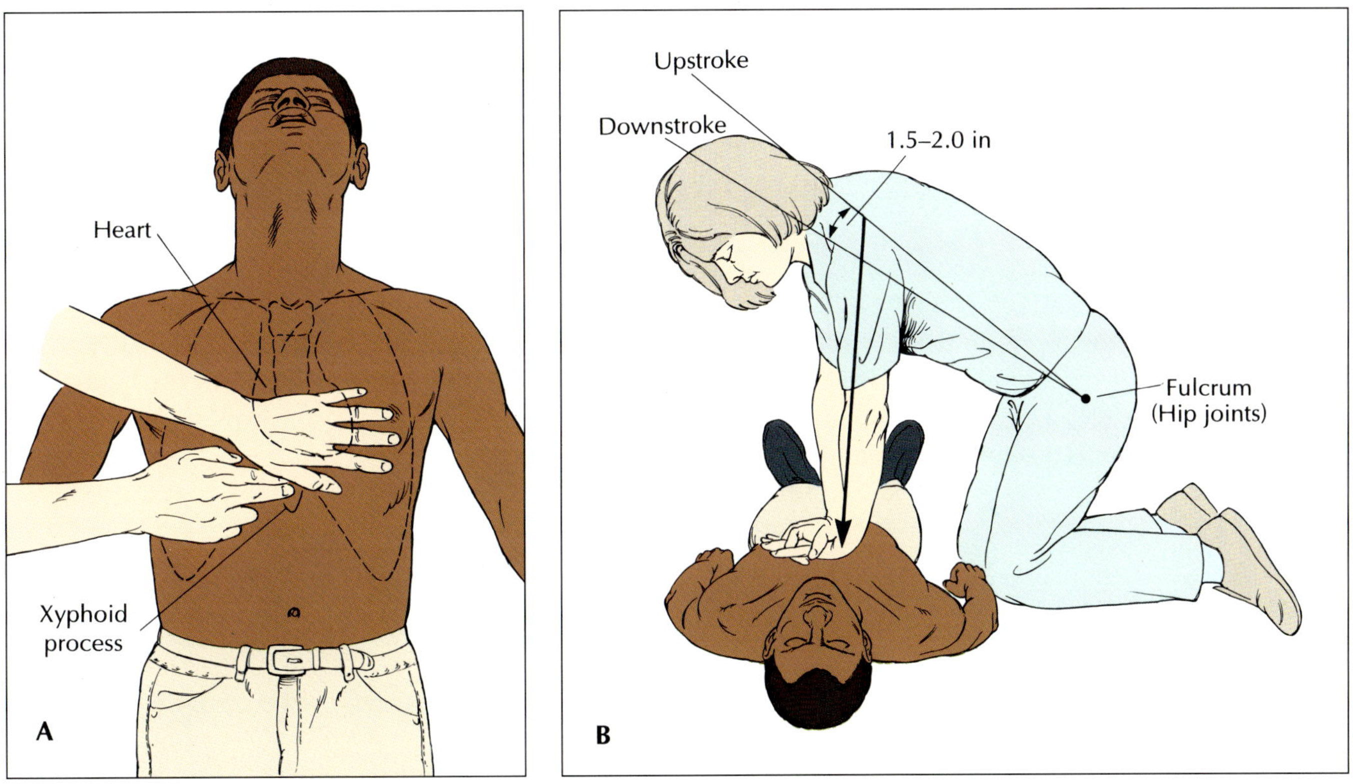

Figure 13-8. Active compressions during standard manual CPR. The technique for standard manual CPR has changed minimally since its first description by Kowenhoven *et al.* in 1960. **A,** Active chest compressions are performed two finger breadths above the xiphoid process. **B,** The American Heart Association recommends that compressions be performed at 1.5- to 2-in depths, 80 to 100 compressions per minute, and a 50% duty cycle (half the time spent in chest compression, half the time spent in chest relaxation). The rescuer's shoulders should be directly over the victim with the palm of one hand over the xiphoid process, the other hand atop it, and the arms outstretched with elbows locked. The hip acts as the fulcrum in the performance of chest compressions. The relaxation or decompression phase is passive. (*Adapted from* American Heart Association [14]; with permission.)

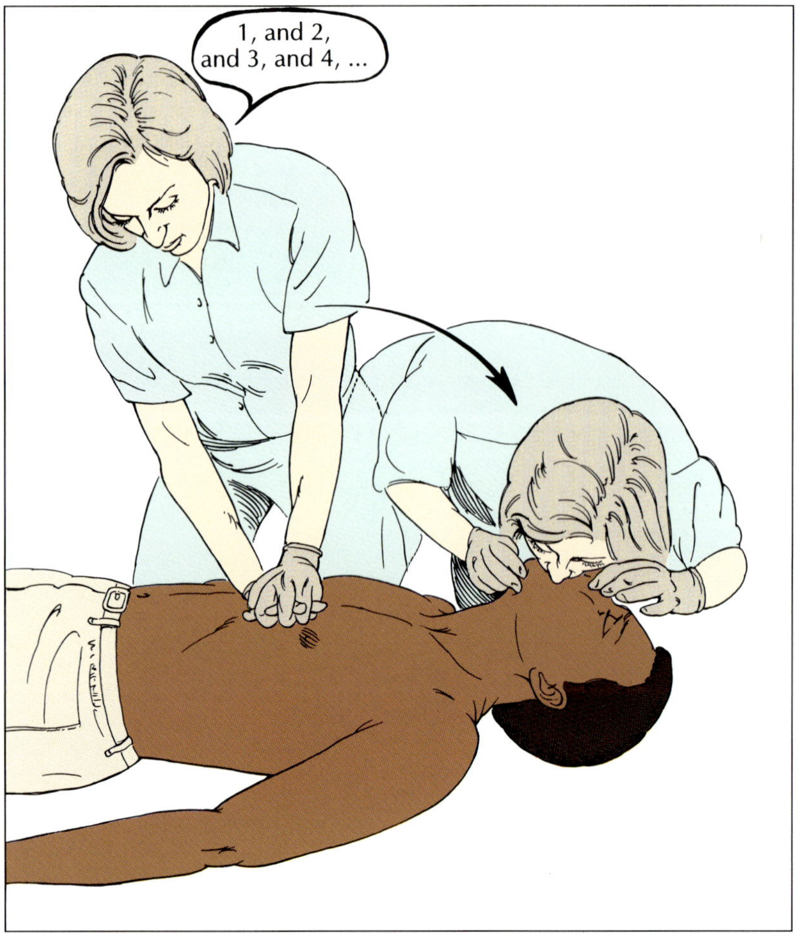

FIGURE 13-9. One-rescuer CPR is performed in a manner such that 15 chest compressions are followed by two ventilations. Approximately six sets, 90 compressions and twelve ventilations, should be performed each minute [14,15].

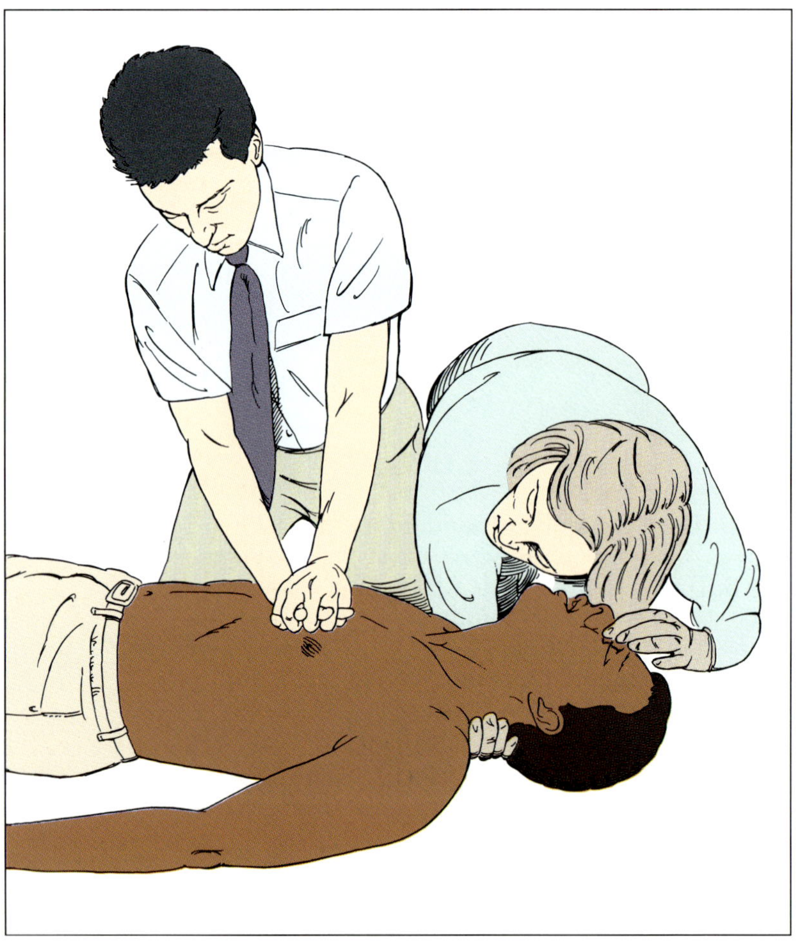

FIGURE 13-10. Two-rescuer CPR is performed in a manner such that one rescuer performs compressions and the other ventilations. Five compressions to one ventilation is the accepted protocol for two-rescuer CPR. The rescuers may synchronously switch positions to prevent fatigue [14,15].

Airway Obstruction

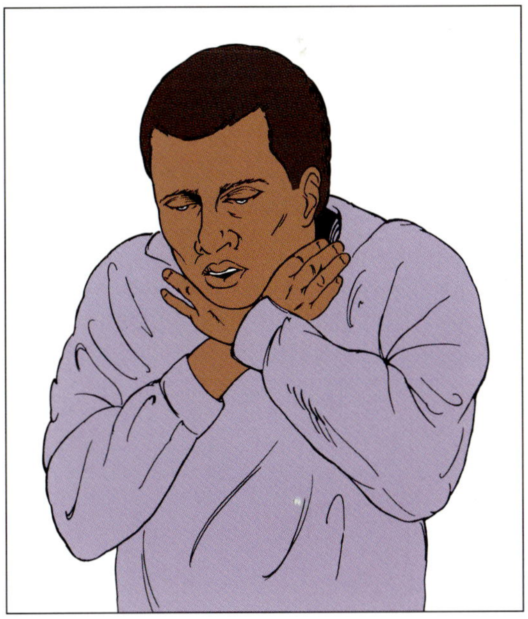

Figure 13-11. The universal distress signal may be observed with a foreign body obstruction of the airway. Victims frequently grab their throat as if they are choking. They may then collapse and emit high-frequency or wheezing sounds. Alternatively, no air flow may be heard or felt with respiratory efforts (seen with chest or diaphragm excursions). It is important to note that with a foreign body caught in the pharynx, one should be careful not to lodge the object deeper. Airway obstruction may be partial or complete. With partial obstruction, some air flow from the oropharynx may be observed. Initial treatment of foreign body obstruction is via the Heimlich maneuver (*see* Fig. 13-12). (*Adapted from* American Heart Association [14]; with permission.)

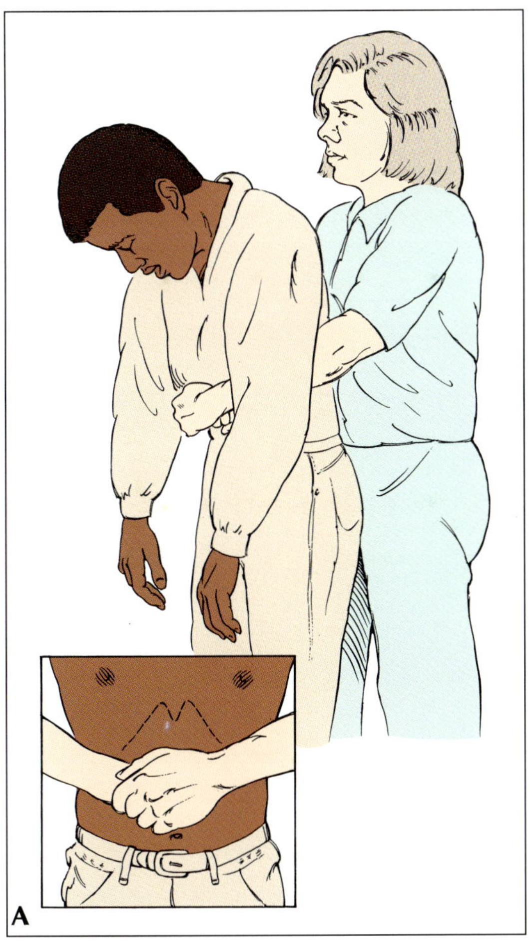

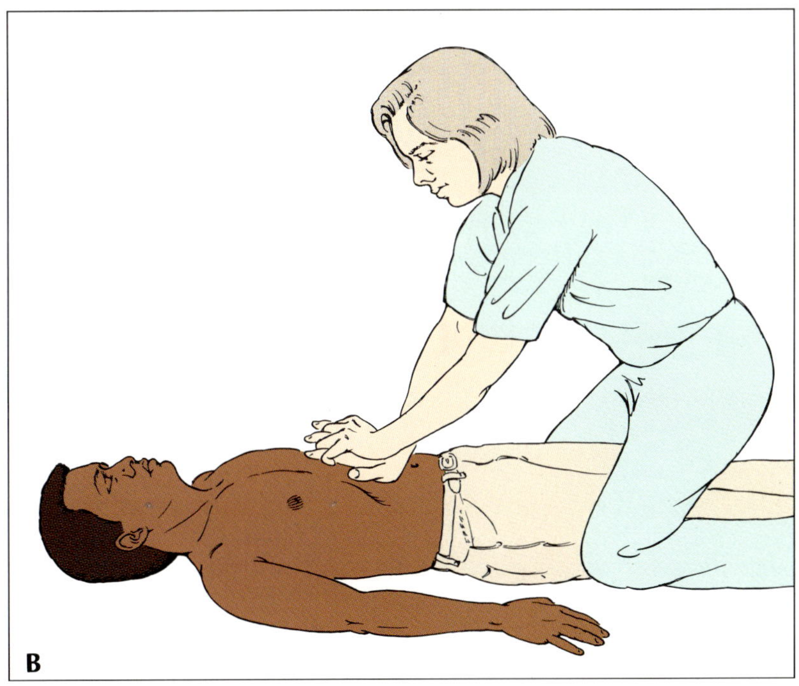

Figure 13-12. The Heimlich maneuver, a response to the universal distress signal, is performed in order to dislodge a foreign body from the airway. **A,** The Heimlich maneuver is typically performed by placing the rescuer's hands around the victim from behind, with the dominant hand held in a fist and the other hand over it, holding the wrist. From below the victim's xiphoid process, the rescuer pushes upward in an attempt to free the foreign body. **B,** Alternatively, this maneuver can be performed by straddling the supine victim and pushing upward from the abdomen to the chest. If no separate rescuer is present, the victim can perform the Heimlich maneuver by using the blunt edge of a chair to perform abdominal thrusts in a similar fashion [9,14–16]. (*Adapted from* American Heart Association [14]; with permission.)

Advanced Cardiac Life Support

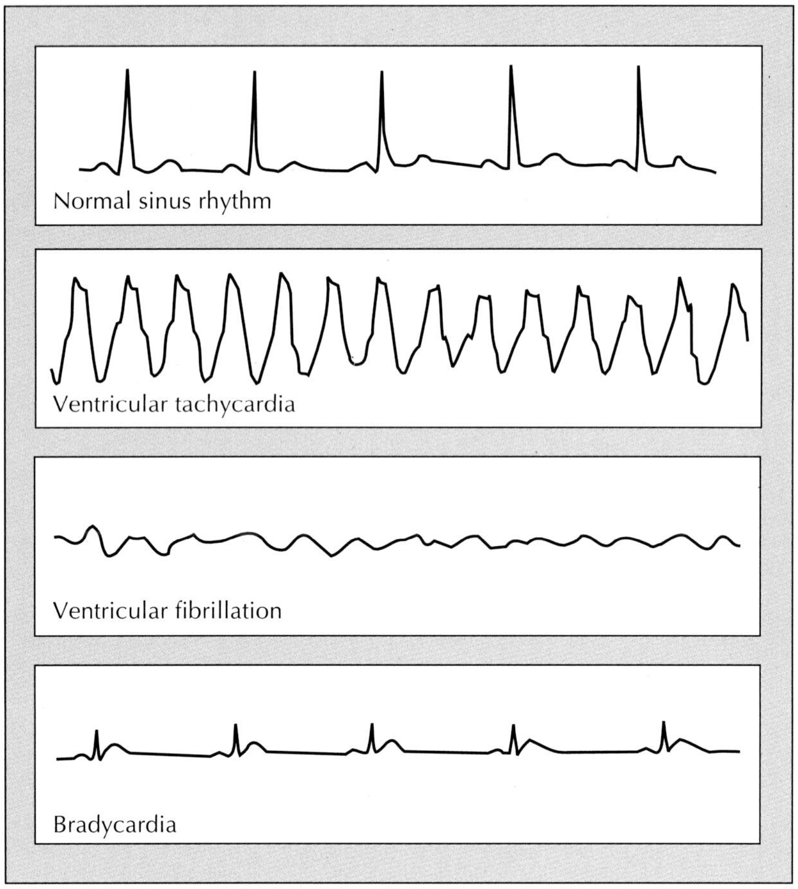

Figure 13-13. In contrast to basic cardiac life support, advanced cardiac life support (ACLS) requires additional training, tools, and certification by the American Heart Association. Techniques include insertion of central venous catheters, pharmacologic and electrical management of cardiac arrhythmias, and treatment of acute myocardial infarction and hypothermia. Personnel providing ACLS must be able to recognize significant arrhythmias, and pattern recognition is an integral part of ACLS training. Difficulty in distinguishing asystole from ventricular fibrillation should be approached initially using the asystole algorithm (*see* Fig. 13-17); if sinus rhythm is not restored, defibrillation should then be performed as a last resort [17].

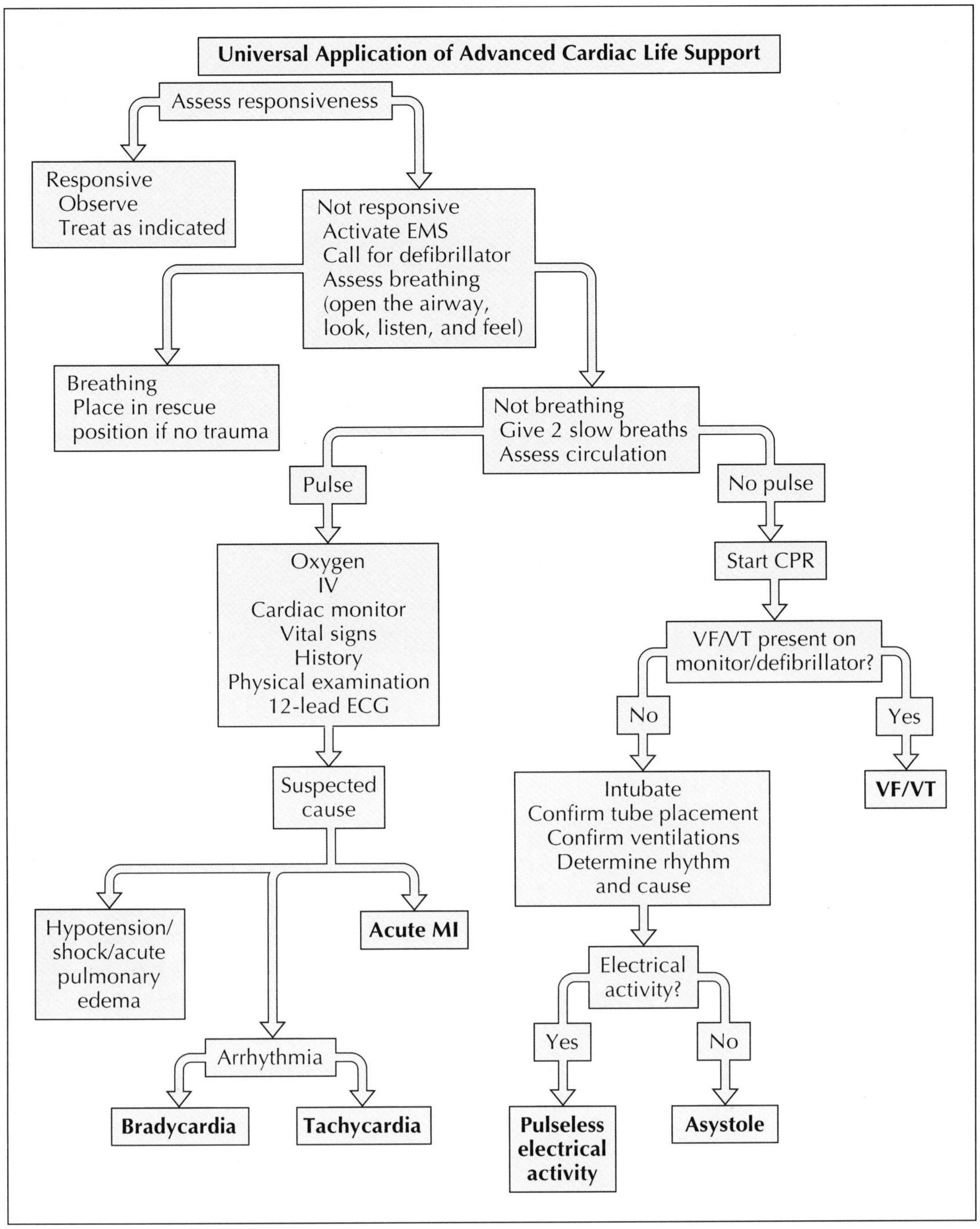

FIGURE **13-14.** Initial approach to advanced cardiac life support (ACLS). With this universal algorithm, rescuers can assess the particular arrhythmia and proceed with the appropriate resuscitative efforts. In addition to this universal algorithm, approaches to specific cardiovascular conditions (*bold print*) and to hypothermia appear in Figs. 13-15 through 13-22. ECG—electrocardiogram; EMS—emergency medical system; IV—intravenous; MI—myocardial infarction; VF—ventricular fibrillation; VT—ventricular tachycardia. (*Adapted from* American Heart Association [14]; with permission.)

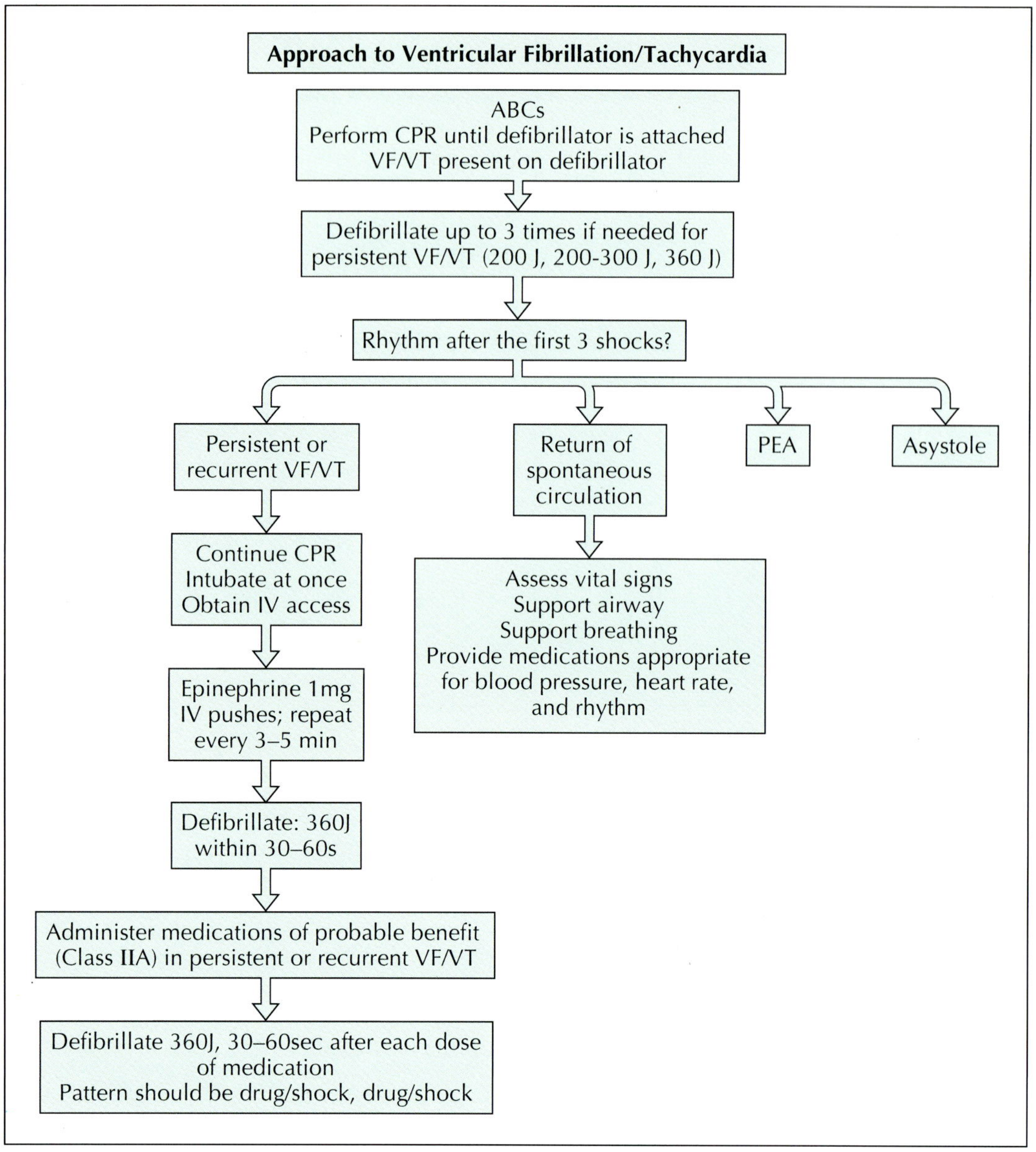

FIGURE 13-15. The third link in the chain of survival is early defibrillation, which is essential to a successful resuscitation. Within 4 minutes of cardiac arrest, central nervous system damage can occur and may be irreversible after 10 minutes. If unstable ventricular tachycardia (VT) or ventricular fibrillation (VF) is detected, the rescuer should deliver as many as three shocks of up to 360 J [14,18–23]. (*See* Figs. 13-16 and 13-17 for approaches to pulseless electrical activity [PEA] and asystole, respectively.) ABC—airway, breathing, circulation; IV—intravenous. (*Adapted from* American Heart Association [14]; with permission.)

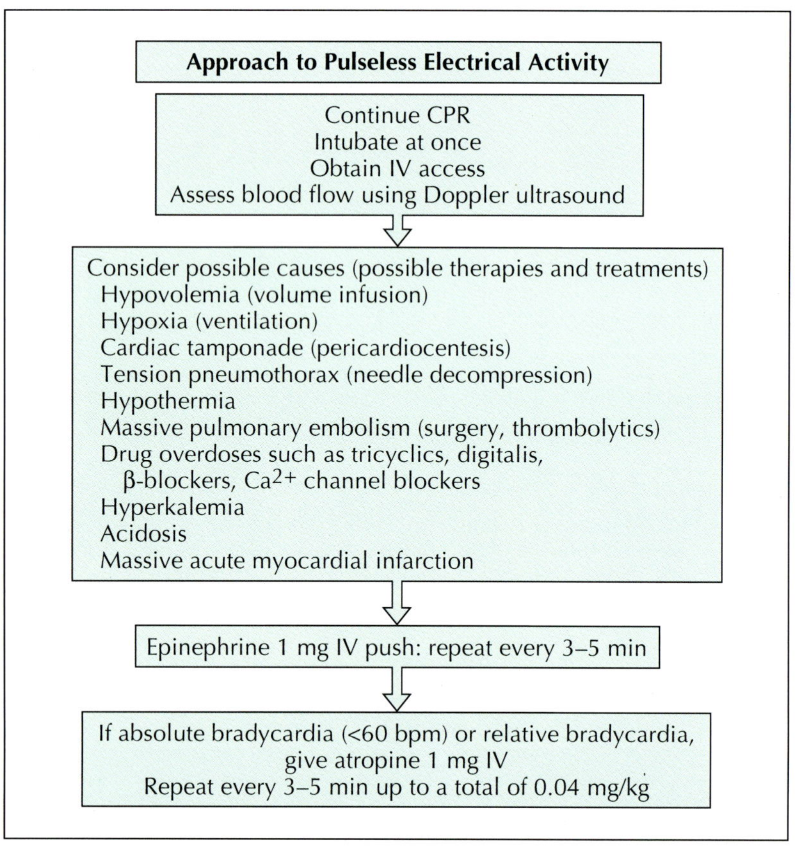

FIGURE 13-16. The absence of a palpable pulse with the presence of electrical activity (not asystole, ventricular tachycardia, or ventricular fibrillation) is known as pulseless electrical activity. This condition has many causes, such as electromechanical dissociation (EMD); pseudo-EMD; and idioventricular, ventricular escape, brady asystolic, and postdefibrillation idioventricular rhythms. When the specific cause is identified, appropriate therapy should be promptly administered [14,16]. IV—intravenous. (*Adapted from* American Heart Association [14]; with permission.)

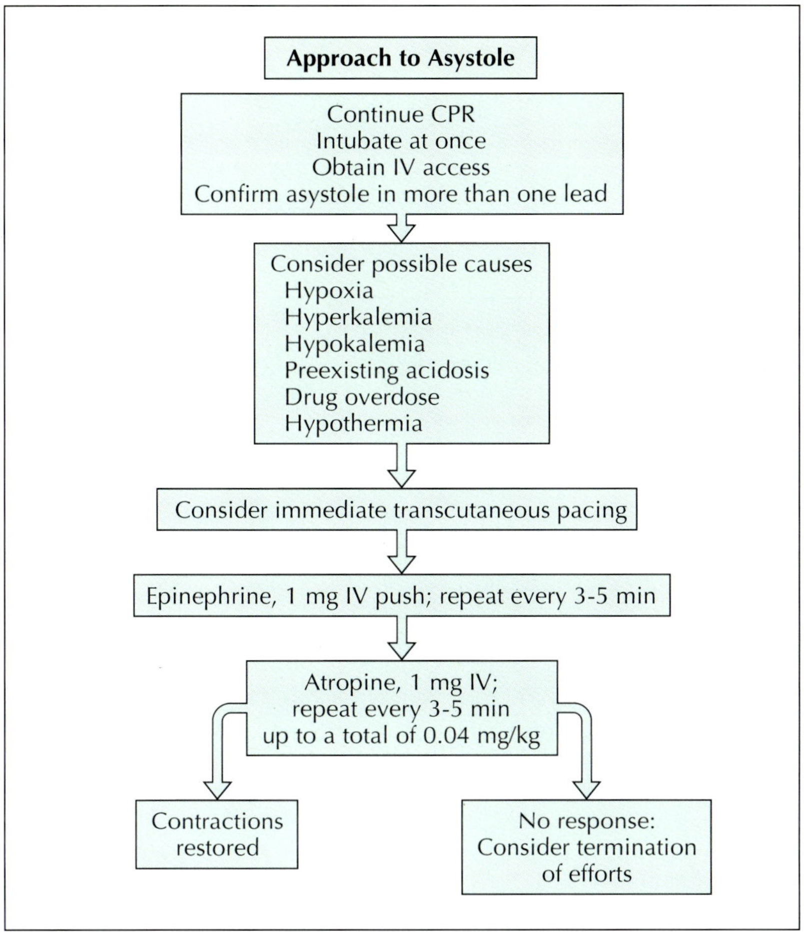

FIGURE 13-17. Asystole requires a rapid diagnosis and aggressive treatment, with atropine being the treatment of choice. If atropine or epinephrine fails to convert asystole, a transcutaneous or transvenous pacemaker may be necessary to provoke effective myocardial contractions. This is possible only if myocardial capture can be achieved. In addition, defibrillation should be considered in light of the possibility that fine ventricular fibrillation was misdiagnosed as asystole. IV—intravenous. (*Adapted from* American Heart Association *[14]; with permission.)*

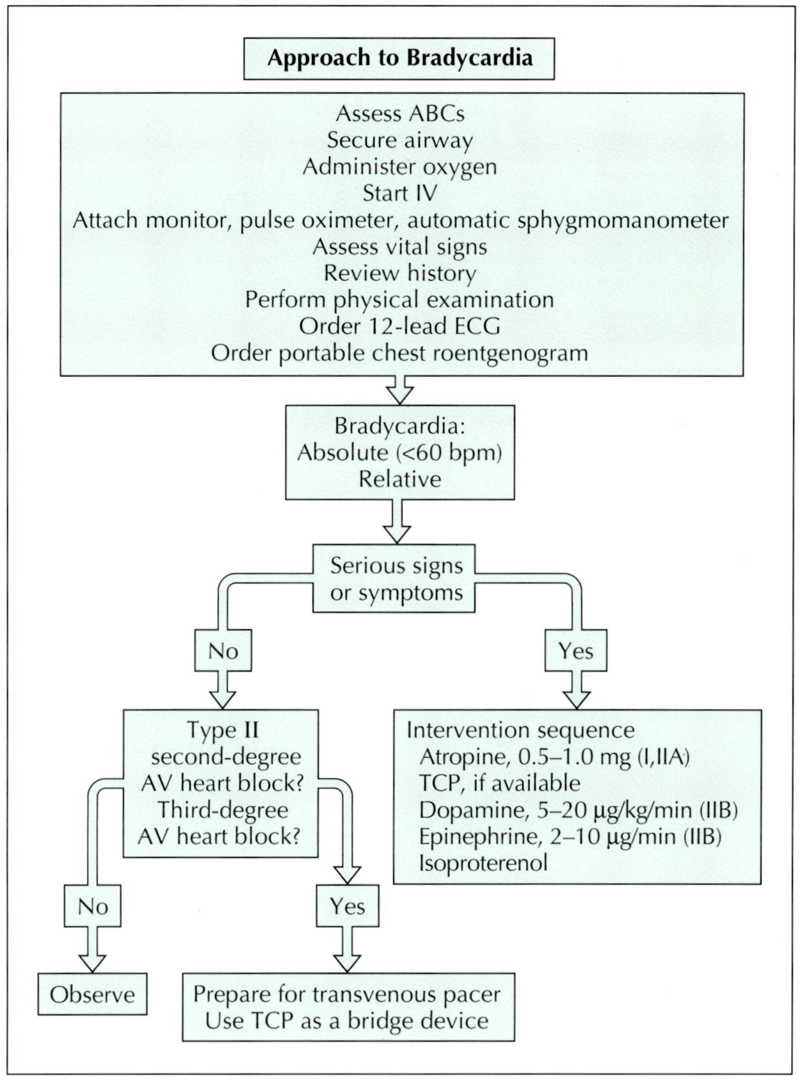

FIGURE 13-18. Advanced cardiac life support distinguishes two different types of bradycardia: absolute and relative. *Absolute* bradycardia is defined as less than 60 heart beats per minute; *relative* bradycardia varies according to the degree of the person's athletic participation. Treatment is initiated when symptoms of hemodynamic instability (fatigue, lightheadedness, dizziness, and syncope) or high-grade atrioventricular (AV) block are present (*ie,* complete heart block or Mobitz type II second-degree AV block). ABC—airway, breathing, circulation; ECG—electrocardiogram; IV—intravenous; TCP—transcutaneous pacing. (*Adapted from* American Heart Association [14]; with permission.)

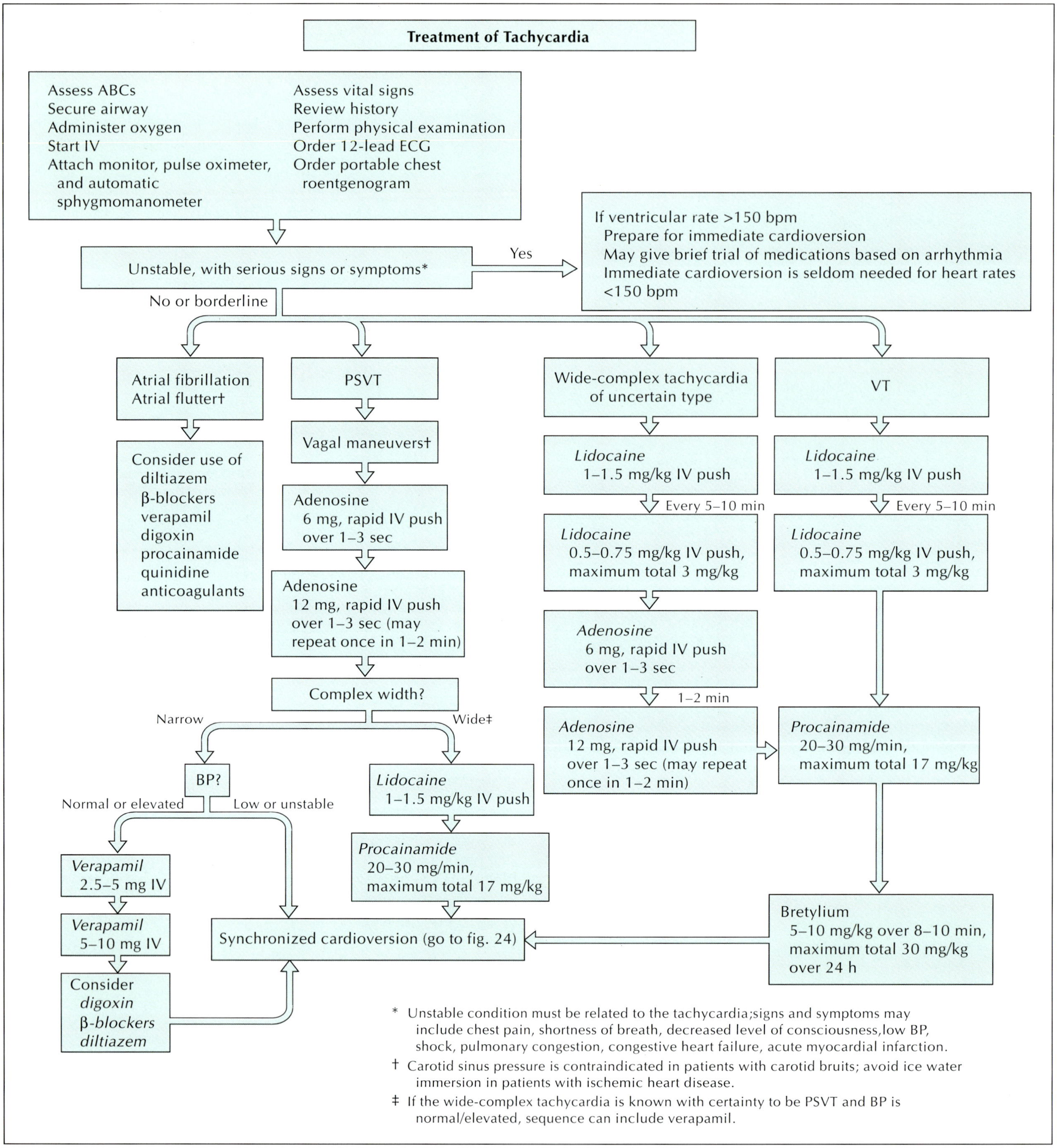

FIGURE 13-19. A comprehensive algorithm can be applied to both supraventricular and ventricular tachycardias (VT). If the tachycardia is unstable, then immediate cardioversion/defibrillation is required. Asymptomatic patients may require pharmacotherapy, antitachycardia pacing, and/or cardioversion depending on the particular arrhythmia. Adenosine can be cautiously administered to help distinguish wide from narrow complex tachycardias. One must realize however, that certain VTs may be adenosine sensitive and therefore terminate after administration. Procainamide also may be useful in terminating a tachycardia of unclear etiology [14,16,24,25]. ABC—airway, breathing, circulation; ECG—electrocardiogram; IV—intravenous. (*Adapted from* American Heart Association [14]; with permission.)

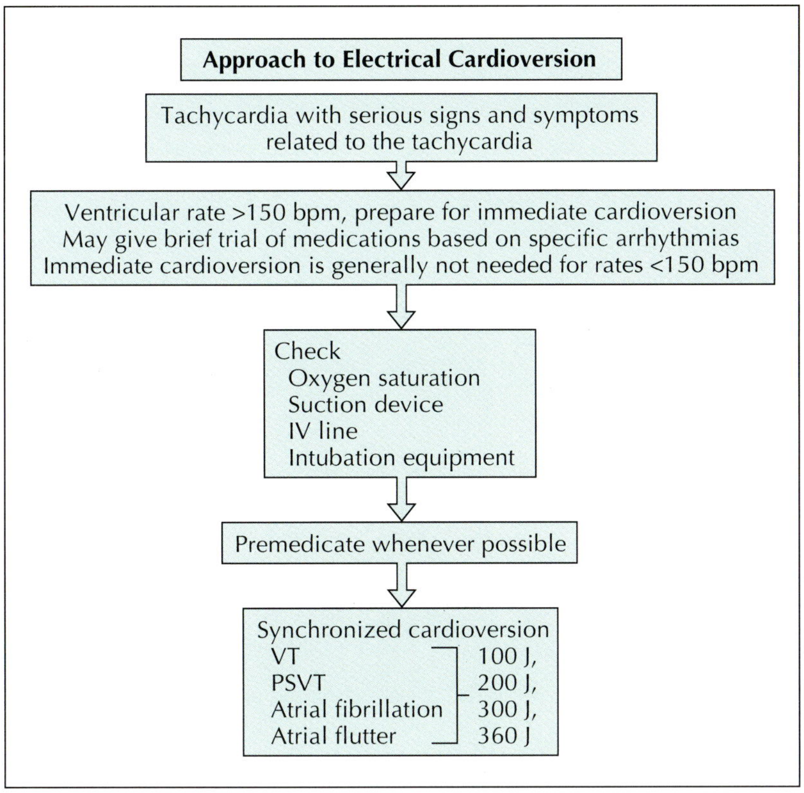

FIGURE 13-20. Cardioversion is the delivery of high-voltage, direct current (energy) synchronized to the R wave. In general, the more organized the rhythm, the less energy is required. For example, ventricular tachycardia (VT) can usually convert at a lower energy level than ventricular fibrillation. Pharmacologic therapy and CPR should continue while preparing for cardioversion/defibrillation. Intravenous (IV) access and electrocardiographic (ECG) monitoring should be performed before cardioversion/defibrillation. This monitoring can be performed with "first-look" or "quick-look" paddles or a standard ECG/telemetry system. Any hemodynamically stable tachyarrhythmia that is refractory to pharmacologic therapy or antitachycardia pacing should undergo cardioversion [14,16,25]. PSVT—paroxysmal supraventricular tachycardia. (*Adapted from* American Heart Association [14]; with permission.)

MEDICATIONS USED DURING ADVANCED CARDIAC LIFE SUPPORT

MEDICATION	INDICATIONS	DOSING	INFUSION RATE	SIDE EFFECTS
Lidocaine	First line Ventricular tachycardia, ventricular fibrillation	1 mg/kg bolus 0.5 mg/kg every 8–10 min; maximum of 3 mg/kg	1–4 mg/min	Nervous system Paresthesias Seizures Confusion
Procainamide	Second line Ventricular tachycardia, ventricular fibrillation	100 mg over 5 min; 20 mg/min until arrhythmia terminates	1–4 mg/min	Hypertension; torsade de pointes
Bretylium	Third line Ventricular tachycardia, ventricular fibrillation	5 mg/kg	If VF persists, 10 mg/kg at 15–30 min intervals; maximum 30 mg/kg	Hypertension initially, then hypotension
Adenosine	Paroxysmal supraventricular tachycardia	6-mg bolus followed by 12-mg bolus in 5 min		Atrial fibrillation; transvenous heart block; dyspnea; chest discomfort
Magnesium	Ventricular tachycardia; ventricular fibrillation	1–2 g (8–16 mEq), over 5–60 min	0.5–1 g (4–8 mEq) over 24 h	Diarrhea
Diltiazem	Second line paroxysmal supraventricular tachycardia	0.25 mg/kg (over 2 min) followed by 0.35 mg/kg (over 2 min) in 15 min if response inadequate	5–15 mg/h	Congestive heart failure; heart block
Verapamil	Second line paroxysmal supraventricular tachycardia	2.5, 5 mg, long bolus		Congestive heart failure; heart block
Atropine	Symptomatic sinus bradycardia/asystole	0.5 mg/min bolus to 2 mg total dose		Heart block; acceleration of tachycardia
Epinephrine	Initial cardiac arrest drug, regardless of rhythm (pressor/α_1, β_1, β_2)	0.5–1 mg bolus may be required every 5 min		Potential for ischemia
Norepinephrine	Pressor support (α_1, α_2, β_1)		0.5–1 µg/min, titrated to effect	Potential for ischemia
Dopamine	Pressor support (α_1, β_1, dopamine)		0.5–10 µg/kg/min, depending on effect	Potential for ischemia

FIGURE 13-21. Drugs that are commonly used as a part of the advanced cardiac life support protocol. A more comprehensive explanation of each medication may be found in the *Physicians Desk Reference* [26] or in Goodman and Gilman's *Pharmacological Basis of Therapeutics* [14,16,27–49].

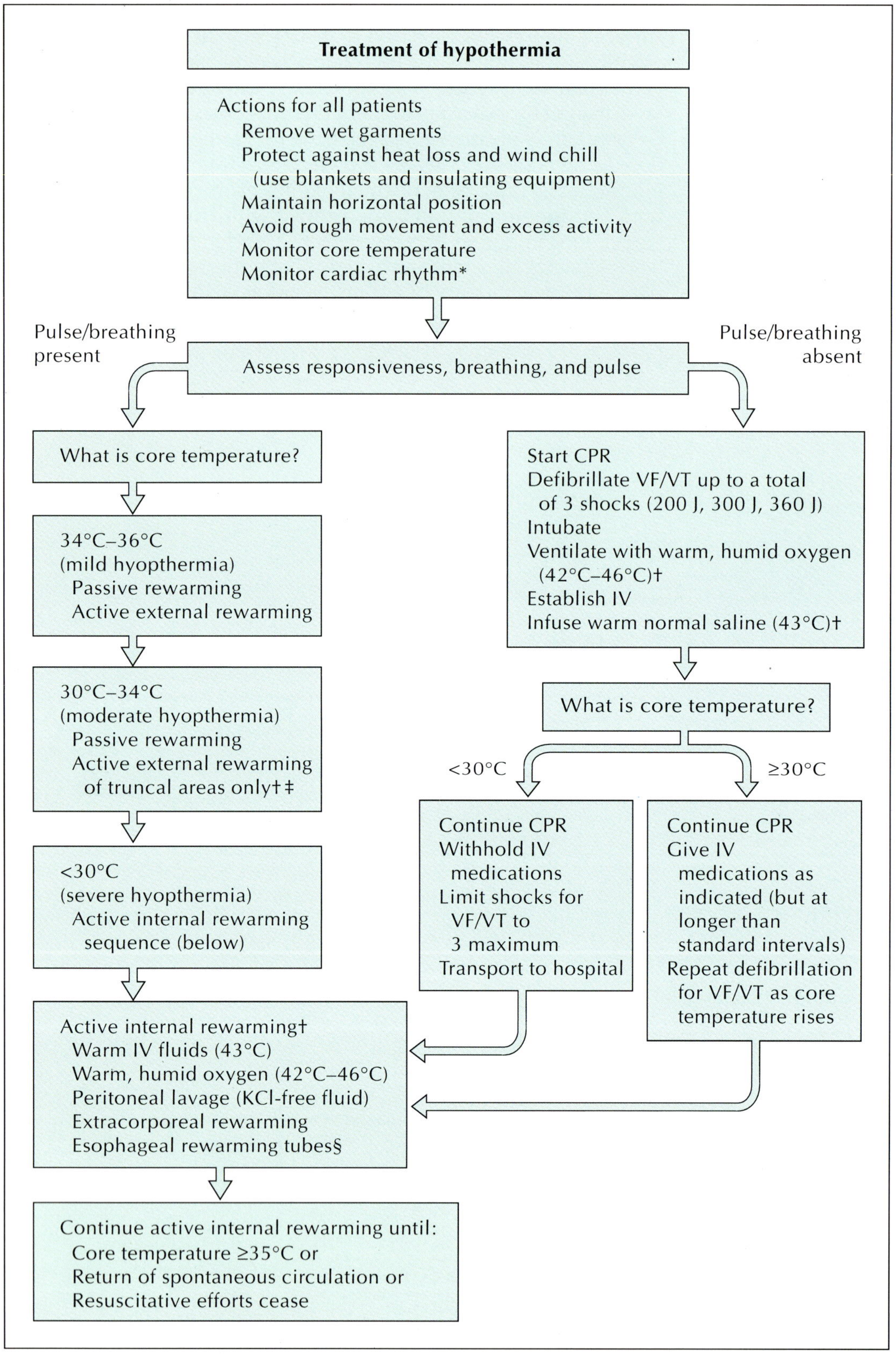

FIGURE 13-22. Hypothermia is defined as the syndrome of circulatory collapse that occurs when the core body temperature drops below 30°C (86°F). Signs include reduced cardiac output, decreased arterial pressure, and a marked depression in cerebral blood flow and oxygen requirement. The electrocardiogram may show characteristic bradycardia with Osborne waves. Despite severely depressed cardiac and pulmonary function at initial assessment, full resuscitative efforts should be performed and may result in a good outcome [14,16]. *Asterisk* indicates that needle electrodes through the skin may be required. *Daggers* highlight interventions that many experts think should be done only in-hospital, although practices vary. *Double daggers* indicate methods such as electric or charcoal warming devices, hot water bottles, heating pads, radiant heart sources, and warming beds. *Section mark* indicates that these are used internationally and should become available in the United States. IV—intravenous; VF—ventricular fibrillation; VT—ventricular tachycardia. (*Adapted from* American Heart Association [14]; with permission.)

INTERPOSED ABDOMINAL COUNTERPULSATION CPR

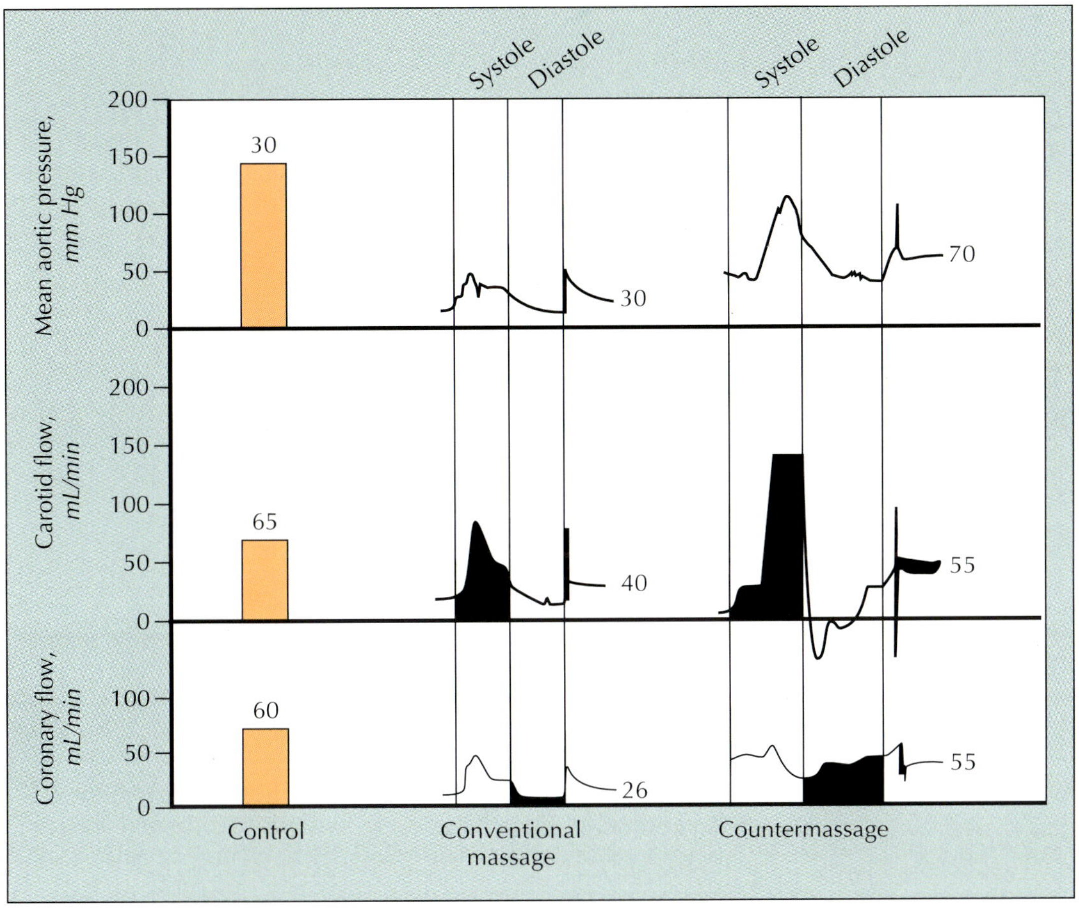

FIGURE 13-23. Many investigators have tried to improve on standard manual CPR over the past three decades. Techniques include military antishock trouser (MAST), high-impulse CPR, cough CPR, mechanical thumper CPR, interposed abdominal counterpulsation CPR, circumferential pneumatic vest CPR, and active compression-decompression CPR. The latter three methods have recently been shown helpful in augmenting cardiopulmonary circulation [11–13,50–72]. Ohomoto *et al.* [11] described a method of CPR in which external compressions would alternate between the chest and abdomen. This method, termed *interposed abdominal counterpulsation CPR* (IAC-CPR), purportedly increases regional perfusion by compressing the abdominal aorta and altering thoracoabdominal pressure. Coronary and carotid arterial blood flow, cardiac output, and aortic pressure were augmented by IAC-CPR when compared with conventional CPR in a canine model. (*Adapted from* Ohomoto and coworkers [11]; with permission.)

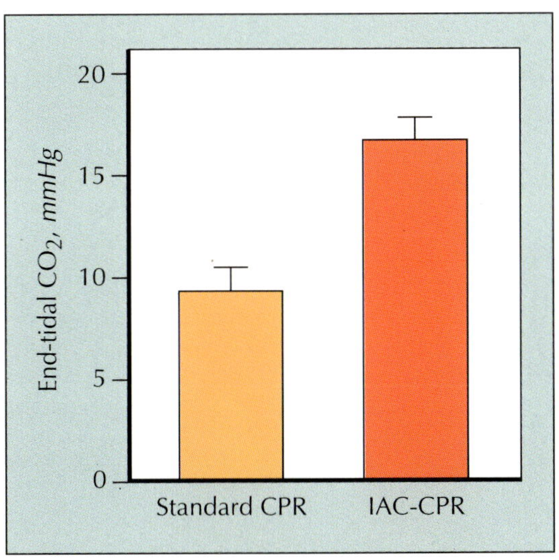

FIGURE 13-24. Ward *et al.* [65] conducted a randomized study comparing end-tidal CO_2 ($ETCO_2$) between patients receiving standard CPR and interposed abdominal counterpulsation CPR (IAC-CPR). $ETCO_2$ is the measure of pulmonary flow which also correlates with increased coronary artery perfusion. This study demonstrated an increase in $ETCO_2$ from 9.6 mm Hg with standard CPR to 17.1 mm Hg with IAC-CPR (an increase of 78%). An improvement in initial resuscitation was seen as well [52,65]. (*Adapted from* Ward and coworkers [65]; with permission.)

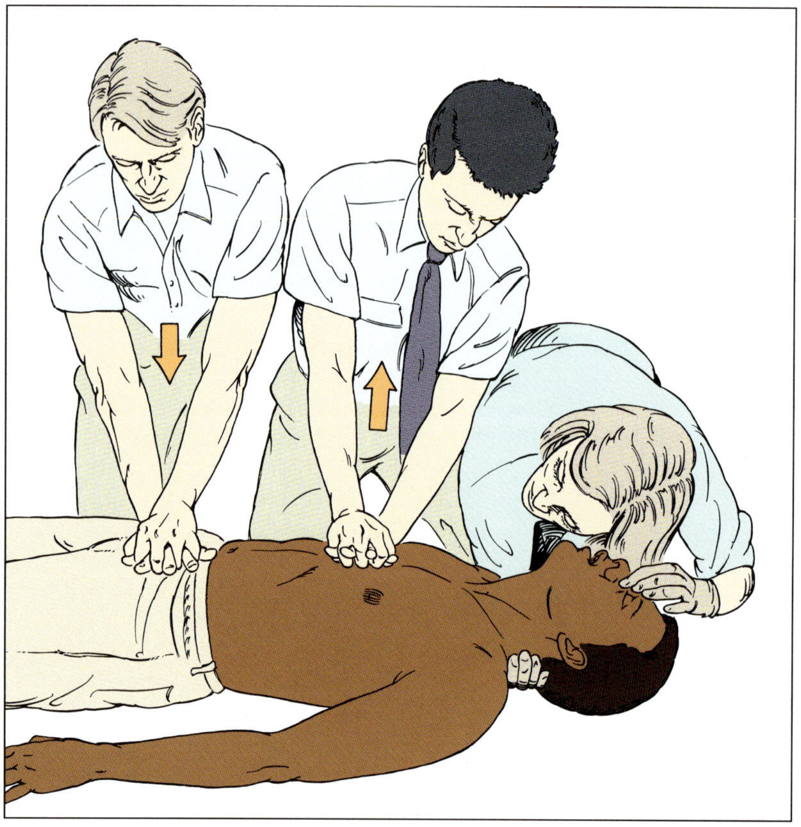

FIGURE 13-25. At least two rescuers are necessary to perform interposed abdominal counterpulsation CPR. One rescuer actively compresses the chest while the other allows for passive decompression of the abdomen. Next the abdomen is actively compressed while the chest is allowed to passively decompress. A third rescuer (or potentially one of the two rescuers) performs ventilation. (*Adapted from* Voorhees and coworkers [66]; with permission.)

CIRCUMFERENTIAL PNEUMATIC VEST CPR

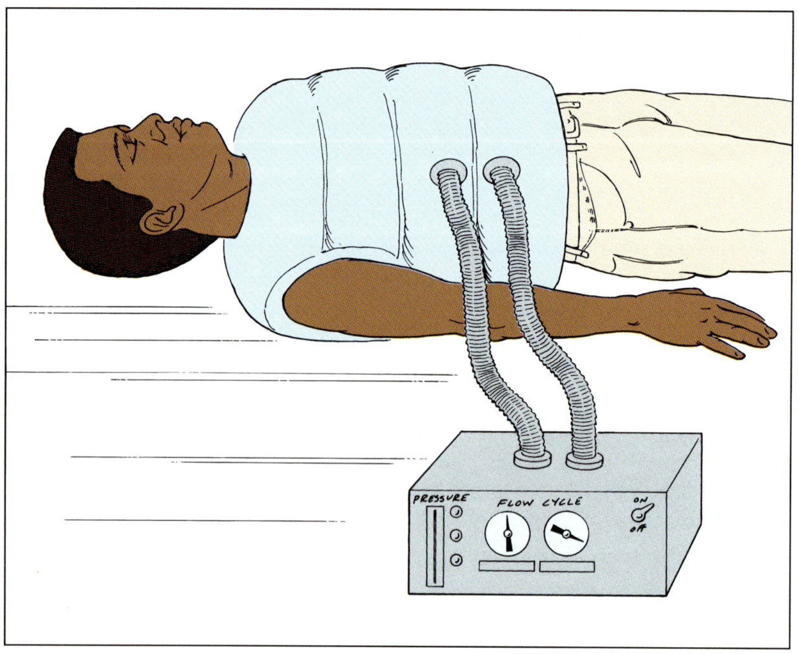

FIGURE 13-26. Halperin *et al.* [12] introduced a method of CPR that produced high intrathoracic pressure without the need for simultaneous ventilation. This method, *circumferential pneumatic vest CPR*, uses a vest that inflates and deflates to change intrathoracic pressure [12,67]. The vest is computer driven and pressure is applied up to 250 mm Hg. As intrathoracic pressures rises, a pressure increase is also seen in the intrathoracic vascular structures. This increase is directly proportional to blood flow. At a vest pressure of 250 mm Hg, cerebral blood flow was maintained at the same levels as before cardiac arrest in a canine model [12].

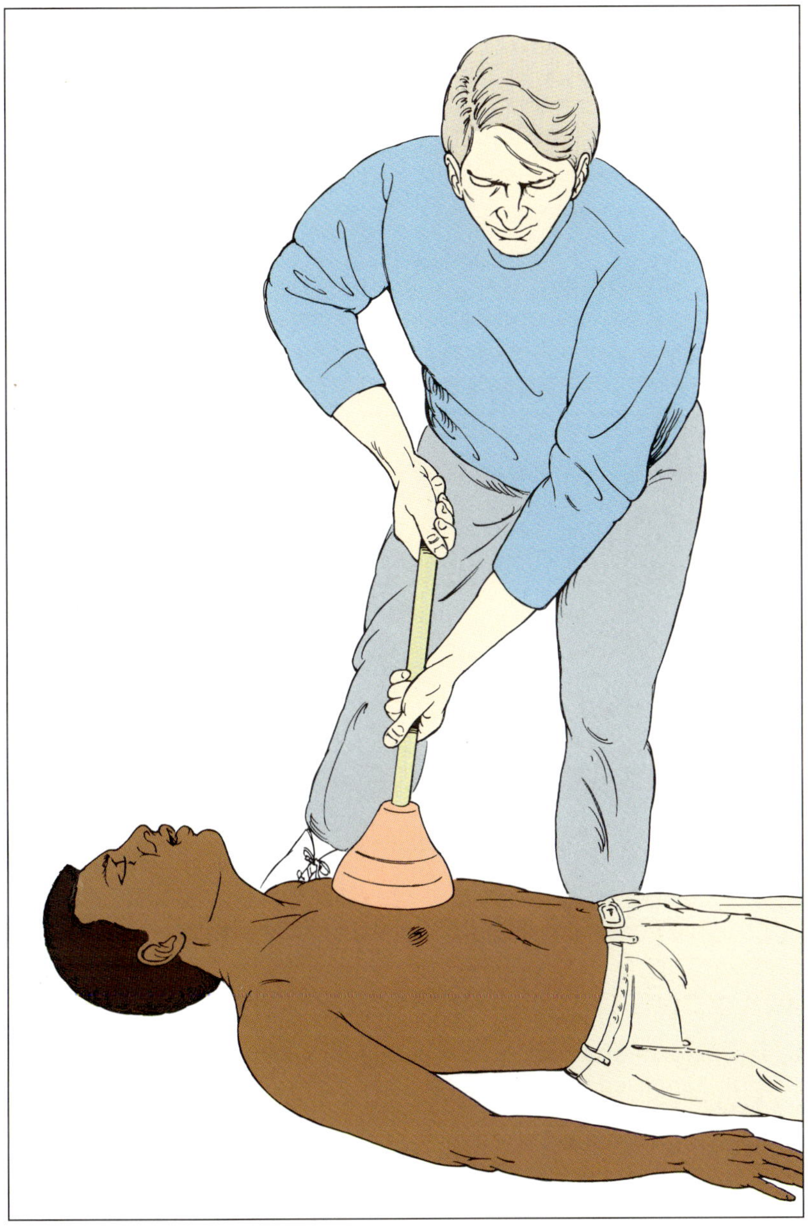

FIGURE 13-27. A third method of CPR was developed after reports of successful resuscitation with a toilet plunger. A 65-year-old man with a history of severe coronary artery disease collapsed. His son attempted manual CPR but was not trained in its use. When his father showed no response, he remembered that 6 months earlier his mother had resuscitated him with a toilet plunger. He then plunged the sternum above his father's heart for 10 minutes until the emergency medical service arrived [12]. This event sparked development of the technique known as *active compression-decompression CPR* (ACD-CPR) [68,69].

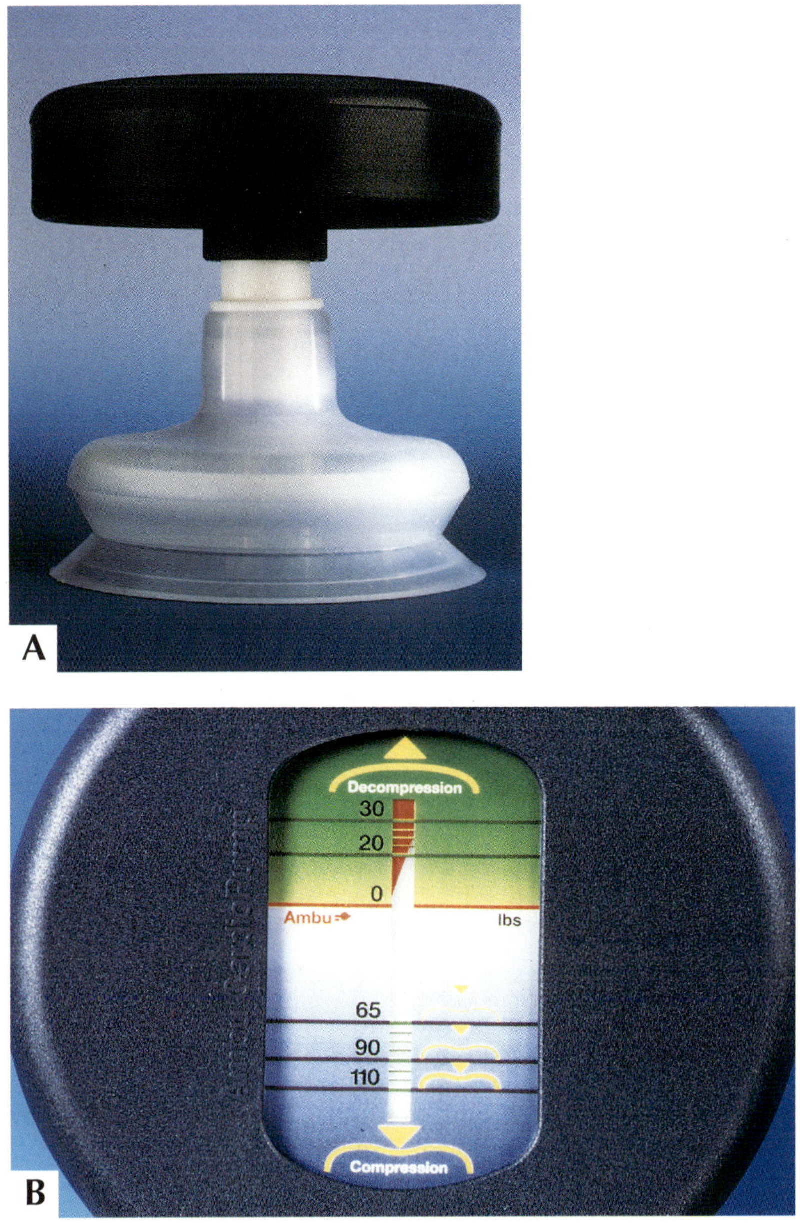

FIGURE 13-28. **A,** Cohen *et al.* [13] designed an active compression-decompression device called the Cardiopump (AMBU International, Copenhagen, Denmark). This device has a suction cup and piston attached to a horizontal undercut handle. **B,** A gauge on top measures the force of compression and decompression and helps guide the rescuer to the proper performance of this technique [13,70,71].

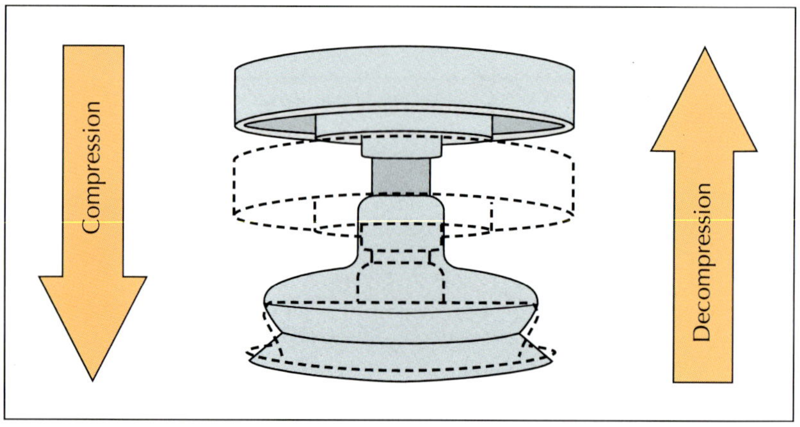

FIGURE 13-29. Active compression-decompression CPR is performed using guidelines for compression that are recommended by the American Heart Association. The Cardiopump is placed midsternum at the level of the nipples. The elbows are outstretched and locked (similar to standard manual CPR), with two hands on the device. Eighty to 100 compressions are performed per minute at 1 1/2- to 2-inch depths [13,70,71].

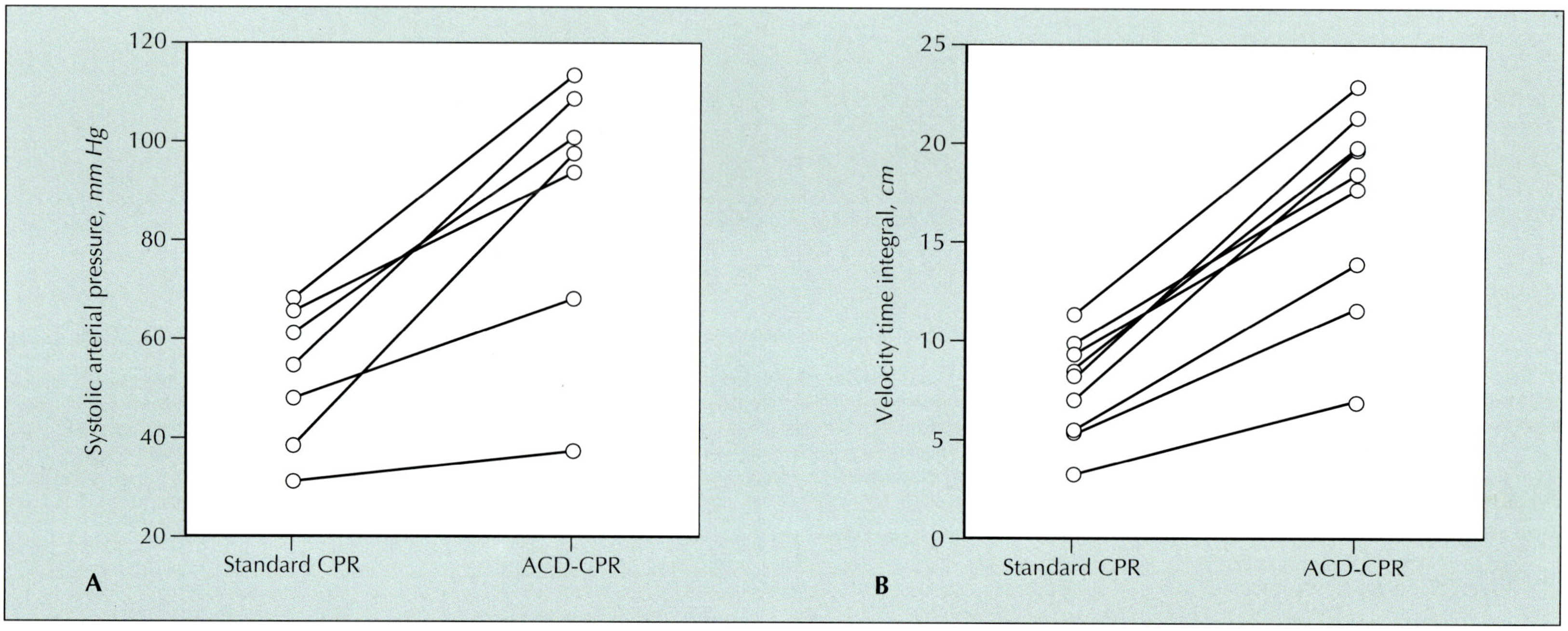

FIGURE 13-30. **A,** Femoral arterial pressures were monitored in nine out of 10 patients enrolled in a study of the effects of active compression-decompression CPR (ACD-CPR) [13]. The systolic arterial pressure showed an increase from 52.5±14.0 mm Hg using standard CPR to 88.9±24.7 mm Hg with ACD-CPR ($P<0.003$). **B,** The velocity time integral, which is a direct analog of cardiac output, increased from 7.3±2.6 cm with standard CPR to 17.5±5.6 cm with ACD-CPR ($P<0.0001$). Values are mean±SD. (*Adapted from* Cohen and coworkers [13]; with permission.)

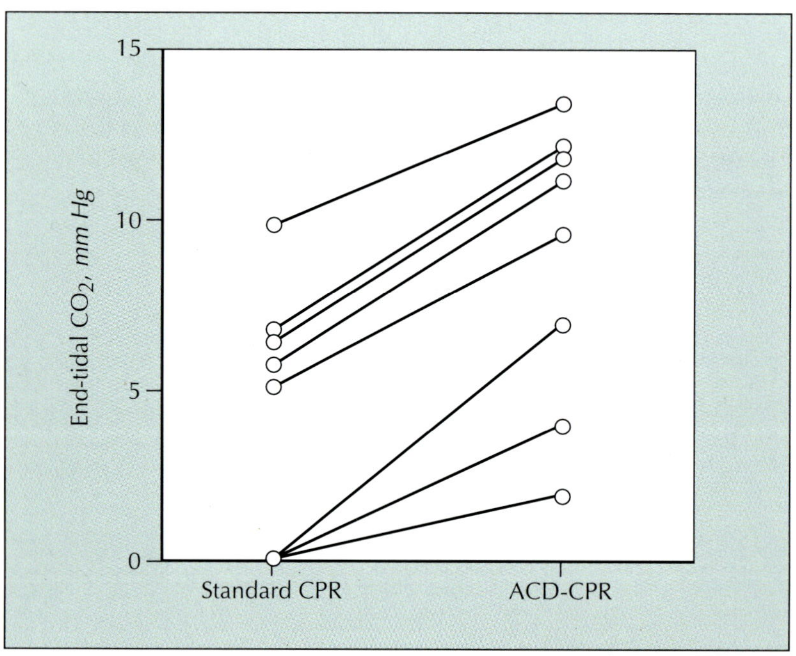

FIGURE 13-31. In the same study, active compression-decompression CPR (ACD-CPR) increased levels of end-tidal CO_2 ($ETCO_2$). With standard CPR $ETCO_2$ was 4.3±3.8 mm Hg as opposed to 9.0±3.9 mm Hg with ACD-CPR ($P<0.0001$). The average ACD-CPR $ETCO_2$ concentration is associated with a 28% chance of initial resuscitation compared with the 1% chance shown by standard CPR. Values are mean±SD. (*Adapted from* Cohen and coworkers [13]; with permission.)

A. ENDPOINTS OF STANDARD VS ACTIVE COMPRESSION-DECOMPRESSION CPR

ENDPOINT	ACD-CPR *N(%)*	STANDARD CPR, *N(%)*	*P* VALUE
Resuscitation	18(62)	10(30)	<0.03
24-h survival	13(45)	3(11)	<0.004
Neurologic outcome, Glasgow Coma Score	8.0±1.3	3.5±0.3	<0.02

B. ENDPOINTS OF STANDARD VS VEST CPR

ENDPOINT	ACD-CPR, *N(%)*	STANDARD CPR, *N(%)*	*P* VALUE
Spontaneous return of circulation	8(47)	3(17.6)	NS
24-h survival	3(18)	1(6)	NS
Hospital discharge	0	0	NS

FIGURE 13-32. A, Summary of the clinical endpoints of a randomized prospective comparison of standard (n=33) versus active compression-decompression CPR (n=29) during in-hospital resuscitation [72]. **B,** Data from a recent trial of standard (n=17) versus circumferential pneumatic vest CPR (n=17) [12].

COMPARISON OF ALTERNATIVES TO STANDARD CPR

VARIABLE	INTERPOSED ABDOMINAL COUNTERPULSATION	CIRCUMFERENTIAL PNEUMATIC VEST	ACTIVE COMPRESSION-DECOMPRESSION
Complexity	++	++++	+
Energy required	++++	++	+++
Set-up time	+	++++	|
Consistency	++	++++	++++
Potential to shock without stopping CPR	0	++++	++++
Need to augment ventilation	+	+	++++
Cost	0	++++	+
Minimum number of operators	++	+	+

FIGURE 13-33. A comparison of standard CPR with its alternatives with respect to complexity, cost, start-up time, and so on. These techniques have shown improved resuscitation and circulation and have proven to be important adjuncts to standard CPR. *Plus signs* indicate relative amounts.

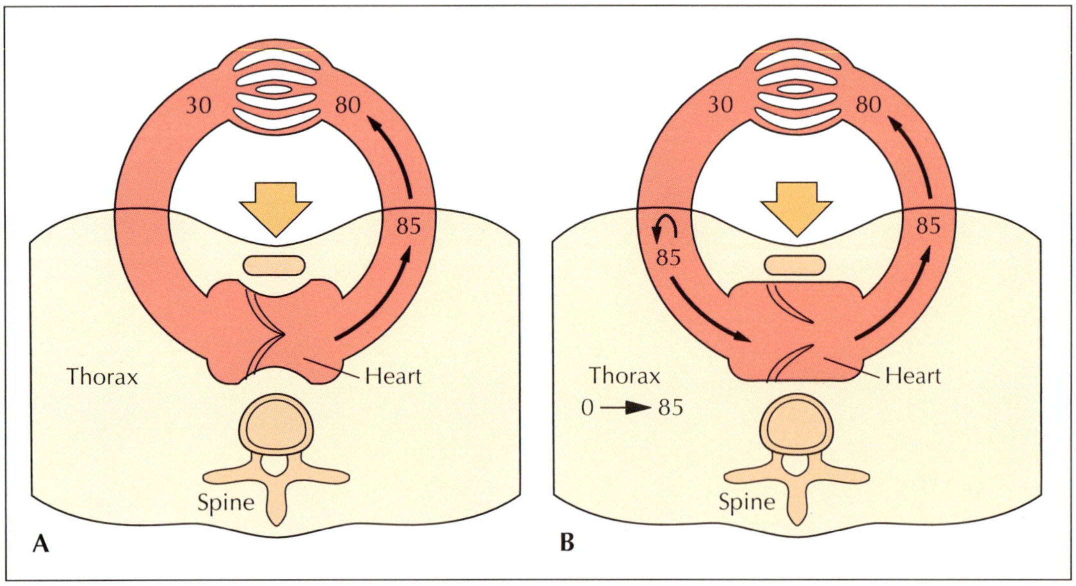

Figure 13-34. The mechanism behind CPR has continually intrigued researchers. In the past 20 years two major theories have been developed to explain this mechanism: the *cardiac pump theory* and the *thoracic pump theory* [73]. **A,** The cardiac pump theory states that compression of the heart between the sternum and spine causes forward blood flow during CPR. This theory claims that direct myocardial compressions provide for forward circulation, which causes closure of the mitral valve and opening of the aortic valve. The ventricles then fill during passive decompression (diastole) [74–76]. **B,** During the past decade research and clinical observations have brought forth an alternative, the thoracic pump theory, which proposes that an increase in intrathoracic pressure caused by chest compression is transmitted to all intrathoracic vessels and coronary chambers. The pressure gradient between the arteries and veins causes forward blood flow. The left side of the heart acts as a passive conduit for blood flow, and the mitral valve remains open during the compression phase [76–80]. Numbers represent theoretical pressures in mm Hg. All the more recent modifications on CPR (active compression-decompression CPR [ACD-CPR], circumferential pneumatic vest CPR, interposed abdominal counterpulsation CPR [IAC-CPR]) appear to augment changes in intrathoracic pressure (thoracic pump model), thus producing improved circulation. The ACD-CPR and vest CPR techniques appear to directly operate by changes in intrathoracic pressure whereas IAC-CPR has been suggested as a "primer for the thoracic pump." Much of the enhancement in ventricular filling appears to occur during chest decompression and is exaggerated with active decompression [13]. (*Adapted from* Higano and coworkers [73]; with permission.)

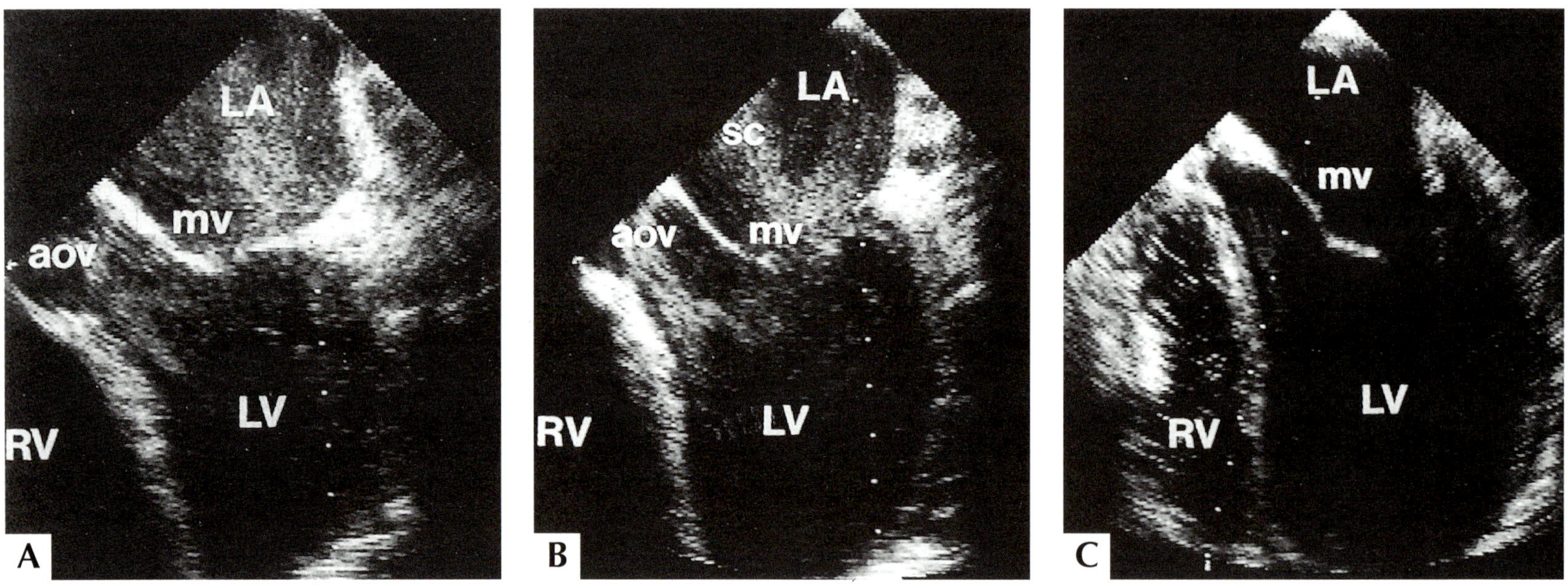

Figure 13-35. In a recent study by Redberg *et al.* [55], transesophageal echocardiography was used to produce images of blood flow during CPR. The findings showed decreased left ventricular (LV) and right ventricular (RV) cavity size, LV volume with compression, mitral valve (MV) closure with compression and opening with release, and aortic valve (AOV) opening with compression systole [55]. This figure shows four-chamber transesophageal echocardiographic views during CPR. **A,** With active compression of the chest, the RV is directly compressed and the AOV and MV are shut. **B,** During passive decompression or relaxation, the tricuspid valve opens (not shown). However, MV opening is minimal, thereby limiting ventricular filling. **C,** With active compression-decompression CPR (ACD-CPR) in the same patient, there is improved atrioventricular valve opening during active decompression, which facilitates ventricular filling. It is the author's belief that both mechanisms are operant. Transesophageal echocardiographic images obtained during standard and ACD-CPR demonstrate that direct myocardial compression does occur (supporting the cardiac pump theory) and that changes in decompression alone can augment ventricular filling, and therefore cardiac output (supporting a thoracic pump theory). Perhaps "cardiothoracic pump" theory might be the most appropriate term. LA—left atrium; SC—spontaneous contrast. (*Adapted from* Cohen and coworkers [13]; with permission.)

EXTERNAL DEFIBRILLATION

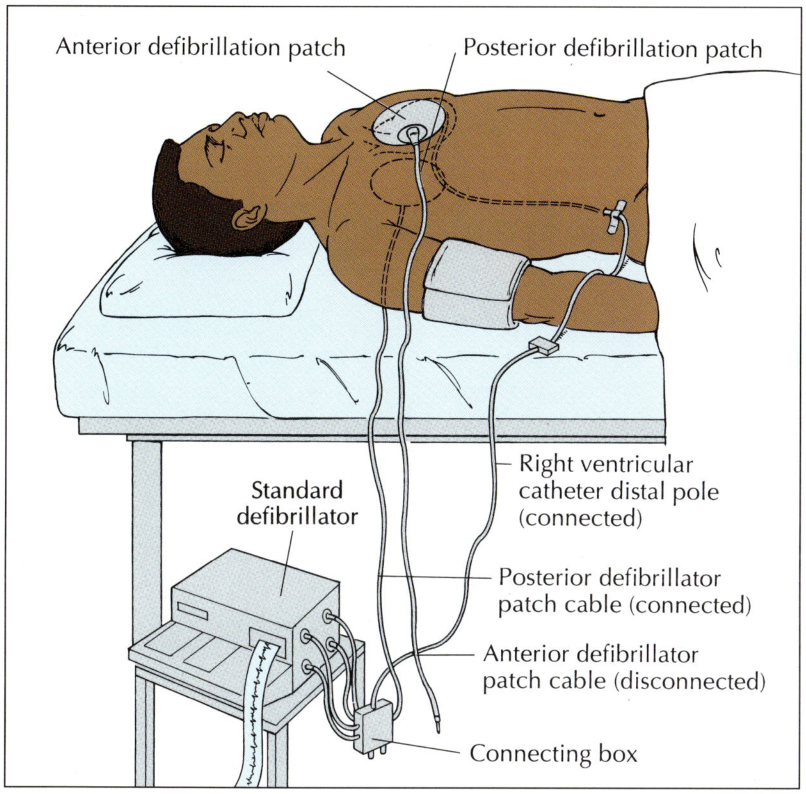

FIGURE 13-36. In 1956, Zoll *et al.* [8] were the first to demonstrate that external defibrillation can terminate ventricular tachycardia during cardiac arrest in humans. Today, external defibrillators provide paramedics and firefighters with the ability to detect and defibrillate ventricular fibrillation in the field. In a multivariate study conducted by Weaver *et al.*, firefighters were trained in the use of automatic external defibrillators. A survival rate of 30% was shown in victims to whom the firefighters delivered initial treatment as compared with 17% when the first defibrillation was performed by the later-arriving paramedics [20]. Standard defibrillators may be configured for hands-off defibrillation by using large skin patches in place of hand-held paddles, a connecting box, and a standard defibrillator. The skin patches are placed anteriorly and posteriorly. Alternatively these patches may be placed across the precordium (apex and sternum). The skin patches lead to the connecting box which, in turn, leads to the defibrillator. This method obviates paddles.

INTRACARDIAC DEFIBRILLATION

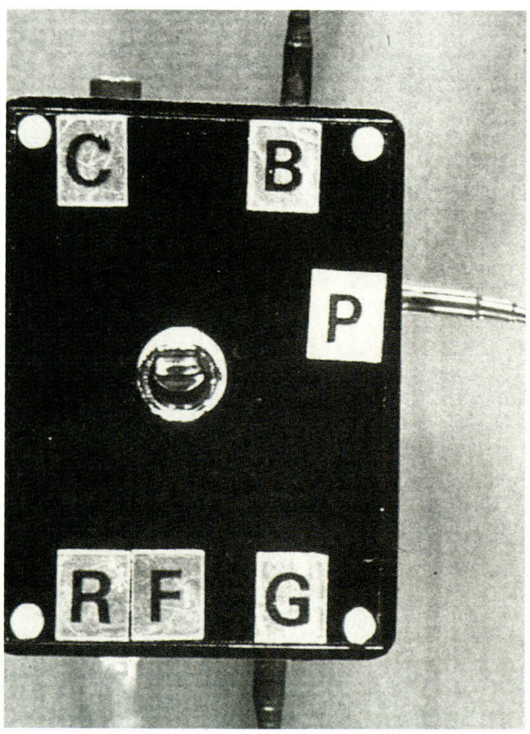

FIGURE 13-37. Intracardiac defibrillation is facilitated transthoracically via a junction box called the "Booker box," after its designer, Booker Pullen. This box is connected in series between standard defibrillation patches and the defibrillator. The switch box (toggle switch) conveys electric current between a single-piece standard right ventricular pacing catheter and the skin patches. The letters on the figure depict the particular attachments for the switch box. This technique was implemented in nine patients in the electrophysiology laboratory, all of whom were in ventricular fibrillation that was terminated with up to 300 J. (*Adapted from* Cohen and coworkers [84]; with permission.)

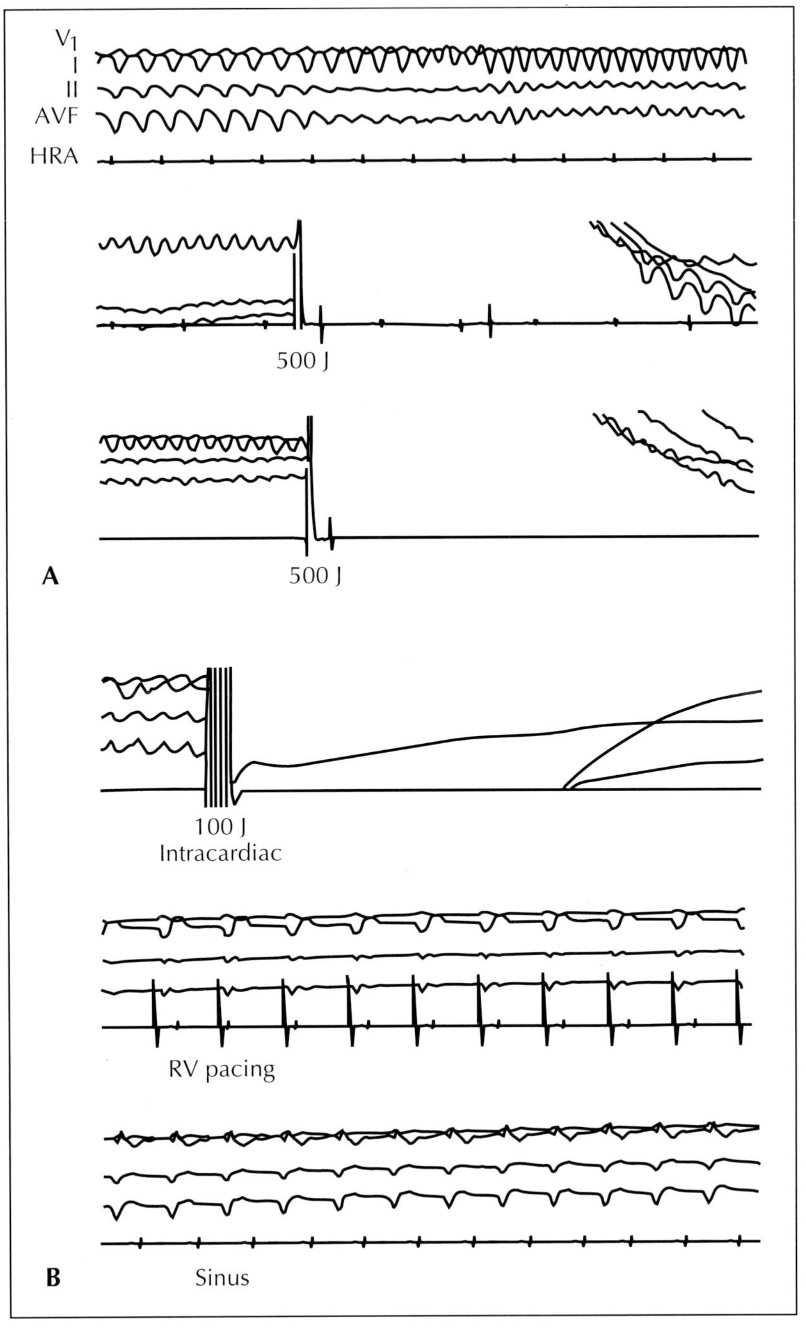

FIGURE 13-38. **A,** Electrocardiograms from a patient who developed ventricular fibrillation that was refractory to multiple standard transthoracic defibrillations. **B,** The delivery of a single intracardiac defibrillation (100 J) successfully terminated the tachycardia [81]. HRA—high right atrium; RV—right ventricular.

TRANSESOPHAGEAL DEFIBRILLATION

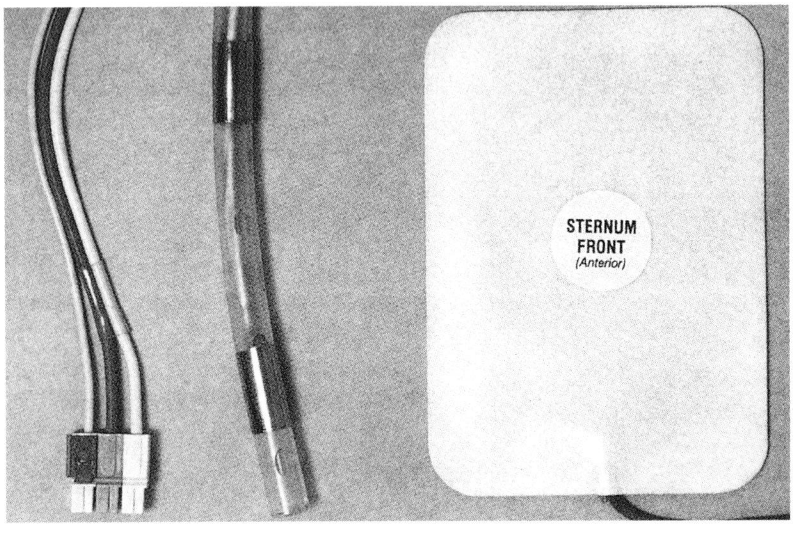

FIGURE 13-39. Transesophageal defibrillation has been described as a method of rescue defibrillation. This method is easy to perform in an intubated patient. The probe is blindly passed down the esophagus to a fixed distance and defibrillation is then performed [82]. The three elements (left to right) represent the defibrillator connector, transesophageal defibrillation probe, and a sternum skin patch, respectively.

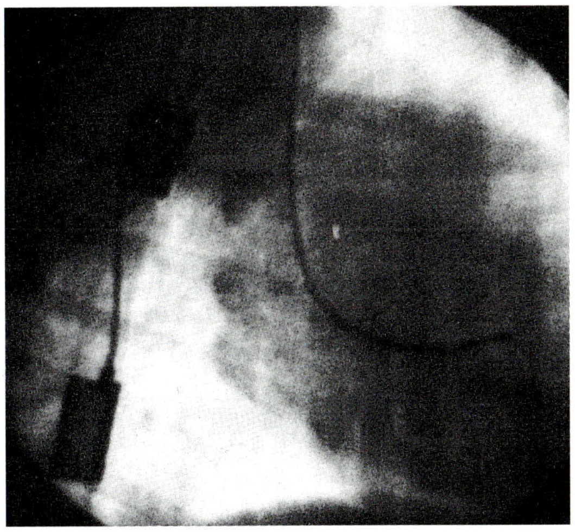

FIGURE 13-40. Transesophageal (TE) defibrillation allows for rapid placement of both proximal (P) and distal (D) electrodes in intubated patients. This technique was successful in terminating ventricular fibrillation (late during cardiac arrest) in five out of five patients. The TE probe is compatible with standard transthoracic defibrillation and pacing equipment. Electrical signals from the atria and ventricles can be recorded and cardiac pacing can be performed from the esophagus. (*Adapted from* Cohen and coworkers [82]; with permission.)

EMERGENCY SIMULTANEOUS TRANSTHORACIC AND EPICARDIAL DEFIBRILLATION

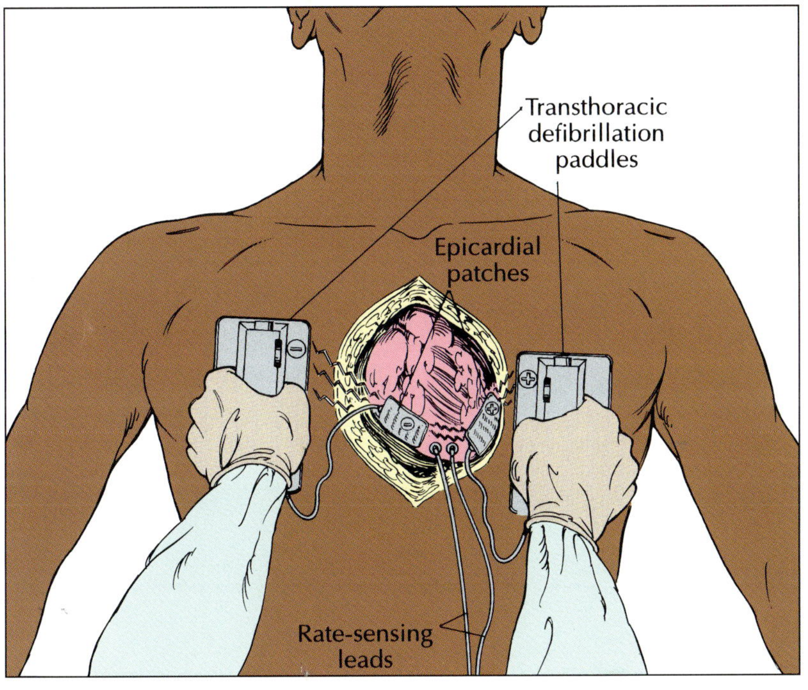

FIGURE 13-41. Emergency simultaneous transthoracic and epicardial defibrillation (ESTED) has been described for refractory ventricular fibrillation (VF) during routine testing of implantable cardioverter-defibrillators [82]. This method is performed by placing the ends of the sensing or patch electrodes against the anterior surface of the chest. Standard transthoracic defibrillator paddles are then positioned approximately 10 inches apart and energy is delivered simultaneously through the thorax to the epicardium. In two cases VF was converted to sinus rhythm with 360 J using the ESTED technique. ESTED provides a simple and effective method for terminating refractory VF in the operating room. (*Adapted from* Cohen and coworkers [83]; with permission.

Sex/Age, *y*	M/54	F/64	M/79	M/63	M/89	M/66	M/40	F/48	F/65	M/55
Substrate	COPD/ IMI	Obese/ ASMI	COPD/ ASMI	Obese/ ASMI	CAD	IDCM	Unknown	Unknown	Unknown	Unknown
Failed transthoracic defibrillations, *n*	15	10	7	5	4	2	7	6	5	5
Rescue technique	Intracardiac	Intracardiac	Intracardiac	Intracardiac	ESTED	ESTED	Trans-esophageal	Trans-esophageal	Trans-esophageal	Trans-esophageal
Energy used, *J*	200, 500	300	100	100, 200	360	360	30	100, 200, 300	100, 200, 300	100, 200, 300

FIGURE 13-42. A summary of clinical data regarding rescue defibrillation techniques that were performed in a variety of hospital settings to terminate refractory ventricular defibrillation in ten patients. Each method was successful. However, transesophageal rescue defibrillation requires further investigation to determine its true practical applications [84]. Importantly, several recent developments in the fields of CPR and defibrillation may provide improvement in overall resuscitation. The simpler the method, the easier it will be to implement on a wide scale. Further research is required to refine these novel techniques and explore other innovations. ASMI—anteroseptal myocardial infarction; CAD—coronary artery disease; COPD—chronic obstructive pulmonary disease; ESTED—emergency simultaneous transthoracic and epicardial defibrillation; IDCM—idiopathic dilated cardiomyopathy; IMI—inferior myocardial infarction.

The author would like to acknowledge the research and dedication of Lisa J. Lehnert in the preparation of this chapter.

References

1. Kouwenhoven WB, Jude JR, Knickerbocker GG: Closed-chest cardiac massage. *JAMA* 1960, 173:1064–1067.
2. Cummins RO, Ornasto JP, Thies WH, Pepe PE: Improving survival from sudden cardiac arrest: the "chain of survival" concept: a statement for health care professionals from the Advanced Cardiac Life Support Subcommittee and Emergency Cardiac Care Committee, American Heart Association. *Circulation* 1991, 83:1832–1847.
3. Lown B: Sudden cardiac death: the major challenge confronting contemporary cardiology. *Am J Cardiol* 1979, 43(2):313–328.
4. Kuller L, Cooper M, Perper J: Epidemiology of sudden death. *Arch Intern Med* 1972, 129:714–719.
5. *Morbidity and Mortality Chartbook on Cardiovascular, Lung and Blood Diseases 1990*. Bethesda, MD: National Heart, Lung, and Blood Institute; 1990.
6. Pantridge JF, Geddes JS: Cardiac arrest after myocardial infarction. *Lancet* 1966, 1:807–808.
7. *1992 Heart and Stroke Facts*. Dallas: American Heart Association; 1991.
8. Zoll PM, Linenthal AJ, Gibson W, *et al.*: Termination of ventricular fibrillation in man by externally applied electric countershock. *N Engl J Med* 1956, 254:727–732.
9. Heimlich HJ: A life-saving maneuver to prevent food-choking. *JAMA* 1975, 234:398–401.
10. Criley JM, Blaufuss AH, Kissel GL: Cough-induced cardiac compression: self-administered form of cardiopulmonary resuscitation. *JAMA* 1976, 236:1246.
11. Ohomoto T, Miura I, Konno S: A new method of external cardiac massage to improve diastolic augmentation and prolong survival time. *Ann Thorac Surg* 1976, 21:284–290.
12. Halperin HR, Tsitlik JE, Gelfand M, *et al.*: A preliminary study of cardiopulmonary resuscitation by circumferential compression of the chest with use of a pneumatic vest. *N Engl J Med* 1993, 329:762–768.
13. Cohen TJ, Tucker KJ, Lurie KG, *et al.*: Active compression-decompression: a new method of cardiopulmonary resuscitation. *JAMA* 1992, 267:2916–2923.
14. American Heart Association: Standards and guidelines for cardiopulmonary resuscitation (CPR) and emergency care (ECC). *JAMA* 1992, 268:2171–2302.
15. White RD: *Clinical Symposia: CPR: Basic Life Support*, vol 34, no 6. NJ:CIBA Pharmaceutical Company; 1982; 34(6):3–30.
16. *Textbook of Advanced Cardiac Life Support*, ed 2. Dallas:American Heart Association; 1987.
17. Dubin D: Rapid Interpretation of EKG's: a programmed course, ed. 4. Tampa Florida: COVER Publishing Co; 1989.

18. Cummins RO, Eisenberg MS: Prehospital cardiopulmonary resuscitation: is it effective? *JAMA* 1985, 253:2408–2412.
19. Pantridge JF: The effect of early therapy on the hospital mortality from acute myocardial infarction. *Q J Med* 1970, 39:621–622.
20. Weaver WD, Hill D, Fahrenbruch CE, *et al.*: Use of the automatic external defibrillator in the management of out-of-hospital cardiac arrest. *N Engl J Med* 1988, 319:661–666.
21. Weaver WD, Copass MK, Bufi D, *et al.*: Improved neurologic recovery and survival after early defibrillation. *Circulation* 1984, 69:943–948.
22. Mayer JD: Paramedic response time and survival from cardiac arrest. *Soc Sci Med* 1979, 13D:267.
23. Eisenberg MS, Copass MK, Hallstrom AP, *et al.*: Treatment of out-of-hospital cardiac arrests with rapid defibrillation by emergency medical technicians. *N Engl J Med* 1980, 302:1379–1383.
24. Swerdlow CR, Winkle RA, Mason JW: Determinants of survival in patients with ventricular tachycardia. *N Engl J Med* 1983, 308:1436–1442.
25. Ewy GA: Cardiac arrest and resuscitation: defibrillators and defibrillation. *Curr Probl Cardiol* 1978, 11:8.
26. *Physicians Desk Reference*, ed 46. Oradell: Medical Economics Corp; 1992.
27. *Goodman and Gilman's The Pharmacological Basis of Therapeutics*, ed. 8. Edited by Goodman A, Gilman, *et al.* New York: Pergamon Press; 1990.
28. Grines CL, Browne KF, Marco J, *et al.*: A comparison of immediate angioplasty with thrombolytic therapy for acute myocardial infarction. *N Engl J Med* 1993, 328:673–679.
29. Rapaport E, Fuster V, Reeves TJ, *et al.*: Guidelines for the early management of patients with acute myocardial infarction: a report of the American College of Cardiology/American Heart Association Task Force on Assessment of Diagnostic and Therapeutic Cardiovascular Procedures (Subcommittee to Develop Guidelines for the Early Management of Patients with Acute Myocardial Infarction). *J Am Coll Cardiol* 1990, 16:249–292.
30. MacMahon S, Collins R, Peto R, *et al.*: Effects of prophylactic lidocaine in suspected acute myocardial infarction: an overview of results from the randomized controlled trials. *JAMA* 1988, 260:1910–1916.
31. Dunn HM, McComb JM, Kinney CD, *et al.*: Prophylactic lidocaine in the early phase of suspected myocardial infarction. *Am Heart J* 1985, 110:353–362.
32. Killip T, Kimball JT: Treatment of myocardial infarction in a coronary care unit: a two-year experience with 250 patients. *Am J Cardiol* 1967, 20:457.
33. Olson DW, Thompson BM, Darin JC, Milbrath MH: A randomized comparison study of bretylium tosylate and lidocaine in resuscitation of patients from out-of-hospital ventricular fibrillation in a paramedic system. *Ann Emerg Med* 1984, 13:807–810.
34. Holder DA, Sniderman AD, Fraser G, Fallen EL: Experience with bretylium tosylate by a hospital cardiac arrest team. *Circulation* 1977, 55:541–544.
35. Haynes RE, Chinn TL, Copass MK, Cobb LA: Comparison of bretylium tosylate and lidocaine in management of out of hospital ventricular fibrillation: a randomized clinical trial. *Am J Cardiol* 1981, 48:353–356.
36. Woods KL, Fletcher S, Roffe C, Haider Y: Intravenous magnesium sulphate in suspected acute myocardial infarction: results of the second Leicester Intravenous Magnesium Intervention Trial (LIMIT-2). *Lancet* 1992, 339:1553–1558.
37. Teo KK, Yusuf S, Collins R, *et al.*: Effects of intravenous magnesium in suspected acute myocardial infarction: overview of randomized trials. *BMJ* 1991, 303:1499–1503.
38. Myerburg RJ, Estes D, Zaman L, *et al.*: Outcome of resuscitation from bradyarrhythmic or asystolic prehospital cardiac arrest. *J Am Coll Cardiol* 1984, 4:1118–1122.
39. Otto C, Yakaitis R: The role of epinephrine in CPR: a reappraisal. *Ann Emerg Med* 1987, 16:743–748.
40. Michael JR, Guerci D, Koehler RC, *et al.*: Mechanisms by which epinephrine augments cerebral and myocardial perfusion during cardiopulmonary resuscitation in dogs. *Circulation* 1984, 69:822.
41. Michael JR, Guerci AD, Koehler RC, *et al.*: Mechanisms by which epinephrine augments cerebral and myocardial perfusion during cardiopulmonary resuscitation in dogs. *Circulation* 1984, 69:822–835.
42. Yakaitis RW, Otto CW, Blitt CD: Relative importance of alpha and beta-adrenergic receptors during resuscitation. *Crit Care Med* 1979, 7(7):293–296.
43. Paradis NA, Koscove EM: Epinephrine in cardiac arrest: a critical review. *Ann Emerg Med* 1990, 19:1288–1301.
44. Callaham M: Epinephrine doses in cardiac arrest: is it time to outgrow the orthodoxy of ACLS? *Ann Emerg Med* 1989, 18(9):1011–1012.
45. Bodon DC: The intracardiac injection of adrenalin. *Lancet* 1923, 1:586–590.
46. Callaham M, Madsen CD, Barton CW, *et al.*: A randomized clinical trial of high-dose epinephrine and norepinephrine versus standard-dose epinephrine in prehospital cardiac arrest [Abstract]. *Ann Emerg Med* 1992. 21:606–607.
47. Otto CW, Yakaitis RW, Redding JS, Blitt CD: Comparison of dopamine, dobutamine, and epinephrine in CPR. *Crit Care Med* 1981, 9:640–643.
48. Lindner KH, Ahnefeld FW, Bowdler IM: Comparison of epinephrine and dopamine during cardiopulmonary resuscitation. *Intensive Care Med* 1989, 15:432–438.
49. Klein NA, Sisking SJ, Frishman WH, *et al.*: Hemodynamic comparison of intravenous amrinone and dobutamine in patients with chronic congestive heart failure. *Am J Cardiol* 1981, 48:170–175.
50. Halperin HR, Tsitlik JE, Guerci AD, *et al.*: Determinants of blood flow to vital organs during cardiopulmonary resuscitation in dogs. *Circulation* 1986, 73:539–550.
51. Paradis NA, Martin GB, Goetting MG, *et al.*: Simultaneous aortic, jugular bulb, and right atrial pressures during cardiopulmonary resuscitation in humans: insights into mechanisms. *Circulation* 1989, 80:361–368.
52. Falk JL, Rackow EC, Weil MH: End-tidal carbon dioxide concentration during cardiopulmonary resuscitation. *N Engl J Med* 1988, 318:607–611.
53. Rudikoff MT, Maughan WL, Effron M, *et al.*: Mechanisms of blood flow during cardiopulmonary resuscitation. *Circulation* 1980, 61:345–352.
54. Sayah AJ, Peacock WF, Overton DT: End-tidal CO_2 measurement in the detection of esophageal intubation during cardiac arrest. *Ann Emerg Med* 1990, 19:857–860.
55. Redberg RF, Kelly TJ, Cohen TJ, *et al.*: Physiology of blood flow during cardiopulmonary resuscitation: a transesophageal echocardiographic study. *Circulation* 1993, 88:534–541.
56. Taylor GJ, Tucker WM, Greene HL, *et al.*: Importance of prolonged compression during cardiopulmonary resuscitation in man. *N Engl J Med* 1977, 296:1515–1517.
57. Feneley MP, Maier GW, Kern KB, *et al.*: Influence of compression rate on initial success of resuscitation and 24 hour survival after prolonged manual cardiopulmonary resuscitation in dogs. *Circulation* 1988, 77:240–250.
58. Kern KB, Sanders AB, Raife J, *et al.*: A study of chest compression rates during cardiopulmonary resuscitation in humans: the importance of rate-directed chest compressions. *Arch Intern Med* 1992, 152:145–149.
59. Shultz JJ, Schwab T, Callaham M, *et al.*: Active compression-decompression CPR improves prehospital cardiopulmonary arrest survival [Abstract]. *PACE Pacing Clin Electrophysiol* 1993, 16:928.
60. Cohen TJ, Goldner B, Tucker KJ, *et al.*: Initial resuscitation and survival in patients receiving active compression-decompression cardiopulmonary resuscitation: results of the ACD-CPR Survival Pilot Study [Abstract]. *Am Rev Respir Dis* 1993, 147(suppl):A613.

61. Sack JB, Kesselbrenner MB, Bregman D: Survival from in-hospital cardiac arrest with interposed abdominal counterpulsation during cardiopulmonary resuscitation. *JAMA* 1992, 267:379–385.

62. Niemann JT, Rosborough JP, Niskanen RA, *et al.*: Mechanical "cough" cardiopulmonary resuscitation during cardiac arrest in dogs. *Am J Cardiol* 1985, 55:199–204.

63. Krischer JP, Fine EG, Weisfeldt ML, *et al.*: Comparison of prehospital conventional and simultaneous compression-ventilation cardiopulmonary resuscitation. *Crit Care Med* 1989, 17:1263–1269.

64. Guerci AD, Chandra NC, Gelfand MI, *et al.*: Vest CPR increases aortic pressure in humans [Abstract]. *Circulation* 1989, 80(suppl II):II496.

65. Ward KR, Sullivan RJ, Zelenak RR, Summer WR: A comparison of interposed abdominal compression CPR and standard CPR by monitoring end-tidal PCO_2. *Ann Emerg Med* 1989, 18:831–837.

66. Voorhees WD, Niebar MJ, Babbs CF: Improved oxygen delivery during cardiopulmonary resuscitation with interposed abdominal compressions. *Ann Emerg Med* 1983, 12:128–135.

67. Nieman JT, Rosborough JP, Niskanen RA, Criley JM: Circulatory support during cardiac arrest using a pneumatic vest and abdominal binder with simultaneous high-pressure airway inflation. *Ann Emerg Med* 1984, 13:767–770.

68. Lurie KG, Lindo C, Chin J: CPR: the P stands for plumber's helper. *JAMA* 1990, 264:1661.

69. Carlson RH: "Plunger" outdoes CPR in human trials. *Cardiol World News* 1992, 8:7.

70. Goldner BG, Cohen TJ: Active compression-decompression: a novel CPR technique. *J Invas Cardio* 1993, 5:114–118.

71. Cohen TJ, Tucker KJ, Redberg RF, *et al.*: Active compression-decompression resuscitation: a novel method of cardiopulmonary resuscitation. *Am Heart J* 1992, 124:1145–1150.

72. Cohen TJ, Goldner BG, Maccaro PC, *et al.*: Comparison of active compression-decompression resuscitation with standard cardiopulmonary resuscitation for cardiac arrests occurring in the hospital. *N Engl J Med* 1993, 329:1918–1921.

73. Higano ST, Oh JK, Ewy GA, Seward JB: The mechanism of blood flow during closed chest cardiac massage in humans: transesophageal echocardiographic observations. *Mayo Clin Proc* 1990, 65(11):1432–1440.

74. Feneley MP, Maier GW, Kern KB, *et al.*: Influence of compression rate on initial success of resuscitation and 24-hour survival after prolonged manual cardiopulmonary resuscitation in dogs. *Circulation* 1988, 77:240–250.

75. Sanders AB, Meislin HW, Ewy GA: The physiology of cardiopulmonary resuscitation. *JAMA* 1984, 252:3283–3286.

76. Chandra NC, Tsitlik JE, Halperin HR, *et al.*: Observations of hemodynamics during human cardiopulmonary resuscitation. *Crit Care Med* 1990, 18:929–934.

77. Garnett AR, Ornato JP, Gonzalez ER, Johnson BE: End-tidal carbon dioxide monitoring during cardiopulmonary resuscitation. *JAMA* 1987, 257:512–515.

78. Criley M, Niemann JT, Rosborough JP: Cardiopulmonary resuscitation research 1960–1984: discoveries and advances. *Ann Emerg Med* 1984, 13:756–758.

79. Rogers MC, Weisfeldt ML, Traystan RJ: Cerebral blood flow during cardiopulmonary resuscitation. *Anesth Analg* 1981, 60:73–75.

80. Kern KB, Ewy GA: Future directions in cardiopulmonary resuscitation. *Learning Center Highlights* 1990, Winter:11–15. Published by the Americn College of Cardiology.

81. Cohen TJ, Scheinman MM, Pullen BT, *et al.*: Emergency intracardiac defibrillation for refractory ventricular fibrillation during routine electrophysiologic study. *J Am Coll Cardiol* 1991, 18:1200–1284.

82. Cohen TJ, Chin MC, Oliver DG, *et al.*: Transesophageal defibrillation: animal studies and preliminary clinical observations. *PACE Pacing Clin Electrophysiol* 1993, 16:1285–1292.

83. Cohen TJ, Scheinman MM, Pullen BT, *et al.*: Emergency simultaneous transthoracic and epicardial defibrillation during routine implantable cardioverter-defibrillator testing in the operating room. *Am J Cardiol* 1993, 71:619–622.

84. Cohen TJ: Innovative emergency defibrillation methods for refractory ventricular fibrillation in a variety of hospital settings. *Am Heart J* 1993, 126:962–968.

INDEX